Color Atlas of Periodontology

Klaus H. & Edith M. Rateitschak
Herbert F. Wolf
Thomas M. Hassell

Forewords by Roy C. Page and Hubert E. Schroeder

804 Illustrations, most in Color

1985
Georg Thieme Verlag Stuttgart · New York
Thieme Inc. New York

The authors:

Dr. Klaus H. Rateitschak
Chairman, Department of Cariology and
Periodontology
and
Dr. Edith M. Rateitschak-Plüss
Senior Instructor
Department of Cariology
and Periodontology

Dental Institute, University of Basle
Petersplatz 14, CH-4051 Basle
Switzerland

Dr. Herbert F. Wolf
Private Practitioner of Periodontics SGP
Zeltweg 63, CH-8032, Zurich; Switzerland

Dr. Thomas M. Hassell
Associate Professor of Anatomy
and Periodontology
Baltimore College of Dental Surgery
University of Maryland, Dental School
666 West Baltimore Street
Baltimore, Maryland 21201 USA

Deutsche Bibliothek Cataloging in Publication Data

Color atlas of periodontology / K. H. & E. M.
Rateitschak ... Introd. by R. C. Page and H. E.
Schroeder. – Stuttgart ; New York : Thieme, 1985.
   Dt. Ausg. u. d. T.: Rateitschak, Klaus H. & Edith M./Wolf, Herbert F.:
   Parodontologie
NE: Rateitschak, Klaus H. [Mitverf.]

Important Note: Medicine is an ever-changing science. Research and clinical experience are continually broadening our knowledge, in particular our knowledge of proper treatment and drug therapy. Insofar as this book mentions any dosage or application, readers may rest assured that the authors, editors and publishers have made every effort to ensure that such references are strictly in accordance with the state of knowledge at the time of production of the book. Nevertheless, every user is requested to carefully examine the manufacturer's leaflets accompanying each drug to check on his own responsibility whether the dosage schedules recommended therein or the contraindications stated by the manufacturers differ from the statements made in the present book. Such examination is particularly important with drugs that are either rarely used or have been newly released on the market.

This book is an authorized translation from the German edition published and copyrighted 1984 by Georg Thieme Verlag, Stuttgart, Germany. Title of the German edition: Parodontologie

© 1985 Georg Thieme Verlag, Rüdigerstraße 14,
D-7000 Stuttgart 30, Germany
Printed in Germany
Typesetting by G. Müller, Heilbronn
Reproductions by K. Porupsky, Stuttgart
Printed by K. Grammlich, Pliezhausen

ISBN 3-13-675001-2 (Georg Thieme Verlag, Stuttgart)
ISBN 0-86577-214-2 (Thieme Inc. New York)   1 2 3 4 5 6

Preface

The purpose of this *Atlas* is to enhance the practical development and improvement of periodontology.

An *Atlas* such as this cannot replace the more traditional textbooks on the subject. Rather, our goal is to provide a clear presentation of *established and proven concepts* of practical periodontal therapy, concepts that can be carried over directly into the operatory.

New knowledge that has emerged from active research laboratories and been substantiated in clinical research programs in recent years is integrated into this *Atlas,* providing an up-to-date presentation of proven concepts and techniques.

consequences than as methods for total elimination of etiologic factors on the root surface.

The authors make no claim to completeness in this *Atlas;* not each and every possible treatment modality is described. The emphasis has rather been on thorough consideration of those standard methods and concepts whose usefulness has been demonstrated in practice and in clinical research studies.
Mention is made throughout this *Atlas* of the limitations and difficulties of treatment techniques; failures are described and areas of therapy that remain nebulous are pointed out as well.

Theoretical principles are presented only insofar as they provide a sound basis for prevention and treatment of the periodontal diseases. The *Atlas* employs internationally accepted nomenclature for the various periodontal disease entities. Related areas in oral pathology are included when they are significant in the differential diagnosis of gingival and periodontal diseases.

Dedicated to our teacher and friend

Hans R. Mühlemann

master Clinician and Scientist

Here at the very outset we must emphasize *our* view that the best "treatment" for periodontitis is *prevention* or regular *maintenance therapy,* which can effectively prevent recurrence.

The authors of this *Atlas of Periodontology* are not only teachers and scientists in the specialty of periodontics, they are also – above all – clinicians and practitioners. We hope that our orientation toward the clinical aspects of our specialty will serve the profession.

The *treatment of periodontitis* is presented very comprehensively. The most important aspects of treatment are presented using practical cases; the procedures are described step-by-step, and the clinical results discussed in a summary section.

Particular emphasis is placed on "causal" therapy, i.e., elimination of the disease process by means of removing the infection. This occurs primarily in the first phase of treatment, initial therapy. Thus, the sometimes unavoidable surgical interventions necessitated in advanced cases of disease may be viewed today less as methods for elimination of symptoms of disease and its

Basle/Zurich/Baltimore, Autumn 1985

Klaus H. & Edith M. Rateitschak
Herbert F. Wolf
Thomas M. Hassell

Foreword – I

Roy C. Page, D. D. S., Ph. D.
Professor, Pathology & Periodontics
University of Washington, Seattle

Disease of the periodontium continues to be one of man's most widespread afflictions. These diseases are taking on an ever increasing importance in dentistry because of the decreasing prevalence of dental caries and the fact that they are prevalent in older people, a segment of our population that is rapidly increasing. Beginning with the early 1970s, there has been a virtual explosion in new basic information about all aspects of the periodontal diseases and this has led to major advances in our understanding. The rate of progress in acquiring new knowledge has greatly outstripped our capacity to integrate the new information into concepts about these diseases and into our methods of diagnosing and treating them. By and large, textbooks and monographs are out of date before they appear on the new book shelves, and all too frequently they fail to incorporate the new information or to apply it to clinical problems. This book is an exception.

The *Color Atlas of Periodontology* is different from existing textbooks and monographs in many ways. Indeed, it is not a textbook but it is far more than an atlas. It is a fresh approach in which the latest information has been integrated into already existing knowledge and presented in a highly effective, easy-to-understand manner using innovative diagrams, drawings, and clinical illustrations.

The publication has numerous strengths. A great deal of thought and planning appears to have been given to the selection of areas to be covered and to their sequencing. Coverage is extraordinarily complete, with sections on structural biology, pathogenesis, host response, epidemiology, diagnosis, therapy, adjunctive therapy, and maintenance. The book also includes sections on areas of dentistry related or allied to periodontics including endodontics, orthodontics, temporary stabilization, occlusal trauma and its management, medications frequently used in the course of periodontal therapy, and fixed and removable restorative treatment for periodontal patients.

The sections on structural biology, microbiology and host response are especially noteworthy because they are based on the most recent research findings and they are presented in a manner that even a beginning student can easily understand. An excellent selection of literature references has been provided. I also liked the section on diagnosis. All of the inflammatory diseases of the periodontium are included and documented using the latest terminology. This is accomplished without the inclusion of peripherally related oral lesions which would dilute and detract from the major diagnostic thrust.

The section on therapy constitutes about two-thirds of the book and is, without doubt, the most outstanding section. Coverage is unusually thorough. Every recognized method and procedure has been included beginning with oral hygiene, scaling, curettage and root planing, and extending through the entire range of resective and reconstructive procedures. For each procedure, the required instrumentation is illustrated, and an excellent clinical example has been chosen. Pretreatment clinical photographs and radiographs are provided along with a step-by-step illustration of the operative procedure and the postoperative results. Although there is a great deal of debate today concerning the relative merits of conservative versus the more extensive surgical methods of treatment, to their credit the authors of this *Atlas* have remained totally objective, showing no favoritism to one school of thought or another.

There has not previously been a comparable publication in the field of periodontology in the United States and there is unlikely to be another in the foreseeable future. The selection, organization, and sequencing of the information and the technical quality of this publication are unsurpassed. The book will be useful to undergraduate and graduate students, teachers, and practicing dentists and periodontists. It will in all likelihood become one of the most widely used and cited publications in our field.

Foreword – II

Hubert E. Schroeder, D.M.D., Dr. odont. h.c.
Chairman, Department of Oral Structural Biology
University of Zurich, Switzerland

This is not a textbook in the usual sense of the term, nor is it merely a picture book of "case reports" and clinical situations. In fact, this book is a guide for practitioners of the periodontal healing arts, an admirable and current compendium of rational practice alternatives based on the contemporary clinical and pathobiological sciences of periodontology.

Although classical literature often provides a relatively clear view of the various diseases of the periodontium, only during the past 20 years has it become possible for periodontal scientists to re-evaluate this picture, and to describe and clarify the etiology and pathogenesis of these diseases. Today, the profession finds itself in the midst of an attempt to utilize the latest scientific discoveries for the improvement of its diagnostic and therapeutic skills. During a lifetime, the periodontium of a clinically healthy human usually undergoes various alterations that relate to physiological, functional, infectious or iatrogenic circumstances.

These alterations manifest themselves in atrophic tissue loss, in the cardinal symptoms of inflammation, in tissue destruction of varying severity and, ultimately, in tooth loss. The most common afflictions of the periodontal supporting structures are the various forms of periodontitis, which are considered today as locally destructive, non-contagious infectious diseases. All types of periodontitis are caused primarily by anaerobic mixed infections, yet susceptibility to these bacterial infections may vary from individual to individual. The infecting bacteria take their origin as a supragingival plaque which extends apically onto the root surface, changing in composition subgingivally. The bacterial attack elicits inflammation, the development of periodontal pockets and abscess formation; the subsequent plethora of host defense mechanisms called into action eventually participates in destroying components of the tissues. Understanding of such host-pathogen relationships as elucidated by recent experimental research, may now provide the framework for modern periodontal therapy which, so-based,

can in many instances lead to clinically successful results.

This *Atlas* is one of the best, most comprehensive, most clinically relevant documentations on the subject of successful practical periodontics, which also illustrates the impact of related dental specialties – endodontics and prosthodontics, for example – upon the success of periodontal therapy. The strength of this book is to be found not only in the ideal integration of theoretical principles with practical considerations and the internal logic of the presentation, but also in the superb clinical photographs and schematic diagrams that weld this text into a coherent, systematic and thoroughly understandable entity. The fact that the authors provide both textual and illustrative emphasis on *prevention* rather than on complicated, expensive and often unnecessary surgical procedures underscores their basic intention, which is to advocate health maintenance, for the patient's benefit. Every basic element of periodontal therapy is portrayed step-by-step by means of coordinated text and illustration; the crucially important elements of therapy are emphasized by repetition; outmoded concepts are either presented in relative terms or discarded entirely.

Each practitioner who peruses this book will come away with the current views of the pathogenesis of periodontal diseases and the essential elements of consequential periodontal therapy. Perhaps the periodontist, above all, will come to realize that for the modern practitioner the biomedical research laboratories in his profession are not merely ivory towers, i.e., remote outposts from which an occasional crumb of a misleading message emanates. In fact, this volume is conclusive proof that many of the research findings from clinical as well as basic scientists have already had direct and immediate impact upon the practice of clinical periodontics today. This book is intended to bring this realization to the practicing professionals of our dental speciality.

Table of Contents

III   **Preface**
IV   **Foreword (I)**
V   **Foreword (II)**
VI   **Table of Contents**
IX   **Acknowledgements**

Basic Principles

1   **Structural Biology**
2   Gingiva
3   Gingival Width – Col
4   Epithelial Attachment
6   Connective Tissue Attachment
8   Physiologic Tooth Mobility

9   **Etiology and Pathogenesis**
10   Accumulated Debris – Microbial Plaque
11   Supragingival Plaque
12   Subgingival Plaque
13   Infection – Bacterial Invasion into Tissues
14   Natural Factors Favoring Plaque Retention
15   Iatrogenic Factors Favoring Plaque Accumulation
16   Bacterial Flora and Types of Disease

18   Histopathogenesis of Gingivitis and Periodontitis
20   Host Response
22   Acute Defense Mechanisms
23   Cyclic Nature of Periodontitis – Attachment Loss – Bone Resorption
24   Cofactors in Etiology and Pathogenesis

25   **Epidemiology and Indices**
25   Epidemiology of Gingivitis
26   Epidemiology of Periodontitis
27   Indices
27   Plaque Indices
29   Gingival Indices
32   Periodontal Indices
32   Indices versus Clinical Findings

Diagnosis

33   **Diseases of the Periodontium**
33   Gingival and Periodontal Diseases, Local Etiology without Systemic Involvement
34   Gingival and Periodontal Diseases, Etiology Partially Local but with Systemic Involvement
35   Gingivitis
38   Mild Gingivitis
39   Moderate Gingivitis
40   Severe Gingivitis
41   Acute Necrotizing Ulcerative Gingivitis (ANUG)
44   Mild ANUG
45   Severe ANUG
46   Gingivitis Modulated by Hormones
47   Mild Pregnancy Gingivitis
48   Severe Pregnancy Gingivitis, Gravid Epulis
49   Gingival Overgrowth, Tumors
52   Autoimmune Diseases, Anomalies of Keratinization, Viral Infections
54   Gingivostomatitis Herpetica
55   Periodontitis
66   Adult Periodontitis (AP)
68   Rapidly Progressive Periodontitis (RPP)
70   Rapidly Progressive Periodontitis (RPP) – Acute Phase

72   Juvenile Periodontitis (LJP) – Initial Stage
74   Juvenile Periodontitis (LJP) – Advanced Stage
76   Periodontitis Ulcerosa – Symptoms
77   Periodontitis Ulcerosa – Acute Phase
78   Prepubertal Periodontitis with Systemic Disease – Papillon-Lefèvre Syndrome
80   Papillon-Lefèvre Syndrome – "An Exception for Every Rule"
81   Recession
84   Recession – Localized
85   Recession – Generalized
86   "Destruction and Shrinkage" – Clinical Situations Resembling Recession

87   **Charting – Diagnosis – Prognosis**
88   Probing Depths and Attachment Loss
90   Furcation Involvement – Root Irregularities
92   Pocket Activity – Subgingival Flora
93   Gingival Recession
94   Radiography
95   Tooth Mobility – Function
96   Diagnostic Charting
98   Prognosis

Prevention

99 **Maintenance of Health – Prevention of Disease**

Therapy

101 **Therapy of Periodontal Diseases**
102 Treatment Planning – Sequence of Treatment
104 Emergency Treatment

107 Initial Therapy
108   Motivation – Information

110 Home Care by the Patient
111   Plaque Disclosing Agents
112   Toothbrushes
113   Dentifrices

114   Toothbrushing Techniques
116   Interdental Hygiene
118   Special Cleaning Aids – Irrigation Devices
119   Chemical Plaque Control – Chlorhexidine (CHX)

121 Professional Care – Creating Conditions that
     Enhance Hygiene
122   Gross Scaling – Supragingival Calculus Removal
         Instruments and Materials
124   Fine Scaling and Polishing
         Instruments and Materials

126   Removal of Iatrogenic Irritants – Amalgam Overhangs
128   Removal of Iatrogenic Irritants –
         Overhanging Crown Margins
129   Correction of Iatrogenic Irritants – Bridge Pontics
130   Removal of Iatrogenic Irritants – Metal Pigmentation

131   Removal of Natural Plaque-Retentive Areas – Extraction
132   Removal of Natural Plaque-Retentive Areas –
         Odontoplasty of Grooves, Ridges, Furcations
134   Reduction of Natural Plaque-Retentive Areas Caused
         by Crowding – Odontoplasty

135 Scaling
     Root Planing
     Curettage
138   Instruments for Root Planing and Curettage
140   Rest Position – Position of the Operator
141   Root Planing and Curettage
         Operative Procedure
146   Treatment of Mild Furcation Involvement (F 1)
147   Treatment of Moderate Furcation Involvement (F 2) –
         Odontoplasty
148   Open Curettage and Root Planing
149   Open Curettage, Root Planing –
         Correction of Undercontoured Crown Margin
150   What Does "Root Planing" Really Mean?

151 Initial Therapy – Possibilities and Limitations

155 Periodontal Surgery
158   Anesthesia

159 Gingivectomy (GV) and Gingivoplasty (GP)
160   Instruments for Gingivectomy / Gingivoplasty
162   Periodontal Dressings and Tissue Adhesives
163   Gingivectomy / Gingivoplasty
         Operative Procedure

170   GV / GP in the Maxilla – Buccal and Palatal
171   GV / GP – Phenytoin-Induced Gingival Overgrowth
172   GV / GP – Corrective Operations, Minor Procedures
174   Gingivoplasty

175 Flap Procedures
176   Instruments for Flap Procedures
178   Needles, Sutures and Suture Knots

179   Partially Reflected Mucoperiosteal Flap
         Modified Widman Procedure (Ramfjord Technique)
180   Principles of the Ramfjord Technique
183   Ramfjord Technique
         Operative Procedure

190   Fully Reflected Mucoperiosteal Flaps
191   Instruments for Osteoplasty
192   Mucoperiosteal Flap without Vertical Incisions
         Osteoplasty – Flap Adaptation
194   Mucoperiosteal Flap with Vertical Incisions
         Osteoplasty – Apical Repositioning of Flap

197 Combined Surgical Techniques
198   Combined Surgical Technique, Schematic Presentation
         Flap (buccal) – GV and Flap (palatal)
199   Combined Surgical Technique
         Flap (buccal) – GV and Flap (palatal) –
         Intraosseous Implant
204   Combined Surgical Technique
         Flap – Extraction – Revision of Adjacent
         Periodontal Structures
         Operative Procedure

209   Surgical Removal of Impacted Third Molar –
         Prevention of a Pocket Distal to Second Molar
210   Wedge Excisions – Surgical Principles
211   Wedge Excision – Most Distal Tooth
         Operative Procedure
214   Wedge Excision – Lone Standing Tooth

Therapy (continued)

215 Transplants and Implants in Infrabony Pockets
216   Instruments for Removal of Autologous Bone
218   Autologous Bone Transplantation
      Operative Procedure
220   Bone Regeneration without Transplantation

221 Surgical Treatment of the Furcation
222   Hemisection in the Mandible – Reconstruction
224   Root Resection in the Maxilla – Reconstruction
226   Root Resection in the Maxilla – No Reconstruction

228 Mucogingival Surgery
    Halting Recession – Covering Denuded Areas
229 Gingival Extension with a Free Gingival Graft (FGG)
230   Instruments for Harvesting a Graft
232   Free Graft – Thickness and Shape
233   Gingival Extension with Free Gingival Graft
      Operative Procedure
240   FGG – Revascularization and Healing
241   FGG – Abutment Teeth
242   FGG over Large Areas – The Mesh Graft

244 Frenotomy, Frenectomy

245 Vestibuloplasty
    Modified Edlan-Mejchar Procedure

246 Edlan Vestibuloplasty
    Operative Procedure
250 Edlan Procedure – Wound Healing

253 Covering Areas of Recession?
254   "Creeping Attachment" after FGG
255   Coronal Repositioning after FGG
      Operative Procedure

259 Periodontics – Endodontics

260 Periodontal Healing
    Reattachment – New Attachment

262 Negative Results of Treatment

263 Medicaments
264 Periodontitis Therapy – Medicaments for Local Use
265 Periodontitis Therapy – Medicaments for Systemic
    Adjunctive Treatment

267 **Maintenance Therapy – Recall**
268 Recall Organization – Recall Effect
269 Recall – Auxiliary Personnel
270 No Maintenance Therapy – Failure

Adjunctive Therapy

271 **Function – Functional Therapy**
272 Occlusal Trauma
273 Idealized Mandibular Border Movements
274 Effective Mandibular Movements with Tooth Contact

276 Goals of Occlusal Adjustment
277 Practical Occlusal Adjustment
    Premature Contacts
280   Working Side
281   Balancing Side
282   Protrusive Movement – Eliminating Interferences
      Reduction of Wear Facets

283 Occlusal Bite Guard – The Michigan Splint

285 **Orthodontics**
286 Space Closure in the Maxillary Anterior Segment
287 Treatment for Protrusion
288 Uprighting the Mandibular Second Molar
290 Treatment of the Malpositioned Cuspid

291 **Splinting – Stabilization**
292 Temporary Splinting
293 Semipermanent Splinting – Anterior Area
295 Semipermanent Splinting – Posterior Area

297 **Reconstruction – Prosthodontics**
298 Fixed Provisional Restoration
299 Removable Provisional Appliance

300 Fixed Prosthetics – Crowns, Bridges, Attachments
301 Removable Prosthetics – Construction of Telescopes
302 Removable Prosthetics – Cast Framework Partial Denture

303 Problems Associated with Prosthetics in the
    Periodontal Patient

Appendix

304 **Conclusion – Periodontology, quo vadis?**

307 **Acknowledgements for Figures**

308 **References**

316 **Index**

Acknowledgements

The authors wish to thank the following individuals:

Dr. BERNHARD GUGGENHEIM, Chairman of Oral Microbiology and Immunology, Zurich, for his advice concerning the chapter on Etiology and Pathogenesis.

Dr. ARTHUR HEFTI, Chairman of Preventive Dental Medicine, Basle, for his assistance in the preparation of the chapter on Etiology and Pathogenesis, as well as for his critical review of the entire manuscript of this *Atlas*.

Dr. MICHAEL MARXER, Periodontist and former Senior Instructor in the Department of Periodontology, Basle, for his preparation of numerous intraoral photographs, particularly surgical series, and for his help in developing the concept for this *Atlas*.

Dr. HUBERT SCHROEDER, Chairman of Oral Structural Biology, Zurich, for his great contribution in the chapter on Structural Biology and for providing a Foreword to this *Atlas*.

The authors gratefully acknowledge the work and talents of Dr. BARBARA LESCO, Private Practitioner of Periodontics, Baltimore, for her editorial and professional guidance and contributions during the preparation of this book.

Furthermore, we wish to thank and acknowledge the following colleagues, who provided us with practical suggestions and sage advice:
- Dr. SANDRA ARCHER, Baltimore
- Dr. GIORGIO CIMASONI, Geneva
- Dr. GEORGE GRABER, Basle
- Dr. HANS GRAF, Bern
- Dr. ALICE KALLENBERGER, Basle
- Dr. NIKLAUS P. LANG, Bern
- Dr. MAX A. LISTGARTEN, Philadelphia
- Dr. FELIX LUTZ, Zurich
- Dr. BENEDIKT MAEGLIN, Basle
- Dr. JEAN-MARC MEYER, Geneva
- Dr. HANS R. MÜHLEMANN, Zurich
- Dr. MARTHA J. SOMERMAN, Baltimore
- Dr. PAUL STÖCKLI, Zurich.

Most of these individuals provided us with photographs from their extensive collections.

Special thanks are due also to the faculty and staff of the Department of Cariology and Periodontology, Dental Institute, University of Basle, and to the co-workers in the private practice of Dr. H. F. WOLF, and to the colleagues in the laboratories fo Dr. T. HASSELL. All of these individuals provided support, encouragement and assistance during the years when this *Atlas* was being prepared for publication.

We would thank especially Mrs. B. KAISER, Departmental Secretary, Basle, for preparation of the extensive manuscript and for editorial assistance, and Mrs. R. LÄUPPI, Zurich, for her noteworthy organizational assistance.

Mr. D. ISCH, Institute Photographer, Basle, merits acknowledgement for his work with the black-and-white illustrations. We thank also Mr. D. HUSER, Dental Laboratory, Wangen bei Olten, and Dr. H. SCHUTZBACH, Basle, for their technical assistance with models.

Mr. B. KÜMIN, Zurich, worked selflessly in developing the concept for the *Atlas*. All illustrations (schematics, tables) were prepared by Atelier Struchen & Partners (Department of Scientific Illustration), Zurich, using drafts provided by author H. F. WOLF.

The following institutions, organizations and companies provided the financial support required for preparation of the illustrations:
- Walter Fuchs Foundation, Basle
- Swiss Society for Periodontology
- Altkliniker, Basle
- Blend-A-Med Research, Mainz
- Elida Cosmetic, Inc., Zurich
- Gaba, Inc., Therwil
- TRISA Toothbrush Company, Triengen
- NIKON Inc., Küsnacht/Switzerland.

Not least of all we offer sincere thanks to Thieme Publishers, New York and Stuttgart, especially to Dr. D. BREMKAMP and Mr. K.-H. FLEISCHMANN, for support during the production of this *Atlas*.

Structural Biology

1 Periodontium – Dictionary definition

periodontium (per" e-o-don' she-um) [Lat. → *peri around* →, Gr. → *odous* tooth]. A *functional* system of different tissues, investing and supporting the teeth, including cementum, periodontal ligament, alveolar bone, and gingiva.
Anatomically, the term is restricted to the connective tissue interposed between the teeth and their bony sockets. Called also *Periosteum alveolare* [Lat.].

periodontology [Gr. → *logos*], the study of the periodontal diseases.

Knowledge of the normal morphology and structural biology of the periodontal tissues is a prerequisite for any understanding of pathological changes in these tissues. Such knowledge is also necessary for an appreciation of the healing processes following therapeutic intervention.

2 Periodontal structures

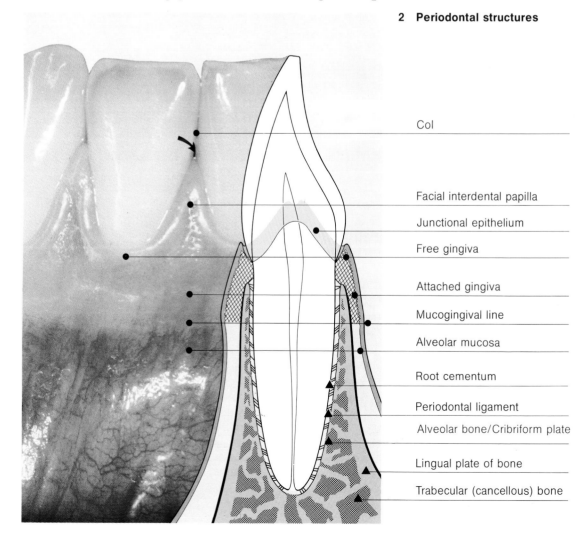

Col

Facial interdental papilla

Junctional epithelium

Free gingiva

Attached gingiva

Mucogingival line

Alveolar mucosa

Root cementum

Periodontal ligament

Alveolar bone/Cribriform plate

Lingual plate of bone

Trabecular (cancellous) bone

Gingiva

The gingiva is one portion of the oral mucosa. It is also the most peripheral component of the periodontium. Gingiva begins at the mucogingival line, covers the coronal aspect of the alveolar process, and terminates as the free marginal gingiva surrounding the cervix of each tooth. By means of a specialized collar of gingival epithelium termed the junctional epithelium, it provides the attachment between gingival soft tissue and the calcified structure of the tooth. Thus the gingiva insures continuity of the epithelial lining of the oral cavity.

The gingiva is demarcated clinically into the free marginal gingiva, ca. 1.5 mm wide, the attached gingiva, which may be of varying width, and the interdental gingiva occupying the embrasures between adjacent teeth.

Healthy gingiva is described as "salmon or coral pink." Healthy gingiva may also be darkly pigmented, most commonly in Blacks, but also occasionally in Caucasians and Orientals. Gingiva is firm in consistency and not mobile upon the underlying structures. The surface of gingiva is keratinized and may also exhibit an orange peel-like appearance called stippling (Schroeder 1982).

3 Healthy gingiva in a young person
The free gingival margin courses parallel to the cementoenamel junction. The interdental gingival papillae completely fill the interdental embrasures. A shallow linear depression, the gingival groove, can be observed in some areas, demarcating the free marginal gingiva from the attached gingiva. The mucogingival line (MGL) is not a distinct structure.

The *radiograph* reveals interdental septa that extend almost to the cementoenamel junction.

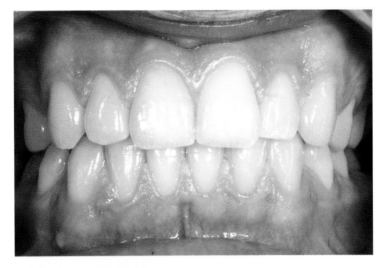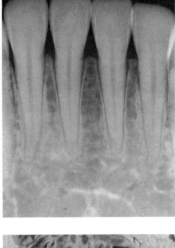

4 Healthy pigmented gingiva
The attached gingiva is deeply stippled and exhibits varying degrees of brownish pigmentation.

This *pigmentation* results from the synthesis of melanin by melanocytes located in the Stratum basale of the epithelium. The melanocytes in this histological section appear as brown spots.

Photomicrograph courtesy of *H. R. Mühlemann*

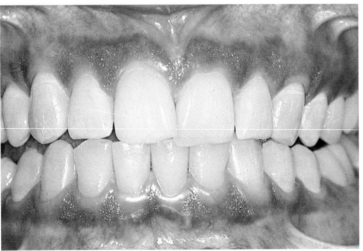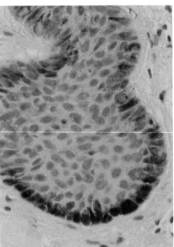

5 Healthy gingiva and severe abrasion / attrition
This 40-year-old male had a long history of clenching and bruxing. Despite the severely abraded teeth, which necessitated occlusal restorations to build up the mandibular posterior segments, the gingiva appears healthy and of normal width and contour.

The *radiograph* reveals slight widening of the periodontal ligament space at the occlusal aspect, but no evidence of pathological changes. Tooth mobility is normal.

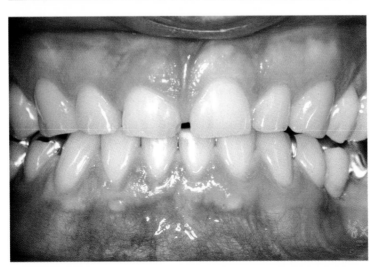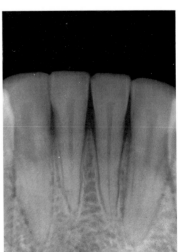

Gingival Width

The attached gingiva becomes wider as a patient ages (Ainamo et al. 1981). It also varies considerably from tooth to tooth and among individuals. Although it was once believed that a minimal width of attached gingiva (ca. 2 mm) was necessary to maintain the health of the periodontium (Lang & Löe 1972), this view has been questioned in recent publications (Wennström 1982, Dorfman et al. 1982, Wennström & Lindhe 1983).

Col

Apical to the contact area between two adjacent teeth, the interdental gingiva assumes a concave form when viewed in labiolingual section (Fig. 8). The concavity, termed the "col," is thus located between the lingual and facial interdental papillae and is not visible clinically. Depending on the expanse of the contacting tooth surfaces, the col will be of varying depth and breadth. The epithelium covering the col consists essentially of the marginal epithelia of the adjacent teeth (Cohen 1959, 1962); col epithelium is not keratinized.

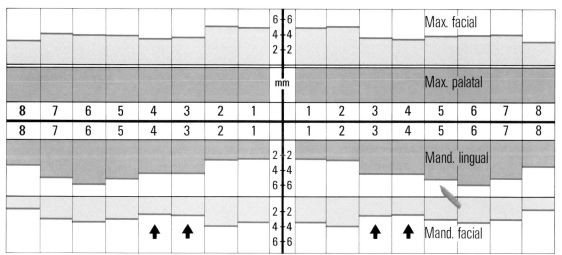

6   Mean width of gingiva
Facial aspect of maxilla:
The gingiva is wide over the incisors but narrower over cuspids and bicuspids.
Palatal aspect of maxilla:
The free gingival margin blends directly into the palatal mucosa without any transition zone.
Lingual aspect of mandible:
The gingiva is narrow in the anterior area and wider in posterior segments.
Facial aspect of mandible:
The gingiva around cuspids and first bicuspids is narrow (arrows) but wider on the lateral incisors.

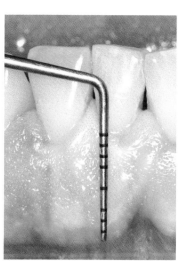
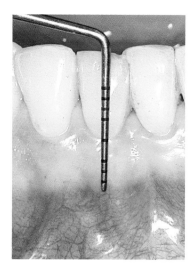
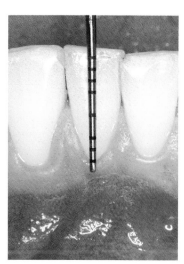

7   Variability of gingival width
The width of attached gingiva can vary dramatically. The three patients depicted here, all about the same age, exhibit gingival width from 1 to 10 mm in the mandibular anterior area.

Staining the mucosa with iodine (*Schiller* or *Lugol* solution) renders the mucogingival line easily visible (right) as the nonkeratinized alveolar mucosa is iodine positive while keratinized gingiva is not (right).

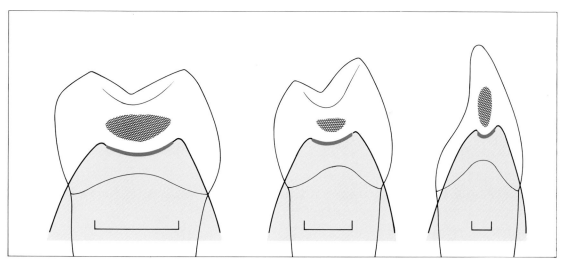

8   Col
Tooth position and tooth morphology, especially the width of the crown, will determine the vestibulo-oral and coronoapical expanse of the interdental contact area (hatched), which in turn accounts for the breadth and depth of the col (red).

If there is no contact between adjacent teeth, i. e., if a diastema is present, the contour of interdental gingiva will lack any concavity, there will be no col *per se,* and keratinization is maintained.

Epithelial Attachment

Junctional epithelium – Epithelial attachment – Sulcus

The specialized junctional epithelium of the free marginal gingiva forms the epithelial attachment of gingiva to the tooth surface. This attachment is continuously being renewed throughout life (Schroeder & Listgarten 1977).

The *junctional epithelium* (JE) is about 2 mm in coronoapical dimension, and surrounds the neck of each tooth. The apical portion of the JE consists of only a few layers of cells, while the coronal JE adjacent to the sulcus may be 15–30 cell layers thick. Immediately subjacent to the sulcus bottom, the JE is about 0.15 mm wide. The JE consists of the Stratum basale, where mitosis occurs, and a Stratum suprabasale. The JE remains undifferentiated; it does not keratinize. The healthy JE does not exhibit rete ridges where it contacts the connective tissue. The basal cells of the JE are intimately connected to the connective tissue by means of hemidesmosomes and an external basal lamina. The cellular turnover rate in the JE is extraordinarily high (4–6 days) compared to oral epithelium (6–12 days; Skougaard 1965, 1970).

9   Marginal periodontium and gingiva in orofacial section
The gingiva consists of three different tissues: The junctional epithelium, the oral epithelium and the underlying connective tissue (Lamina propria).

The *junctional epithelium* assumes a key role in health maintenance of the periodontium: It creates the firm attachment of soft tissue to hard tissue; it is quite permeable, and thus serves as a pathway for diffusion of the metabolic products of plaque bacteria (toxins, chemotactic agents, antigens/mitogens etc.). Even when the gingivae do not appear inflamed clinically, the JE is transmigrated by polymorphonuclear leukocytes (PMNs) moving toward the sulcus (see Etiology and Pathogenesis, p. 18).

The three red arrows indicate the path of movement of JE cells from the Stratum basale toward the gingival sulcus.

The circled areas **A–C** are depicted in detail on page 5.

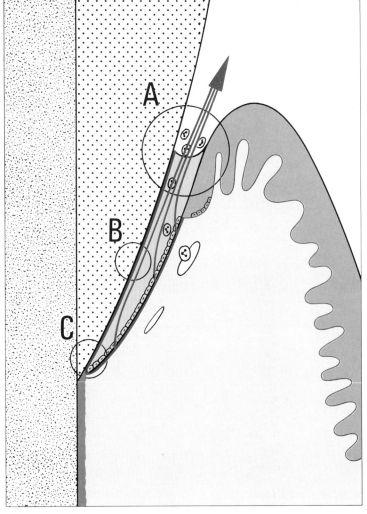

Structure of the junctional epithelium (JE)
Height: 2 mm
Coronal width: 0.15 mm

A. Normal gingival sulcus (GS)
Histological
    depth: 0–0.5 mm
Width: 0.15 mm
Clinical depth: 0.5–3 mm
                         (due to probe
                         penetration of
                         JE; see Fig. 219)

B. Internal basal lamina (IBL) "Epithelial attachment"
Thickness: 350–1400 Å
(1 Å = 0.000 000 1 mm)

C. Apical extent of the junctional epithelium

The *epithelial attachment* to the tooth provided by the JE consists of an internal basal lamina and hemidesmosomes. The attachment of JE to hard tooth structure can occur on enamel, cementum or dentin in exactly the same manner. The basal lamina and hemidesmosomes of the epithelial attachment are structural analogs of their counterparts that comprise the junction between epithelium and subjacent connective tissue.

All of the cells of the JE are in continual coronal migration, even those cells in immediate contact with the tooth surface. Such cells must constantly dissolve and re-establish their hemidesmosomal attachments. Between the basal lamina and the tooth surface, a 0.5–1 µm thick dental cuticle is frequently observed. This cuticle is probably a synthetic product of JE cells.

The *gingival sulcus* is a narrow groove surrounding the tooth, about 0.5 mm deep. The bottom of the sulcus is comprised of the most coronally located cells of the JE, which are in the process of being sloughed. One lateral wall of the sulcus is made up of the tooth structure, the other wall is the oral sulcular epithelium (Lange & Schroeder 1971).

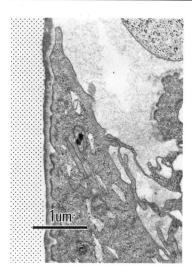

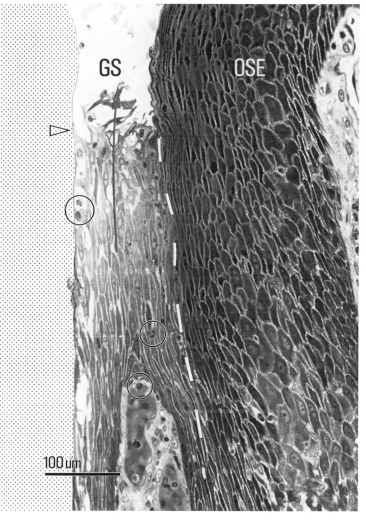

10 Gingival sulcus – Junctional epithelium

The spindle shaped cells of the junctional epithelium (JE) are oriented parallel to the tooth surface and are sharply demarcated (broken line) in this histologic section from the more deeply staining cells of the oral sulcular epithelium (OSE). All JE cells originate at the Stratum basale and migrate toward the sulcus bottom (red arrow) where they are sloughed into the sulcus. The Stratum basale can be 1.5–2 mm long, yet the sulcus bottom may be only 100–150 µm across, emphasizing the bottleneck through which JE cells must pass. Observe the polymorphonuclear leukocytes (circled), which emigrate from venules in the subepithelial connective tissue (CT) and transmigrate the JE.

In the *enlargement* (left), a portion of the most coronal JE cell at the sulcus bottom (open arrow, right) is shown still manifesting hemidesmosomes and an internal basal lamina attaching it to the enamel surface (dot pattern).

TEMs courtesy of *H. E. Schroeder*

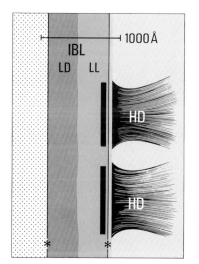

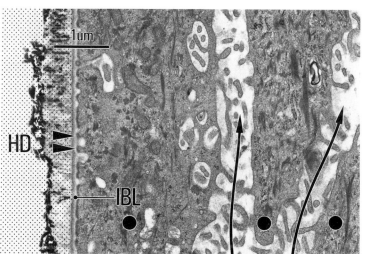

11 Internal basal lamina and hemidesmosomes

Each JE cell adjacent to the tooth surface forms hemidesmosomes (HD) that enable the cell to attach to the internal basal lamina (IBL) and ultimately to the surface of the tooth. Remnants of enamel crystals are visible at the left (black spots). The black arrows indicate intercellular space between JE cells. Portions of three JE cells are observed (black dots).

The *internal basal lamina* is comprised of two layers: the Lamina lucida (LL) and the Lamina densa (LD; see schematic at left).

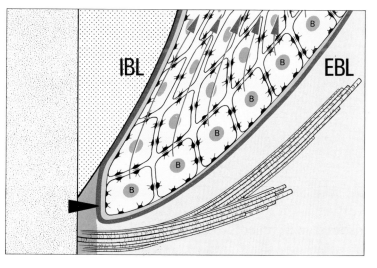

12 Most apical portion of the junctional epithelium

In a young, healthy patient the JE ends at the cementoenamel junction. Daughter cells of the cuboidal basal cells (B) migrate toward the sulcus (red arrows). If a JE cell comes into contact with the tooth surface, it establishes the attachment mechanism described above. The internal basal lamina (IBL) is continuous with the external basal lamina (EBL) around the apical extent of the JE (arrow).

Immediately below the JE, the first dentogingival collagen fiber bundles are seen.

Connective Tissue Attachment

Gingival and periodontal fiber groups – Cementum – Alveolar bone

The components of the connective tissue compartment provide the connection of the tooth to the alveolar bone as well as each tooth to its neighbor.

Gingival fiber bundles
Within the gingiva, collagen fiber bundles course in various directions (see Figs. 14 and 15). It is these bundles

of fibrous connective tissue that provide the gingiva with resiliency and resistance to external forces. These fibers stabilize the positions of individual teeth and unite the teeth of each arch into a functional entity (Fig. 14).

The *periodontal ligament* (PDL) is also composed primarily of fibrous connective tissue. Collagenous PDL fiber bundles (Fig. 16) secure the tooth within its alveolus (Feneis 1952).

13   Gingival and periodontal fiber bundles, cementum, alveolar bone
The major portion of the connective tissue compartment of free marginal and attached gingiva is comprised of collagen fiber bundles (**A**). These splay from the cementum of the root surface into the gingiva. Other fiber bundles course more or less horizontally within the gingiva and between the teeth, forming a complex architecture (see Figs. 14, 15). In addition to collagen fibers, one may also observe a smaller number of reticular (argyrophilic) fibers.

The periodontal ligament space (**B**) in adults is ca. 0.15–0.2 mm wide. About 60% of the space is occupied by collagen fiber bundles of ca. 4 µm thickness. The periodontal ligament fiber bundles traverse from cementum to the alveolar bone (**C**).

Approximately 28,000 fiber bundles may be detected in 1 mm² of cementum surface!

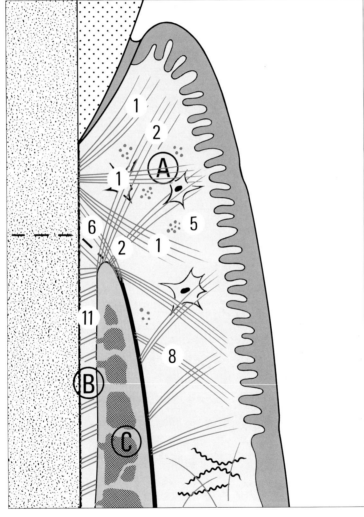

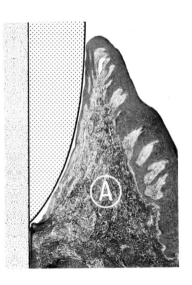

A   Gingival fibers

B   Periodontal ligament fibers

C   Alveolar bone

The *cementum* covers the entire root of each tooth. Anatomically, cementum is part of the tooth; functionally it belongs to the tooth-supporting structures because the gingival and periodontal fibers are anchored in cementum as Sharpey's fibers. The cementum becomes thicker from the coronal (50–150 µm) extent. In the apical third of the root (200–600 µm), cementum containing viable cells (cementocytes) entrapped in lacunae is often observed.

Cementum resembles bone in its physical properties. It is always covered by a very thin, uncalcified layer of cementoid substance that is synthesized and secreted by resident cementoblasts.

The *alveolar bone* is part of the alveolar processes of the maxilla and mandible. The process can be divided anatomically into: 1) The alveolar bone proper, also called the cribriform plate and observed radiographically as the Lamina dura. It is a thin layer of bone lining each socket, and exhibiting numerous perforations through which blood vessels, lymph channels and nerves pass. 2) The supporting alveolar bone is that portion of the alveolar process that surrounds the alveolar bone proper. It has two major components, cortical bone that comprises the heavy facial and oral plates of the process, and cancellous bone located between the cortical plates and the alveolar bone proper.

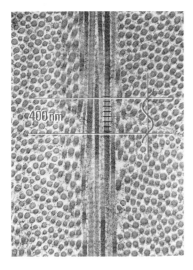

Fiber bundles

Gingival:
1. Dentogingival
   – coronal, horizontal, apical
2. Alveologingival
3. Interpapillary
4. Transgingival
5. Circular / Semicircular
6. Dentoperiosteal
7. Transseptal
8. Periostogingival
9. Intercircular
10. Intergingival

Periodontal:
11. Alveolodental
    – horizontal, oblique, apical, interradicular

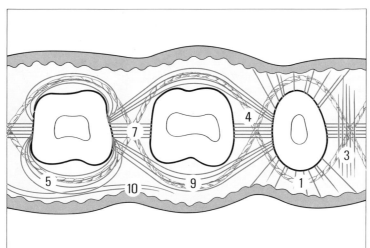

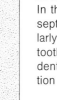

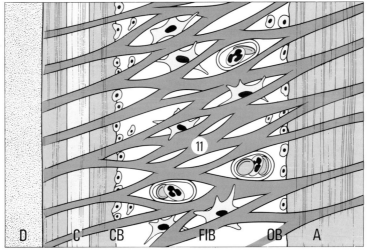

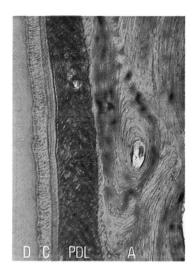

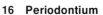

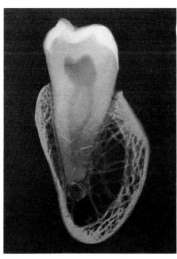

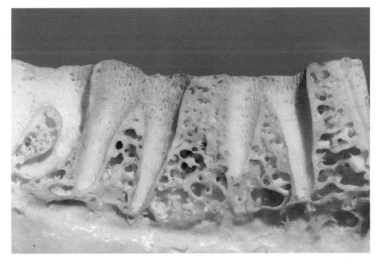

14 Gingival fiber architecture in horizontal section

The spatial arrangement of especially important fiber bundles is depicted schematically. The numbers refer to the list adjacent to Figure 15.

The *basic element* of fiber bundles is the *collagen fibril* (shown at left in both horizontal and longitudinal section), which is secreted by fibroblasts. Such fibrils exhibit a periodic banding pattern of 64 nm intervals; for comparison, the wave length of blue light = 400 nm.

TEM courtesy of *H. E. Schroeder*

15 Fiber bundles viewed in mesiodistal section

In the interdental area, the transseptal fibers course supraalveolarly from one tooth to the adjacent tooth. These fibers stabilize the dental arch in a mesiodistal direction (H & E, × 10).

Photomicrographs courtesy of *N. P. Lang*

The descriptive names of *all* gingival and periodontal fiber groups are given in the list at left.

16 Periodontium

The collagen fiber bundles are intertwined, coursing primarily in a coronoapical direction from the alveolar bone (A) to the cementum (C) where they insert as Sharpey's fibers. Osteoblasts (OB) line the surface of the bone on one aspect of the periodontal ligament space, while cementoblasts (CB) line the root surface on the other aspect. Numerous fibroblasts (FIB) are found within the substance of the periodontal ligament.

Histologic section (Azan, × 50): Periodontal ligament (PDL), cementum (C), alveolar bone (A).

17 Alveolar bone – Cribriform plate

In this mesiodistal section through the mandible after removal of all teeth, the cribriform plate and the trabecular structure are clearly revealed.

In an *orofacial section* (radiograph, left) one may observe the massive cortical plates, the trabecular bone and the thin cribriform plate.

Physiologic Tooth Mobility

The manner in which a tooth is supported within its alveolus, and the elasticity of the entire alveolar process provide for a measurable physiologic tooth mobility in horizontal, vertical and rotational directions (Mühlemann 1967). Physiologic tooth mobility varies within a 24-hr cycle: The teeth are more mobile in the morning than in the evening (Himmel et al. 1957). Variation in tooth mobility also exists among healthy individuals; this is referred to as the normal physiologic range. Nevertheless, each type of tooth will exhibit characteristic mobility depending upon the *surface area* available for insertion of periodontal ligament fibers, and this in turn will depend upon number of roots, root length and root diameter.

Tooth mobility may increase as a result of occlusal trauma or quantitative bone loss due to periodontitis. However, *elevated tooth mobility is not a criterion for periodontal health or pathology.*

18 Physiologic tooth mobility with increasing force (force p = gram)

A. After orofacial loading with **100 gm,** the collagen fibers of the periodontal ligament are stretched: Initial tooth mobility.

B. Loading with **500 gm** force reversibly deforms the entire alveolar process (blue): Secondary tooth mobility.

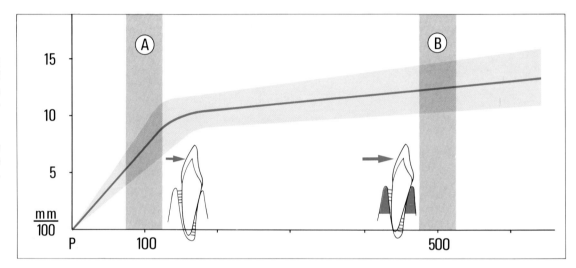

19 Tooth mobility – Mean values of various tooth types

| I – Incisors
| C – Cuspids
| P – Bicuspids
| M – Molars

The values depicted here represent *mean mobility figures in health,* after application of a constant heavy force (500 gm) to elicit secondary tooth mobility.
    These values would be scored as zero in clinical charting (see Tooth Mobility – Function, p. 95).

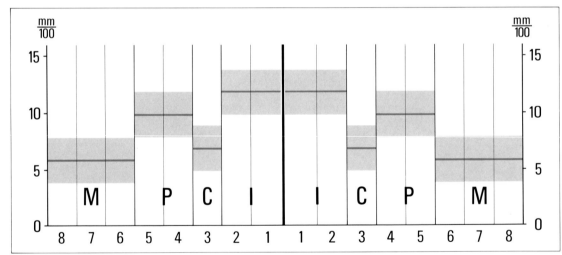

Initial tooth mobility (A)

This is defined as the first phase of movement after application of a 100 gm force to a tooth in a labiolingual direction. The tooth moves relatively easily within the alveolus. Some periodontal ligament fiber bundles are stretched, others relaxed, but there is no significant deformation of the alveolar process.
    The initial tooth mobility is relatively high and depends entirely upon the width of the periodontal ligament space and the histologic structure of the periodontium. Depending upon the tooth being assessed, initial tooth mobility will range from 5–10 mm $\times 10^{-2}$.

Secondary tooth mobility (B)

This is measured after application of 500 gm of force to a tooth in a labiolingual direction. At this magnitude of force, the entire alveolar process is deformed and any further movement of the tooth would require much higher forces.
    Variations in secondary tooth mobility in a healthy periodontium result from the quality, thickness and elasticity of the alveolar bone. Secondary tooth mobility may range from 8–15 mm $\times 10^{-2}$.

Etiology and Pathogenesis

Health◄————————►**Gingivitis**————————►**Periodontitis**

Gingivitis and periodontitis are inflammatory diseases of bacterial origin.

Gingivitis may persist for many years without progressing to periodontitis. With good oral hygiene and effective removal of plaque and calculus, gingivitis is completely reversible.

The etiology of *periodontitis* is not yet completely understood, but it is likely the result of an *opportunistic infection*. An increase in the number of pathogenic plaque microorganisms, their ability to invade into tissue, and the individual host response (resistance, immune status) to the infection appear to be the determining criteria. Even after professional treatment, the destruction caused by periodontitis is only partially reversible (see Reattachment, New Attachment, p. 260). The *Status quo ante* will never be achieved.

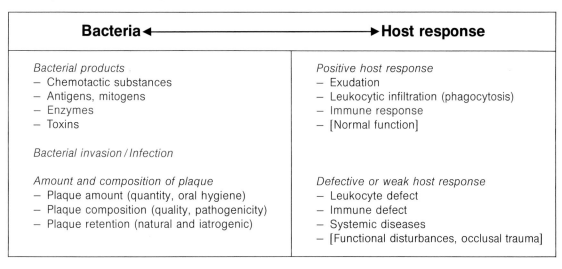

Bacteria◄————————————►**Host response**	
Bacterial products – Chemotactic substances – Antigens, mitogens – Enzymes – Toxins *Bacterial invasion / Infection* *Amount and composition of plaque* – Plaque amount (quantity, oral hygiene) – Plaque composition (quality, pathogenicity) – Plaque retention (natural and iatrogenic)	*Positive host response* – Exudation – Leukocytic infiltration (phagocytosis) – Immune response – [Normal function] *Defective or weak host response* – Leukocyte defect – Immune defect – Systemic diseases – [Functional disturbances, occlusal trauma]

20   Bacterial attack and host response
The strength of bacterial attack depends on amount and composition of plaque, ability of the organisms to invade tissues, and metabolic products.

The effectiveness of the host response to bacterial challenge will determine the severity of an ensuing gingivitis, the initiation of periodontitis, and the rapidity with which destruction of periodontal tissues proceeds.

An absolutely plaque-free condition in the oral cavity is unachieveable, an illusion, and probably even unphysiologic. Nevertheless, gingival and periodontal health can be maintained if the plaque contains few virulent organisms and if an effective host response is mounted.

The most important bacterial products in terms of inflammation and tissue destruction are antigens, mitogens and chemotactic substances. If bacteria invade the tissue directly, one may speak of a true infection.

Bacterial enzymes and various toxins can probably cause tissue injury and destruction directly, without an immediate host response. Bacterial products including hyaluronidase, chondroitin sulfatase, proteolytic enzymes as well as cytotoxins in the form of organic acids, ammonia, hydrogen sulfide and bacterial endotoxins (lipopolysaccharide, LPS) can be demonstrated in tissues.

Accumulated Debris – Microbial Plaque

Food debris cling only lightly to the teeth and oral mucosa, and can be easily rinsed away with water.

Food impaction may occur in interdental spaces when fibrous foodstuff become trapped, but can be removed mechanically.

Microbial plaque is a structured, resilient, yellowgrayish substance that adheres tenaciously to teeth. It is comprised of bacteria in a matrix of salivary glycoproteins and extracellular polysaccharides like glucans

(e.g., dextrans, mutans) and fructans (e.g., levan). This matrix makes it impossible to rinse plaque away with water; it must be removed mechanically by means of hand instruments, the toothbrush or other oral hygiene aids. Supragingival plaque and subgingival plaque are two distinct morphological and microbiological entities.

Further, one can distinguish between adherent plaque and nonadherent subgingival plaque. The pathogenicity of bacterial strains within plaque varies considerably. Plaque adhering to the tooth surface can become calcified.

21 Initial supragingival plaque colonization – Healthy appearing gingiva
A disclosing agent reveals the initial, extremely thin layer of plaque.

The gingiva is still relatively free of inflammation as observed clinically. Gingival Index (GI) and Papilla Bleeding Index (PBI) scores are zero.

This initial accumulation of plaque is only a few cell layers thick, and consists primarily of gram positive cocci.

Gingival health can be maintained with this amount of plaque accumulation!

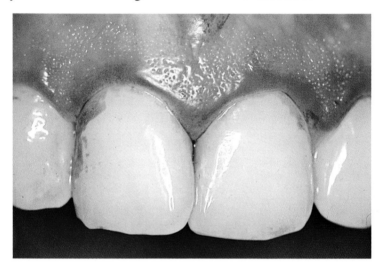

22 Initial gingivitis
In 1965 Löe et al. published the classic experimental proof of the bacterial etiology of gingivitis. In plaque-free subjects and manifesting inflammation-free gingiva, plaque begins to accumulate if all oral hygiene is ceased. For the first few days this plaque is composed of *gram-positive* ⊕ cocci and rods, then later of filamentous organisms and finally of Spirochetes (*gram-negative* ⊖). Within a few days, a mild gingivitis ensues (GI = 1).

If the plaque is removed, the gingiva returns to a state of health.

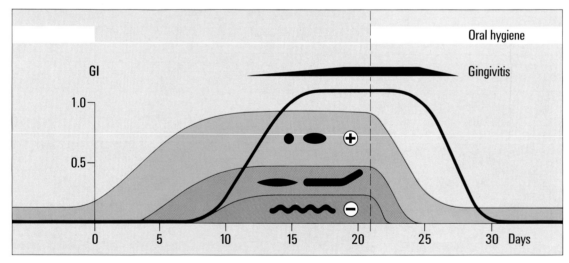

23 Plaque accumulation – Gingivitis
Whenever there is an accumulation of plaque, gingivitis will develop. As accumulation continues, the percentage composition of various organisms in plaque changes. Gram-negative anaerobes increase in frequency; these are more pathogenic than the earlier-appearing gram-positive cocci and rods. The gingiva reacts to both the quantitative and qualitative plaque changes with inflammatory reactions of differing intensity.

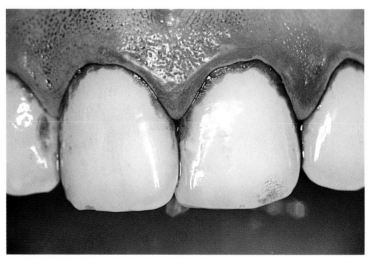

Supragingival Plaque

Accumulation – Alteration of composition

Within minutes to hours, an absolutely clean tooth is covered by a 0.1–0.8 µm thick pellicle composed of salivary glycoproteins. Upon this pellicle, primarily gram-positive colony-forming bacteria (Streptococcus and Actinomyces species) become established within 24 hr.

During the course of the next few days, the plaque increases in quantity as gram-negative cocci as well as gram-positive and -negative rods and filaments gain a foothold.

After 3 weeks, there is a significant increase in filamentous organisms, especially at the gingival margin (Listgarten et al. 1975; Listgarten 1976a). The metabolic products of the plaque microorganisms provoke an elevated level of PMN migration and sulcus fluid flow in the host tissues. This is the host's attempt to wall off invading bacteria. As gingivitis increases in severity, the junctional epithelium loses some of its resiliency, permitting the ingress of bacteria between the tooth and the epithelium. A gingival pocket develops.

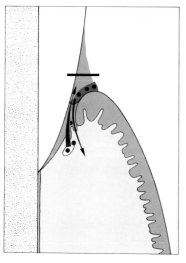

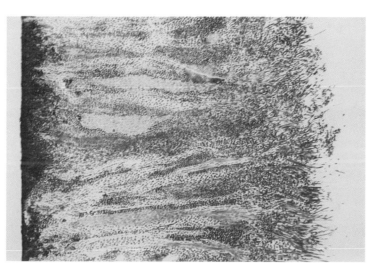

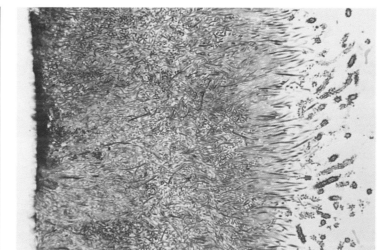

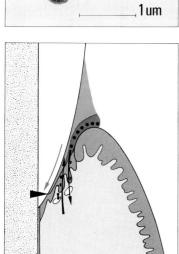

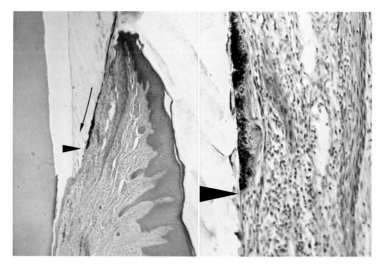

24 1-week-old plaque – Metabolic interactions
The newly formed plaque exhibits column-like structured colonies of coccoid organisms, with overlying rods and filaments.

Diagram: Initial host response to plaque microorganisms (blue, gram-positive; red, gram-negative). Increased migration of PMNs (thick arrow), with formation of a wall of leukocytes. Chemotactic substances from plaque (thin arrow).

The black horizontal line indicates the level from which the section of plaque was taken.

25 3-week-old plaque – "Corn cobs"
The composition of the supragingival plaque has changed markedly. Filamentous organisms now predominate. Conspicuous forms resembling corn cobs are observed at the plaque surface.

In the *electron photomicrograph* at left, the structure of such a corn cob is revealed. At the center is a filamentous organism (F), surrounded by gram-positive cocci (C).

Photomicrographs and TEM courtesy of *M. Listgarten*

26 Expansion of supragingival plaque – Gingival pocket
Diagram: The weakening of the attachment between tooth and JE permits apical immigration of gram-positive plaque bacteria (blue) in a thin layer, forming a gingival pocket. Gram-negative anaerobic bacteria (red) are observed mainly on the soft tissue aspect of the sulcus, and elicit an enhanced host response.

The lateral arrowheads in the two histological sections and the diagram (left) indicate the apical extent of bacterial progression.

Photomicrograph, *G. Cimasoni*

Subgingival Plaque

Adherent flora – Nonadherent flora

In the subgingival region it is possible to differentiate between *adherent* and *nonadherent* plaque. A dense plaque layer of varying thickness adheres to the tooth (root) surface. The composition of this adherent layer resembles the supragingival plaque associated with gingivitis: some *gram-positive* cocci but primarily filaments and Actinomyces species. The adherent plaque can become mineralized to form subgingival calculus.

Near the soft tissue surface are observed freely moving bacterial accumulations ("swimmers") comprised almost exclusively of *gram-negative* anaerobes: cocci, spirochetes and rods (Bacteroides species, especially B. gingivalis). These nonadherent, partially motile, gram-negative, pathogenic anaerobes increase sharply in number in acute inflammatory lesions. They appear to play an important role in the progression of periodontitis (Listgarten 1976a; Slots 1979; Page & Schroeder 1982; Lindhe 1983).

27 Subgingival flora
On the tooth surface (left side of histologic section) is a thin layer of adherent, primarily gram-positive plaque bacteria (blue-violet).

Within the pocket exudate are observed larger loose accumulations of gram-negative anaerobic bacteria. Inset: Accumulations resembling test tube brushes also appear. Courtesy of *M. Listgarten.*

Diagram: Adherent plaque shown as blue; nonadherent bacteria (swimmers) shown as red. Black bar represents level from which the depicted plaque was taken.

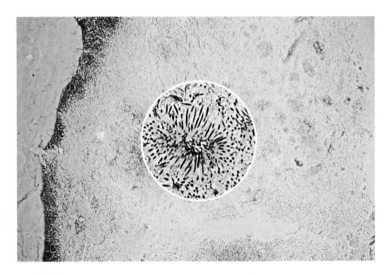
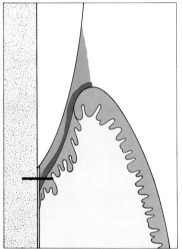

28 Adherent plaque – Root surface
Within a pocket, the root surface of a tooth manifesting periodontitis is covered with a densely intertwined bacterial colonization composed of many different bacterial forms (scanning electron photomicrograph).

Adherent plaque predominates, with an occasional swimmer from the nonadherent plaque.

The morphology of the bacteria permits neither a determination of the species nor any clues concerning pathogenicity.

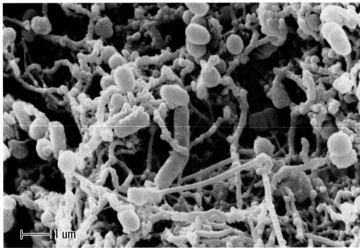

29 Microorganisms of the nonadherent plaque
In a streaked preparation (dark field) motile rods and spirochetes predominate, while cocci and filaments are rare: Typical sign of an active pocket (exacerbation).

Right: Intact phagocytes (PMNs) in the pocket exudate do not lose their capacity for phagocytosis. Arrow depicts a spirochete being engulfed.

Photomicrographs courtesy of *B. Guggenheim*

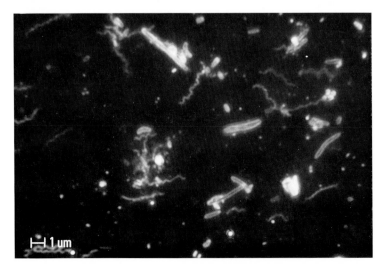
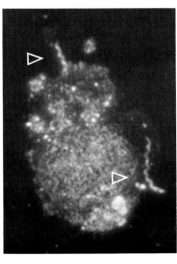

Infection − Bacterial Invasion into Tissues

In cases of periodontitis, especially the rapidly progressive (RPP) and juvenile (LJP) forms, bacteria may traverse the pocket epithelium and invade the subepithelial connective tissue. This usually occurs only in the depth of a pocket where the organisms can avoid the massive inflammatory infiltrate that is located marginally. It is probable that the invading bacteria secrete protective leukotoxins that can momentarily either inhibit or neutralize the chemotactic substances guiding phagocytic host defense cells (PMNs) to the area. In the end, the host defense cells do recognize and kill the bacteria. If the number of invading organisms is small, necrotic areas will be left within the tissue; if the bacterial invasion is massive, a purulent abscess with external drainage may be created.

It is not yet completely clear whether the resulting tissue damage is due primarily to direct toxicity of the bacteria or their products, or whether the destruction is caused by products of the host's own immune system, or both (Frank 1980; Saglie et al 1982; Gillet & Johnson 1982; Allenspach-Petrzilka & Guggenheim 1983; Genco & Slots 1984).

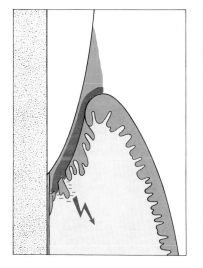
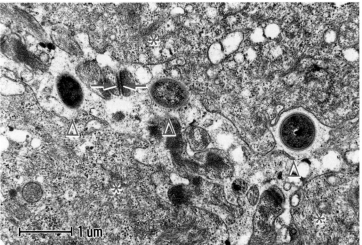

30 Bacteria in the pocket epithelium

During an exacerbation, bacteria (open arrows) traverse the widened intercellular spaces of the pocket epithelium. Three epithelial cells (*) and one desmosome (arrows) are observed.

Diagram: Ulcerated epithelium is found in the depth of an active periodontal pocket. Bacteria are capable of penetrating such epithelia to reach the connective tissue compartment. In this phase, components of the nonadherent subgingival plaque (red) assume prime importance.

31 Bacterial invasion − Infection

In electron photomicrographs of *active* periodontal pockets, bacteria of various species are frequently observed within the connective tissue (arrows). Tissue damage (* = degraded collagen) may result, or the tissue may reamin completely healthy in appearance.

Left: A gram-negative bacterium (G⊖) is observed in the midst of otherwise essentially intact collagen fibrils.

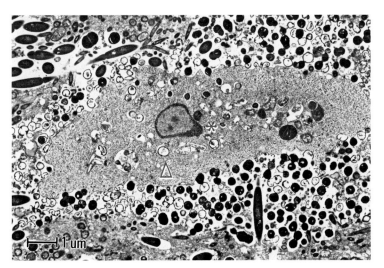

32 Necrosis − Suppuration

Almost the entire photomicrograph is filled by a dead phagocytic cell (*). The cell contains phagosomes, some of which exhibit digested material (arrow).

The dead phagocyte is surrounded by likewise dead bacteria and bacterial cell walls.

This pus must either be resorbed by the tissue or expelled.

TEMs courtesy of *B. Guggenheim*

Natural Factors Favoring Plaque Retention

The most important naturally occurring plaque-retentive factors or "nitches" include:

- Supra- and subgingival calculus
- Crowding of teeth in the arch
- Enamel projections, pearls, CEJ
- Mouth breathing.

Calculus is dead, calcified plaque. By itself it is not pathogenic, but due to its rough surface it is an ideal substrate for retention of pathogenic microorganisms.

Crowding leads to increased accumulation of plaque because self-cleansing mechanisms are foiled and because oral hygiene is more difficult.

Rough areas at the *cementoenamel junction* enhance plaque retention. On molars one often observes enamel projections or enamel "pearls" that may extend into the furcation.

Mouth breathing leads to dehydration of the oral cavity, rendering the plaque tougher and stickier. The protective function of saliva is reduced.

33 Supragingival calculus
The lingual surfaces of mandibular incisors and the buccal surfaces of maxillary molars are typical areas for supragingival calculus. These areas are near the duct orifices of salivary glands, where the minerals for calcification derive.

Right: TEM of old supragingival calculus. Calcified plaque (A) is observed close to the tooth surface (arrow). Visible also is the calcification of plaque bacteria both *inter-* and *intracellularly.* Note cell-free accumulation of hexagonal *monocrystals* (B).
Courtesy of *H. Schroeder*

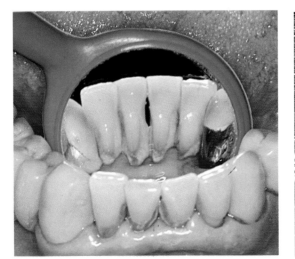
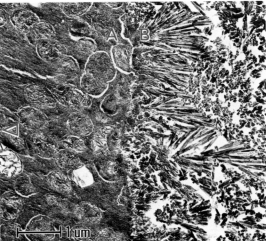

34 Subgingival calculus
In this patient with long-standing periodontitis the gingiva has receded. Calculus that was formerly subgingival is now supragingival (left).

Subgingival calculus is observed clinically after deflecting the gingival margin (right). Subgingival calculus is usually dark in color. It is also harder than the more loosely structured supragingival calculus. The cementoenamel junction is indicated by a dashed line.

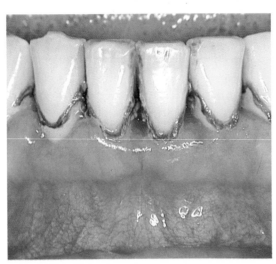
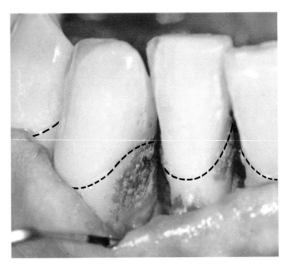

35 Crowding
The lingually displaced mandibular incisors do not benefit from the natural self-cleansing action of the lower lip. Oral hygiene is also made more difficult.

Enamel projection (+ pearl)
The furcation on this molar is filled by a projection of enamel that ends in a bulbous pearl. When a pocket forms in such an area, plaque control is particularly difficult.

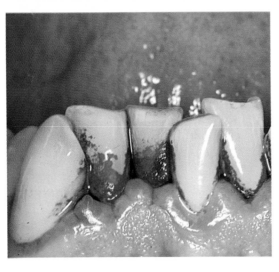
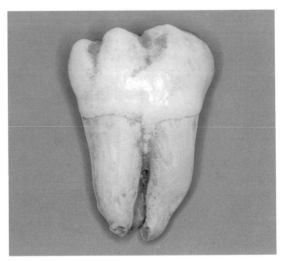

Iatrogenic Factors Favoring Plaque Accumulation

Restorative dentistry – from a simple restoration to a full-mouth reconstruction – if performed improperly can do more harm than good to the patient's oral health.

Fillings that appear to be perfect clinically and macroscopically almost always exhibit deficiencies at the margins when viewed microscopically. Thus, when filling margins are located subgingivally they are always an irritation for the marginal periodontium (Renggli 1974; Hammer & Hotz 1979).

Overhanging margins of restorations and crowns accumulate additional plaque. Gingivitis ensues. The composition of the plaque changes. The number of gram-negative anaerobes, those mainly responsible for the initiation and progression of periodontitis, increases rapidly (Lang et al. 1983).

Gross iatrogenic irritants such as poorly designed clasps and prosthesis saddles may exert a direct traumatic influence on periodontal tissues.

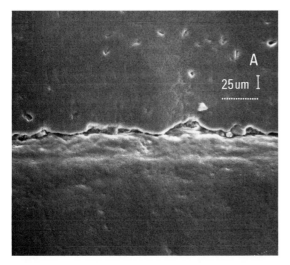
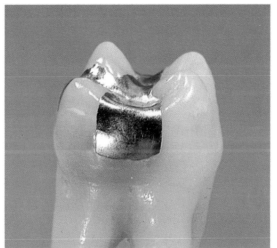

36 Amalgam restoration
A clinically acceptable proximal restoration (right) exhibits a clearly visible margin defect when viewed with the scanning electron microscope (left). Such a defect is a perfect nitch for the accumulation of plaque. A = amalgam.
The white dots under the 25 µm legend are representative of the size of coccoid microorganisms (ca. 1 µm)!

Courtesy of *F. Lutz*

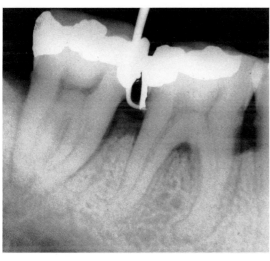
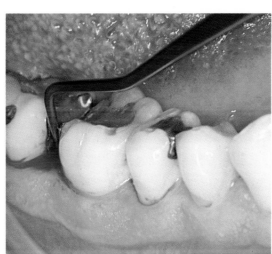

37 Amalgam restoration with overhang
Gross overhangs such as this, located subgingivally, invariably lead to plaque accumulation and to gingivitis (note hemorrhage). The plaque accumulated beneath an overhang changes in its composition: Pathogenic gram-negative anaerobes (e. g., Bacteroides species) increase markedly in number.

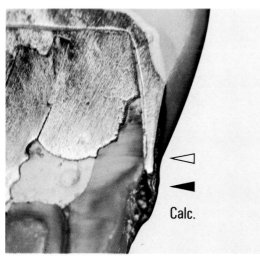
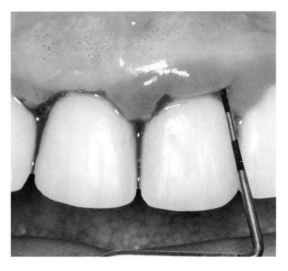

38 Crown margin overhang and open margins
Right: The cement that was used to cement this porcelain jacket crown has begun to extrude from the open margin. The massive retention of plaque between the crown and the prepared tooth led to severe gingivitis with establishment of a pathogenic bacterial flora.

Left: Section through a porcelain-fused-to-gold crown with a margin that is both overhanging (arrows) and open. Darkly stained calculus is observed apical to the poor crown margin.

Bacterial Flora and Types of Disease

The intensity of gingivitis and periodontitis is determined by the quantity and quality of the microorganisms. When plaque accumulation is great and gram-negative anaerobes increase, gingivitis develops. From this, slowly progressive adult periodontitis (AP) can develop. In the rapidly progressive form of periodontitis (RPP) and in juvenile periodontitis (LJP), specific forms of gram-negative anaerobes appear to play the most important role, combined with some type of altered host response (Listgarten 1976a; Slots 1979; Lindhe 1983; Palenstein-Helderman 1981).

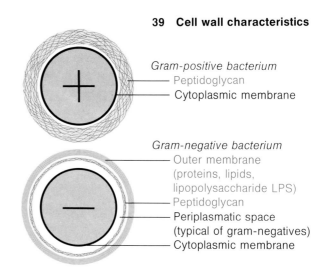

39   Cell wall characteristics

Gram-positive bacterium
— Peptidoglycan
— Cytoplasmic membrane

Gram-negative bacterium
— Outer membrane
  (proteins, lipids,
  lipopolysaccharide LPS)
— Peptidoglycan
— Periplasmatic space
  (typical of gram-negatives)
— Cytoplasmic membrane

40   Healthy gingiva

Clinically healthy gingiva can persist even in the presence of a thin (60 μm), adherent layer of plaque that is a few cell layers thick.

The pie slices depicted below *do not* represent plaque *quantity*; rather, they depict the *qualitative* relationships between aerobes/anaerobes and gram+ / gram−.

41   Gingivitis – Adult periodontitis (AP)

When gingivitis is manifest clinically, one generally observes plaque layers 400 μm and more thick. This *quantitative* increase in plaque plays an important role in the development of gingivitis. Alterations in the *qualitative* composition of plaque occur simultaneously. The gingivitis plaque (present supragingivally) is similar to that of quiescent, slowly progressing adult periodontitis (AP).

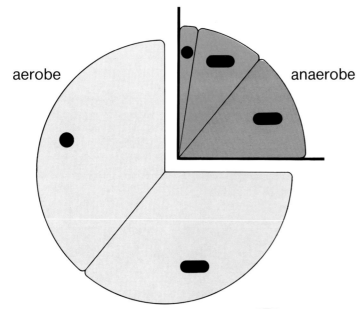

aerobe   anaerobe

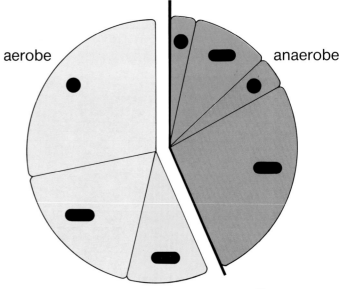

aerobe   anaerobe

Composition of dental plaque with healthy gingiva
The size of the pie slices represents the percentage composition of classifiable cocci and rods. In the extremely thin plaque, gram-positive aerobic cocci and rods predominate (75%). These appear to be relatively nonpathogenic to the periodontal tissues.

Light blue: gram + aerobes
Dark blue: gram + anaerobes

Light red: gram − aerobes
Dark red: gram − anaerobes

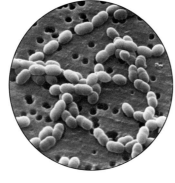

Streptococcus mutans (SEM)
Streptococcus species
Actinomyces viscosus
Actinomyces naeslundii
Rothia dentocariosa
Bacteroides intermedius
Capnocytophaga species

Composition of plaque in gingivitis (and AP)
Especially in sites where plaque accumulates, gram-negative anaerobic organisms begin to predominate at the cost of gram-positive aerobic cocci and rods. In particularly black pigmented types of Bacteroides and various forms of Spirochetes begin to predominate.

This plaque composition is also observed in the quiescent phases of AP, while plaque from an active AP lesion resembles that of RPP.

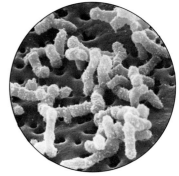

Actinomyces viscosus (SEM)
Actinomyces species
Streptococcus species
Bacteroides melaninogenicus
Capnocytophaga gingivalis
Eikenella corrodens
(Spirochetes)

		GRAM ⊕ POSITIVE		GRAM ⊖ NEGATIVE	
		Facultative anaerobes	Anaerobes	Facultative anaerobes	Anaerobes
COCCI ●		**STREPTOCOCCUS** S. mutans, S. mitis **STAPHYLOCOCCUS** **MICROCOCCUS**	**STREPTOCOCCUS** S. intermedius **PEPTOSTREPTOCOCCUS** **PEPTOCOCCUS**	**NEISSERIA** **BRANHAMELLA**	**VEILLONELLA** **ACIDAMINOCOCCUS**
RODS ▬		**ACTINOMYCES** A. naeslundii A. viscosus **BACTERIONEMA** **ROTHIA** **LACTOBACILLUS**	**ACTINOMYCES** A. israelii **ARACHINA** **EUBACTERIUM** **BIFIDOBACTERIUM** **PROPIONIBACTERIUM** **CLOSTRIDIUM**	**ACTINOBACILLUS** A. actinomycetemcomitans **CAPNOCYTOPHAGA** C. gingivalis C. ochracea C. sputigena **EIKENELLA** E. corrodens **CAMPYLOBACTER** **HAEMOPHILUS**	**BACTEROIDES** B. gingivalis B. melaninogenicus B. ss. intermedius B. ss. melaninogenicus **FUSOBACTERIUM** F. naviforme F. nucleatum **LEPTOTRICHIA** **SELENOMONAS** **WOLINELLA**
SPIROCHETES 〜					**TREPONEMA** T. denticola, T. vincentii T. macrodentium, T. oralis

42 Classified organisms of dental plaque

The known pathogenic organisms and several subtypes (species) of the most frequently isolated plaque microorganisms are presented in the Table according to their Gram staining and respiratory (aerobes or anaerobes) characteristics.

The *color code and symbols* are the same as those in Figures 40, 41, 43 and 44. These summarize the relative percentage of the individual groups of microorganisms (adapted from *Lindhe* 1983; *Slots* 1976, 1979).

43 Rapidly progressive periodontitis (RPP)

In cases of RPP, the composition of nonadherent subgingival plaque exhibits a markedly different composition. Supragingival plaque in such cases may be minimal, and is generally similar to supragingival plaques found in the presence of healthy gingiva or gingivitis.

44 Juvenile periodontitis (LJP)

In localized juvenile periodontitis (incisor-molar type), the nonadherent subgingival pathogenic plaque is different from that found in rapidly progressive adult periodontitis. However, in LJP one seldom observes microorganisms adherent to the root surface.

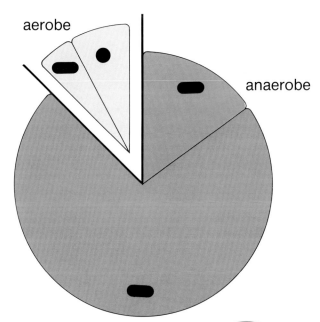

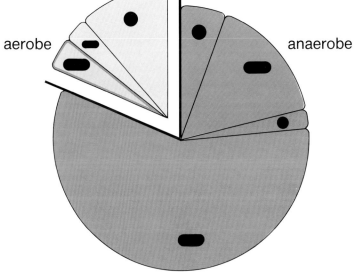

Composition of the plaque in RPP (subgingival)

Almost 3/4 of the entire subgingival plaque consists of gram-negative anaerobic motile rods and spirochetes. Among these are likely to be found the specific causative organisms for this form of periodontal disease. Gram-positive cocci and rods (Actinomyces) are present in small quantity, and are most often observed in the plaque adherent to the root surface.

SEMs courtesy of *B. Guggenheim*

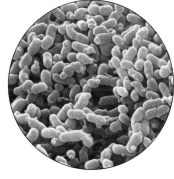

Bacteroides gingivalis (SEM)
Bacteroides species
Fusobacterium nucleatum
Spirochetes (Treponema species)

Composition of plaque in LJP (subgingival)

Considerably more than half of the microorganisms are gram-negative anaerobes. The bacterial species and their percentage composition are somewhat different from the rapidly progressive adult form. Remarkable is the invariable presence of the facultative anaerobe *Actinobacillus actinomycetemcomitans* (AaC), against which unusually high titers of circulating antibodies are found in the blood of LJP patients.

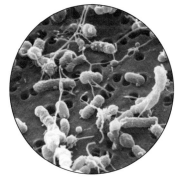

Actinobacillus actinomycetemcomitans (SEM)
Capnocytophaga ochracea
Bacteroides species
Fusobacterium
(Spirochetes)

Histopathogenesis of Gingivitis and Periodontitis

The fine line demarcating healthy gingiva from gingivitis is difficult to discern. Even gingiva that appears quite healthy clinically will exhibit a few polymorphonuclear leukocytes within the junctional epithelium when viewed histologically. These PMNs have emigrated from the subepithelial vascular plexus and end their journey by being shed into the gingival sulcus. Very small quantities of gingival sulcus fluid may therefore be considered physiologic (Cimasoni 1983).

Page and Schroeder (1976) described the temporal sequence of gingivitis and periodontitis development,

based on their own research and a thorough literature review.

As plaque begins to accumulate, *healthy gingiva* begins to exhibit the histological features of the *"initial lesion,"* followed by an *"early lesion"* that persists for a few days, and then an *"established lesion."* The clinically observable gingivitis in adults is always an established gingivitis, whose intensity, however, may vary considerably. The initial and early lesions are actually nothing

45   Healthy gingiva (A)
Absence of plaque or very little accumulation; normal junctional epithelium (pink); minimal sulcus depth (red arrow). A few PMNs (blue dots) transmigrate the JE in the direction of the sulcus bottom. Dense collagenous fiber system; intact fibroblasts.

46   Initial / Early gingivitis (B)
Early plaque accumulation. In the *initial* lesion, increased transmigration of PMNs (blue dots) within the JE.

As the *early* lesion develops, the PMNs create within the slightly deepened sulcus (red arrow) a wall against the plaque bacteria. A lymphocytic infiltrate (black dots) occurs in the subepithelial tissues.

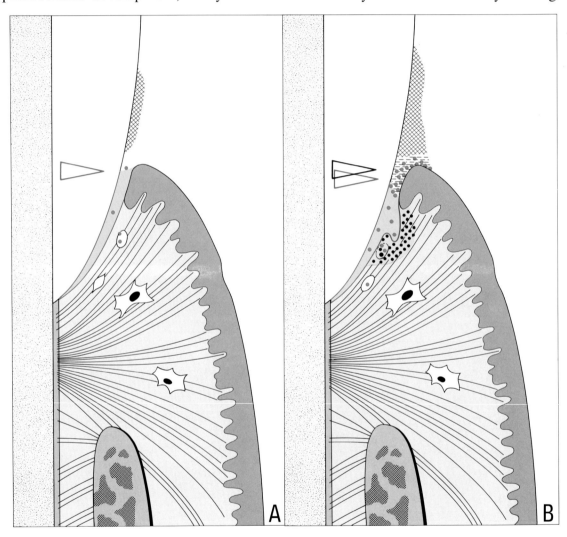

Plaque	Little, primarily gram +, aerobic	Primarily gram +, aerobic
Junctional epithelium/ pocket epithelium	Normal junctional epithelium without rete ridges	Initial alteration and lateral proliferation of the junctional epithelium in coronal region
Vessels Inflammatory cells, infiltrate, exudate	Few *PMNs* from subepithelial vasculature in junctional epithelium, very minimal exudate from the sulcus	Vasculitis, exudation of serum proteins, *PMN migration,* accumulation of *lymphoid* cells, very few plasma cells; appearance of immunogloblins and complement
Fibroblasts, connective tissue, collagen	Normal	Cytopathic alterations of fibroblasts; collagen loss in infiltrated connective tissue areas
Alveolar bone	Normal	Normal
Course of disease	—	*Initial lesion* 2–4 days after plaque accumulation, *early lesion* 4–7 days

more than histologic precursors for the established lesion. In adults, the initial and early lesions last but a few days. In children, however, the "early lesion" can persist for extended periods of time as a clinical entity.

The *established lesion* in adults can persist unchanged for years, perhaps even decades, without progressing to periodontitis. Adult gingivitis appears to be the result less of specific microorganisms than of quantity of plaque and plaque products.

The progression of gingivitis into *periodontitis*, on the other hand, may well be due to some alteration of the pathogenic potential of the plaque (Palenstein-Helderman 1981, Figs. 26 & 43). Periodontitis may manifest clinically in various forms.

The histopathologic characteristics of the development of the gingivoperiodontal lesions are summarized in the table below.

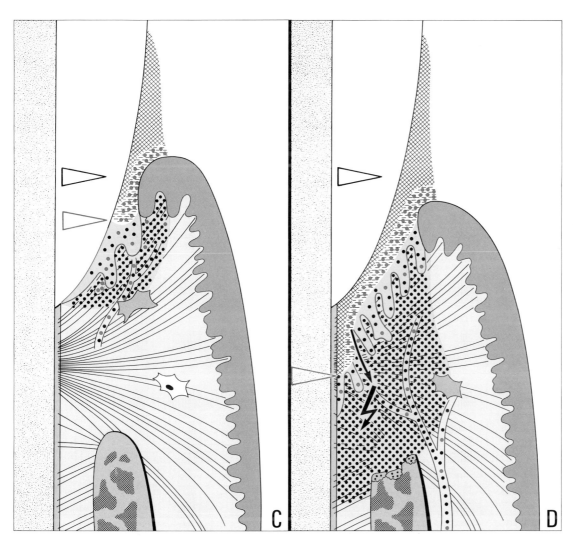

47 Established lesion (C)
The gingiva responds to a massive accumulation of plaque. All of the characteristics of gingivitis are manifest but may be more or less pronounced both clinically and histologically. The junctional epithelium, i. e., the epithelial attachment, may actually be displaced somewhat apically as a consequence of the advancing front of accumulating plaque, resulting in the formation of a gingival pocket (distance between red and black arrows). Nevertheless, at this stage there is no loss of connective tissue attachment. The differentiated inflammatory infiltrate protects the deeper structures of the periodontium.

48 Periodontitis (D)
The most important histological differences between gingivitis and periodontitis are bone resorption, apical proliferation and ulceration of the junctional (pocket) epithelium (red arrow indicates base of pocket), and progressive loss of connective tissue attachment.
   In acute phases there may be bacterial invasion of the tissue, with resultant micro- or macroabscesses.

Gram + and gram − (gingival pocket)	Adherent gram +, nonadherent gram− (pocket)	**Plaque**
Lateral proliferation of JE, deepening of sulcus with formation of gingival pocket or pseudopocket	Apical proliferation of pocket epithelium, true pocket formation; ulceration of pocket epithelium	**Junctional epithelium/ pocket epithelium**
Acute inflammatory alterations; *predominance of plasma cells; immunoglobulins in connective tissue, JE and gingival sulcus; increased sulcus exudate*	Acute inflammatory alterations as in gingivitis; *predominance of plasma cells;* copious exudate often suppurative; expansion of the inflammatory and immunopathologic reactions	**Vessels Inflammatory cells, infiltrate exudate**
Severe fibroblast injury, further loss of collagen, continued infiltration	Further collagen loss in the infiltrated tissues, fibrosis in peripheral gingival regions	**Fibroblasts, connective tissue, collagen**
Normal	Loss of alveolar bone (attachment loss)	**Alveolar bone**
Manifest 1 week after plaque accumulation, can persist for years without progressing	Periods of quiescence and exacerbation. Progression: AP = slow; RPP & LJP = rapid	**Course of disease**

Host Response

The task of the immune system is to intercept agents that would be injurious to body surfaces and tissues. However, if the host immune response is excessive, destruction of host tissue may result. The various immune mechanisms may act singly or in a coordinated manner depending on the challenge. The very basis of immune defense is to be found in the capability of leukocytes to recognize and eliminate a foreign substance. According to Bainton (1980), the primary components of the immune system include:

1. *Phagocytes:* Neutrophilic polymorphonuclear granulocytes (PMN) and monocytes/macrophages ingest foreign substances and destroy them.

2. *Cellular immunity:* T-lymphocytes elicit a delayed hypersensitivity reaction by production of various *lymphotoxins* and *lymphokines* that influence the activation and migration of macrophages and the proliferation of lymphocytes. Examples include macrophage chemotactic factor (MCF), macro-

Cell type	Characteristics	Function
Polymorphonuclear granulocyte (PMN)/Microphage (PMN)	– produced in bone marrow – lifespan: 2–3 days – 5–10 µm diameter – IgG (F_c) receptors – esterase-2-positive	– chemotaxis – *phagocytosis* ⟨ adherence / phagolysosome formation / degradation – microbicidal processes *(cytotoxicity)* – release of microbicidal enzymes, neutral proteases, acid hydrolases, etc.
Monocyte/Macrophage (MΦ) MΦ	– produced in bone marrow – lifespan: months – 12–20 µm diameter – IgG (F_c) receptors – esterase-1-positive	– *phagocytosis,* pinocytosis – microbicidal processes *(cytotoxicity)* – antigen processing and presentation – regulation of lymphocyte function – production and release of biologically active substances: interferon, prostaglandins, complement components, neutral proteases, acid hydrolases
T-Lymphocyte T	– stem cell from bone marrow, thymus-dependent maturation (**T**) – lifespan: months – 6–7 µm diameter – no surface immunoglobulins – stimulation – lymphoblast	– *cell mediated immunity* – helper T-cells: interaction with B-cells, leading to antibody production – suppressor T-cells: inhibit B-cell response – killer T-cells – lymphokine production, e.g., MCF, MIF, MAF, LMF, interferon, lymphotoxin *(cytotoxicity)*
B-Lymphocyte/ Plasma cell B	– stem cell from bone marrow, maturation bursa-equivalent (**B**) – lifespan: months – 6–7 µm diameter, activated (plasma cell) 10–15 µm – surface Ig as antigen receptor	– *humoral immunity, immunoglobulin synthesis* – B-lymphocyte: immunoglobulin, antigen-specific, variable Ig classes – plasma cell: immunoglobulin, antigen- and class-specific

Antibodies (Ab) Immunoglobulins
 	
Approximate molecular weights   IgG 150,000
           IgM 900,000
           IgA 300,000
	– 5 classes: **IgA, IgD, IgE, IgG, IgM**
	– basic molecule: heavy and light polypeptide chains
	– F_{ab} fragment with antigen-binding regions
	– F_c fragment: complement activation, adherence to cell surface (opsonization)
		– antigen-antibody reaction: Ag-Ab complex
		– agglutination ⎫ *toxin neutralization*
		– precipitation ⎭
		– opsonization
		– *cytotoxicity*
		– complement activation

Complement system Cascade C_1–C_9	– activation via *classical pathway* (**CPW**) by antibodies that aggregate with antigen (Ag–Ab) – activation via *alternate pathway* (**APW**) antibody-independent, elicited by microbial polysaccharides, which leads to splitting off of C_3 and activation of C_5, chemotaxis	– immune adherence – elevated capillary permeability – anaphylotoxin – PMN chemotaxis – irreversible, structure-dependent and functional membrane damage (= *cytotoxicity*) – B-cell transformation

(vertical label between columns: INFILTRATE)

phage migration inhibition factor (MIF), macrophage activation factor (MAF) and lymphocyte mitogenic factor (LMF).

3. *Humoral immunity:* Under the influence of antigens, B-lymphocytes proliferate and subsequently differentiate into plasma cells. Activated B-cells produce immunoglobulins (antibodies) of all classes while differentiated plasma cells produce and secrete antibodies of only a single class.

These three basic protective immune mechanisms may be modulated by additional leukocytes (eosinophils, basophils, mast cells), by the clotting system and platelets, by the complement system, and by the kinins to provide an enhanced defensive response to particular antigenic or other challenge to the host. The natural, nonspecific, immediately available immunity is enhanced on demand by the specific (acquired) immunity.

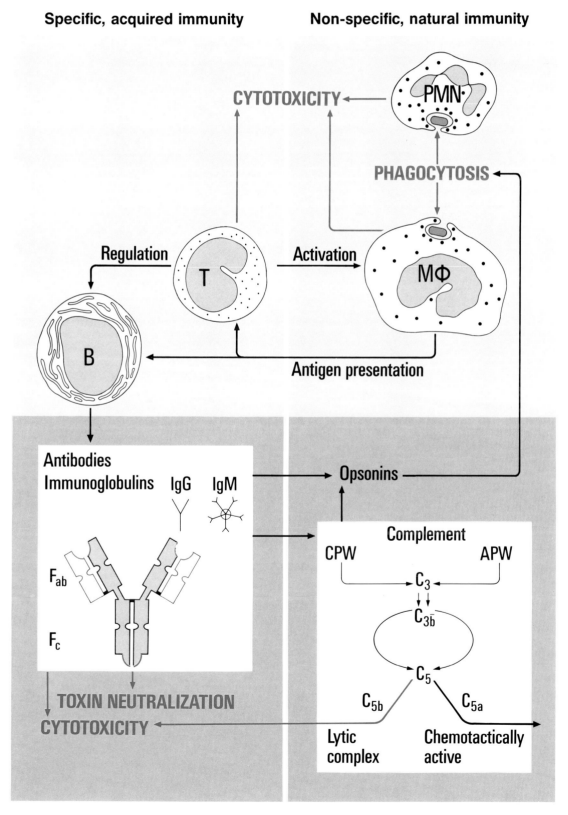

Specific, acquired immunity   **Non-specific, natural immunity**

49   Adaptive relationship between natural and acquired immunity

Cellular

– *PMN granulocytes:*
   This dynamic element provides the initial acute reaction within the junctional epithelium and in the gingival sulcus. The PMN is short-lived; upon cell death, lysosomal enzymes are released. These may inflict damage upon host periodontal tissues *(cytotoxicity).*
– *Macrophages* (MΦ), *T- and B-lymphocytes, plasma cells:*
   These are static elements that represent coordinated and regulated defense mechanisms adapted to the specific situation. Associated with chronic defense and sulcus infiltrate.
Certain lymphocytes (killer cells) with F_c receptors can recognize and kill invading cells *(cytotoxicity).*

Humoral

– *Antibodies IgM, IgG, (IgA, IgD, IgE):*
   Secretion product of B-cells and plasma cells. Biologically active only in combination with or through activation by other effector systems.
   Active in *toxin neutralization.*
– *Complement cascade:*
   May be activated initially via the alternate pathway (APW), independent of antibodies. Subsequent activation of the complement cascade by antibodies, over the classical pathway (CPW). Activation products from complement can affect cell lysis *(cytotoxicity)* through membrane destruction. Activation products also can be chemotactic and may make it easier for phagocytes to engulf and destroy antigens.
Modified from *Playfair* et al. 1974; *Roitt & Lehner* 1980)

Acute Defense Mechanisms

Function of polymorphonuclear leukocytes (PMNs)

Granulocytes in the circulating blood are attracted to a site of host defense via chemotactic mechanisms elicited by metabolic products of plaque microorganisms and by the invasion of these bacteria into tissue. PMNs initially adhere to the vessel lumen ("pavementing"), then exit the vessel by migrating between endothelial cells. The ameboid migration of PMNs is target oriented toward the particle to be phagocytosed. Recognition of the tar-

get is made easier when the foreign substance or bacteria are marked by opsonins. Examples of opsonins are the C_{3b} fragment released upon complement activation and the F_c fragment of immunoglobulin G. When the receptor on the PMN comes into contact with the opsonized particle (adherence), the phagocytic process begins. Phagolysosomes begin to form within the PMN, and these fill with enzymes, which digest the phagocytosed microorganisms. The process of phagocytosis is characterized by the activation of microbicidal mechanisms, e.g., production of hydrogen peroxide.

50 Polymorphonuclear granulocyte (PMN)
This mature, functional phagocytic cell (microphage) has taken up several bacteria (arrows), which are killed in phagolysosomes. Portions of the PMN's segmented nucleus (N) are visible.

Upon the death of the short-lived PMN, the contents of its lysosomes are released and can inflict injury to host tissues.

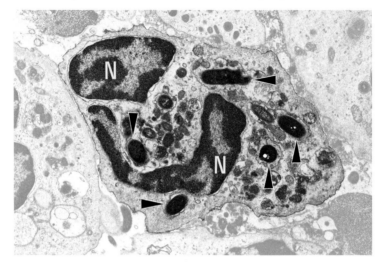

Neutrophil defects

Defects of PMN function can significantly reduce host defense capabilities against infection. PMN functions that may be compromised include:

- Chemotaxis
- Adherence and phagocytosis
- Microbicidal activity.

Systemic diseases characterized by *granulocyte defects* are well known (e.g., Lazy leukocyte syndrome, Che-

diak-Higashi syndrome, diabetes mellitus, chronic granulomatosis, Crohn's disease, Down syndrome). These are usually accompanied by severe periodontal disease.

Granulocytes in most patients with prepubertal, juvenile (LJP) or rapidly progressive periodontitis (RPP) exhibit more or less severely compromised functions.

Host defense can be further compromised by the *"left shift"* of PMNs (young, immature cells) as observed in all infections.

51 Possible defects of polymorphonuclear granulocytes
Defective phagocytes diminish acute defense capacity. Normal PMN function may be blocked at various sites. Chemotactic defects are most common, but inadequate adherence to bacteria, defective phagocytosis and impaired ability to digest engulfed substances may also occur.

Immature granulocytes (left shift during infection) represent a compromised first line of defense that leads to diminished effectiveness of the host response.

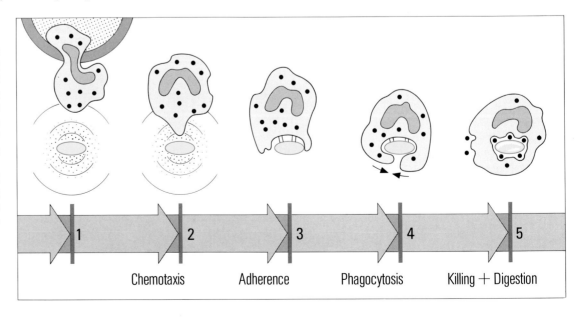

1	2	3	4	5
	Chemotaxis	Adherence	Phagocytosis	Killing + Digestion

Cyclic Nature of Periodontitis – Attachment Loss – Bone Resorption

Contrary to earlier concepts, periodontitis is not a purely chronic, steadily and evenly progressing disease. Rather, acute episodes of tissue destruction (exacerbation, active lesion) alternate with periods of relative dormancy (quiescence, inactive lesion). Active disease progression seldom occurs simultaneously in all areas of the dentition. Active lesions may pervade a quadrant or sextant, or may be present only on a single tooth, or even on a single root surface.

When an acute episode begins, gram-negative anaerobic motile bacteria quickly become predominant. A direct invasion (infection) of the tissues by microorganisms occurs. The tissue responds with a massive acute defense reaction, specifically the formation of micronecroses or suppurating abscesses. Periodontal tissue is lost during each such active episode, i.e., loss of attachment occurs (Goodson et al. 1982; Schroeder 1983).

The acute infection sets in motion the mechanisms that lead to *bone destruction.* Products of both humoral and cellular immunity can cause bone loss, as can bacterial products. Important mediators in this regard are

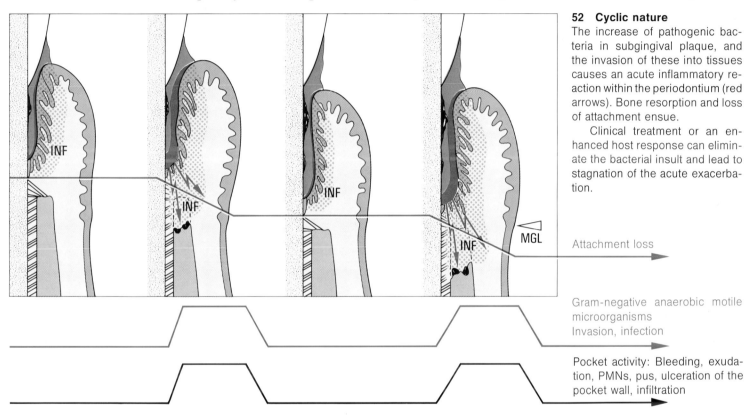

52 Cyclic nature
The increase of pathogenic bacteria in subgingival plaque, and the invasion of these into tissues causes an acute inflammatory reaction within the periodontium (red arrows). Bone resorption and loss of attachment ensue.

Clinical treatment or an enhanced host response can eliminate the bacterial insult and lead to stagnation of the acute exacerbation.

Attachment loss

Gram-negative anaerobic motile microorganisms
Invasion, infection

Pocket activity: Bleeding, exudation, PMNs, pus, ulceration of the pocket wall, infiltration

osteoclast activating factor (OAF) and prostaglandin PGE_2; the latter also mediates bone resorption induced via the complement cascade. Collagen synthesis by osteoblasts is reduced by PGE_2 as well. The resorption-stimulating effect of bacterial lipopolysaccharides (LPS, from gram-negative bacteria) is probably also mediated via PGE_2 and macrophages.

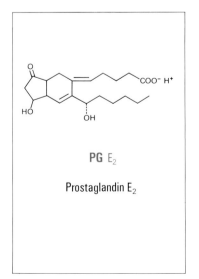

PG E_2

Prostaglandin E_2

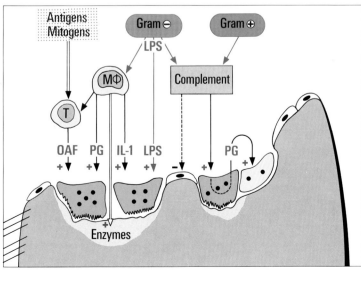

53 Mechanisms of bone destruction
Activated osteoclasts demineralize bone and destroy noncollagenous matrix.

Collagen fibrils are phagocytosed by mononuclear or fibroblastlike cells.

Active bone resorption can occur independent of prostaglandins by way of osteoclast activating factor (OAF, from T-cells), interleukin (IL-1, from macrophages), or bacterial lipopolysaccharides (LPS).

Prostaglandin E_2 (see chemical structure, left) may also be an important mediator substance.

Cofactors in Etiology and Pathogenesis

The bacterial insult and the host response to it may be modified by various cofactors that can alter the clinical course of gingivitis and periodontitis.

Local: – Saliva quantity and composition
– Mouth breathing
– Mechanical, chemical, thermal, allergic and actinic irritation
– Functional disturbances, occlusal trauma, orofacial muscular parafunctions (clenching, bruxism), parafunctions related to occupation.

General: – Severe systemic disease
– Endocrine disturbances
– Stress
– Medicaments
– Nutrition
– Age.

The saliva has a protective function. Salivary mucin (a glycoprotein) lines the oral mucosa as a protective film. Depending on flow rate and viscosity, saliva may exert a greater or lesser cleansing effect. The content of bicarbonate, phosphate and minerals will determine saliva's buffering capacity and its remineralizing potential. Secretory immunoglobulins (sIgA) as well as lysozyme, catalase, lactoperoxidase and additional enzymes help to determine the antimicrobial activity of saliva.

Mouth breathing leads to dehydration of the oral mucosa, cancelling the protective functions of saliva. Dryness allows plaque to cling even more tenaciously to the tooth surface.

Exogenous irritants of various types may be injurious to the oral mucosa, gingiva and periodontium.

Mechanical injuries resulting from eating or from improper use of the toothbrush or other oral health aids may elicit acute inflammatory reactions, which are usually of short duration. If periodontitis is already present, such irritation may cause an acute exacerbation to an active lesion.

Chemical irritations resulting from excessive concentration of locally applied medicaments or acids lead, like *thermal* effects, to damage to mucosa and gingiva, which is usually reversible. In more severe cases, necrosis may be the consequence.

Allergic reactions may exhibit a range of clinical manifestations from erythema to painful blistering. These may be caused by topical medicaments, dentifrices, oral rinses, dental materials etc.

Radiation burns (actinic irritation) may occur subsequent to X-ray therapy for tumors in the head and neck area. Damaging consequences of such therapy are xerostomia and altered saliva composition that result from devastation of the salivary glands. Only intensive radiation therapy will cause direct injury to mucosa or bone (hemorrhage, ulceration, osteoradionecrosis).

Functional disturbances (occlusal trauma) cannot cause either gingivitis or periodontitis. However, if an active periodontitis is already present, its progression may be accelerated by damaging and unphysiological forces (see Function, p. 271).

Functional disturbances and orofacial muscle phenomenae *(oral parafunctions)* such as tongue thrusting, lip biting etc., as well as parafunctions related to one's occupation (e.g., playing a wind instrument, holding nails or pins in the teeth etc.), may lead to drifting of teeth, particularly in patients with periodontal disease.

Severe systemic diseases, disturbances in hormonal balance and the *side effects of drugs* that elicit or enhance gingivitis or periodontitis are dealt with in the chapter on Diseases of the Periodontium (p. 33).

Improper or inadequate nutrition by itself will not elicit gingivitis or periodontitis. However, since starvation and a diet deficient in one or more of the basic food groups will cause a decrease in host response to marginal infection, gingivitis and periodontitis will develop more quickly and progress more rapidly. Of special importance in this regard are pronounced deficiencies of vitamins, minerals and trace elements, and particularly protein deficiency in poorly nourished individuals.

Locally, nutrition (e. g., sugar) can also modify both quantity and composition of plaque (Rateitschak-Plüss & Guggenheim 1982).

Age does not necessarily predispose one to periodontal diseases, although the histologically detectable biochemical alterations in connective tissue may be age related. Clinically, one may observe a certain involution of the healthy periodontium. This is, however, likely to be less an age-related phenomenon than the result of years of exposure to exogenous factors such as intensive oral hygiene, chronic inflammation, or iatrogenic irritants (Gorman 1967; Hansen 1973; Sauerwein 1983).

Epidemiology and Indices

Descriptive epidemiology deals with the occurrence, the severity and the distribution of diseases, invalidity and mortality in a population.

Analytic epidemiology seeks furthermore to discern the causes of a disease and to evaluate any public health consequences with regard to prevention and therapy.

In periodontology, epidemiology is concerned with the prevalence of gingivitis and periodontitis as well as microbial plaque, which is the most important etiologic factor in this family of diseases. Today, the results of the classical epidemiological studies dealing with the prevalence of periodontitis are no longer generally accepted (p. 26).

In epidemiological investigations, the incidence of plaque accumulation and the severity of gingivitis and periodontitis are not determined by collecting individual findings from vast numbers of patients, but rather from the systematic collection of indices from selected populations.

Epidemiology of Gingivitis

For decades, throughout the world, innumerable epidemiological studies have been performed, especially in children and adolescents. The morbidity figures (percentage of those examined who exhibit the disease) reported from such studies range from very low to 100 percent (Page & Schroeder 1982). In addition, the severity of gingivitis as reported in these investigations exhibits differences from study to study. These differences result from use of non-standard methods of investigation, i.e., the indices employed were seldom the same. Additional reasons for the large interinvestigation differences include the varying levels of oral hygiene (plaque control) within the populations examined, as well as geographic, social and ethnologic factors. The incidence and severity of gingivitis can vary within even a single population examined repeatedly at short intervals (Suomi et al. 1971). Furthermore, gingivitis is to some extent reversible in the short term, even without professional treatment. The severity of gingivitis can also change when present for a long period of time: In adolescents reaching puberty it achieves its maximum, then recedes somewhat (Mühlemann & Mazor 1958; Curilović et al. 1977). All of these factors have to be considered in constructive epidemiological studies.

In those studies in which both parameters – gingivitis and plaque – are considered, a clear relationship between oral hygiene and severity of gingivitis has emerged (Silness & Löe 1964; Koivuniemi et al. 1980; Hefti et al. 1981).

Nevertheless, it can be demonstrated that gingivitis prevalence is indeed high in the deciduous dentition, as well as in the permanent dentition in adolescents and adults.

The existence of gingivitis cannot be taken as evidence that periodontitis will eventually develop in an individual (Page & Schroeder 1982; Listgarten et al. 1985).

Epidemiology of Periodontitis

From many nations of the world, numerous epidemiological studies of periodontitis have been reported. The results of these studies – as in gingivitis – must be interpreted with caution. Particularly the figures concerning morbidity must be considered suspect. A figure of 100 percent incidence in a population can hardly be considered to be of public health significance if the attachment loss is minor and isolated to only a few interdental areas. Only data concerning the *severity* of the disease process will permit any meaningful statement, and even then cautious statements.

Periodontitis is seldom a generalized disease. The periodontal supporting structures of individual teeth, maxillary molars and mandibular anteriors, for example, may manifest severe destruction while other teeth such as cuspids and lower bicuspids exhibit no loss of attachment (Socransky et al. 1984). The *average* degree of severity for individual patients and that of entire populations provides no clear picture of the periodontal condition of the patient under study.

Only very few investigators have attempted to study the rapidity of attachment loss in a single population longitudinally over a course of years. In one large study,

Löe and coworkers (1978) recorded the course of attachment loss over several years in one group of Norwegian students and academicians, and another group of laborers in a Sri Lankan tea plantation. The investigators then compared the findings from these two exceedingly different racial and socioeconomic groups. The results demonstrated that in the Norwegian group the average annual loss of attachment was 0.1 mm, while in the Sri Lankan population this figure was 0.2–0.3 mm. Löe and his colleagues then accounted for this significant difference in attachment loss by pointing up the excellent motivation and awareness of prevention on the part of the Norwegians, as compared to the virtual absence of oral hygiene in the Sri Lankan laborers.

In general, epidemiological studies seldom make any differentiation between the less frequently occurring forms of periodontal disease such as the rapidly progressive and localized juvenile periodontitis, and the more frequent but slowly progressive adult periodontitis.

Despite these limitations in the interpretation of epidemiological studies, it is clear that periodontitis is a

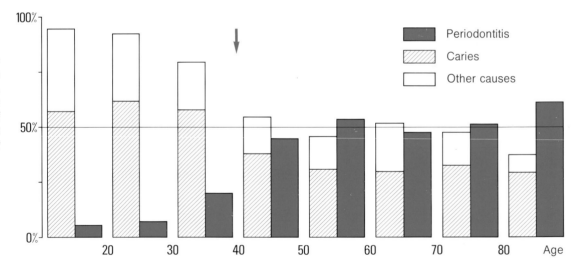

54   Causes of tooth loss with increasing age (adapted from Curilović 1977)
From the fifth decade of life on (arrow), more teeth are lost due to periodontitis than from caries. Overall, however, even in the very elderly, not more than 50% of tooth loss is due to periodontitis as compared to caries and "other causes" (e.g. prosthetics).

Legend: Periodontitis / Caries / Other causes

very widespread disease which may manifest itself in very different clinical courses.

The loss of periodontal supporting structure (attachment loss) increases with age and can lead to tooth loss. One study from Switzerland revealed that from the fifth decade of life on, more teeth are lost to periodontal disease than to caries (Curilović 1977). Nevertheless, periodontitis cannot be relegated to the category of age-dependent diseases.

Future epidemiological investigations should not study simply "periodontitis" but rather should differentiate

between the various disease entities (LJP, RPP, AP; see p. 33). The differences in susceptibility of individual teeth must also be taken into consideration. The causes for exacerbation, stagnation and remission need to be clarified (Socransky et al. 1984). Average values from the entire dentition of an entire population are effectively *worthless*.

Indices

Value and possibilities for use

- Plaque indices
- Gingival indices
- Periodontal indices.

Alterations in the gingiva and the periodontium, as well as the main cause of these diseases – microbial plaque – may be assessed and quantitated through use of *indices.* These are useful primarily for epidemiological studies, but may also comprise part of an individual patient examination.

Indices are numerical expressions of defined diagnostic criteria. An alteration, a disease or severity of a disease is expressed by assessing a numerical value. In simplified indices, only the presence or absence of a symptom or an etiological factor may be recorded as yes or no. For example, after probing a gingival sulcus, a plus (+) signifies "bleeding," a minus (–) signifies "no bleeding."

A good index should be able to provide quantitative and qualitative expression of the criteria under study. Furthermore, an index should be simple, objective, reproducible, quick and practical. It should be easy enough for auxiliary personnel to use (e.g., dental assistant or hygienist) and should be amenable to statistical evaluation.

Although indices were developed primarily for use in epidemiological studies, and continue to be used mainly for such studies, it is difficult to achieve any degree of standardization among various international scientific groups. It is therefore often impossible to compare the results obtained in one epidemiological study to those obtained in another investigation.

For the past several years, indices have come to be used in the dental practice on individual patients. The numerical quantitation of plaque and gingivitis can be performed particularly well. By recording indices throughout the course of a preventive program or a treatment regimen, it is often possible to document success (or failure) objectively for both the practitioner and the patient. The change (improvement) in the index can also help to motivate a patient.

In the following pages, a few of the indices that are used internationally in epidemiological studies are described, with emphasis on those that are well suited for use in the periodontal practice.

Plaque Indices

A plaque index should provide a *quantitative* assessment. Criteria such as "good" or "poor" oral hygiene are gross and not sufficiently objective. They cannot provide enough information to accurately draw any correlation between the degree of oral cleanliness (or lack of it) and the severity of any gingival disease.

For epidemiological studies, the relatively gross indices such as the Plaque Index (PI, see Fig. 55; Silness & Löe 1964) are usually sufficient. Such indices may even be adequate when applied only to certain selected teeth such as the six "Ramfjord teeth" (see Fig. 67), to provide a quick and representative picture of the level of oral hygiene in a population.

In private practice, on the other hand, the collection of a plaque or hygiene index is not intended to determine the average plaque accumulation, but to record the distribution of plaque in the oral cavity, i.e., to determine the *"plaque picture"* of an individual patient. Some areas of a patient's dentition may be cleaned quite effectively, while others, e.g., the lingual surfaces of mandibular molars, remain routinely uncleaned. Right-handed persons usually clean the left facial tooth surfaces better than the right, and exposed tooth surfaces are cleaned better than interdental areas. A plaque index for patients in private practice should also make it possible to record any improvements (or the opposite) in cleaning efficacy during the course of therapy or during the recall interval. This is possible only through the use of a sensitive index that evaluates all tooth surfaces. Examples are the indices proposed by O'Leary (1972) and Lindhe (1983). In these indices the quantity of plaque on individual teeth is not recorded; rather, it is simply noted whether or not plaque is present along the gingival margin on the four surfaces of each tooth (compare yes/no decision; Hygiene Index, HI, Fig. 57).

In recent years attempts have been made to diagnose the *qualitative* bacterial composition of plaque, especially subgingival plaque, in addition to recording the quantity and distribution. This has been done through use of dark field or phase contrast microscopy. This type of analysis of the various microorganisms will not only help to demonstrate the general dependency of gingivitis/periodontitis on plaque, but will also help to provide a more precise diagnosis of the gingivitis forms and particularly the various types of periodontitis (see p. 16, Figs. 40–44).

55   Plaque Index (PI) of Silness and Löe

The most important consideration in the Plaque Index is the *thickness* of plaque along the gingival margin, because only this plaque in direct contact with the gingival tissue plays any role in the etiology of gingivitis. To visualize plaque, teeth are dried with air. Plaque is not stained.

The PI is relatively time-consuming. It is indicated for *epidemiological studies* in which the Gingival Index (GI) is recorded simultaneously. It is less useful for routine charting.

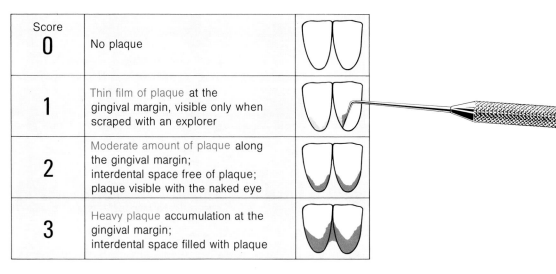

Score		
0	No plaque	
1	Thin film of plaque at the gingival margin, visible only when scraped with an explorer	
2	Moderate amount of plaque along the gingival margin; interdental space free of plaque; plaque visible with the naked eye	
3	Heavy plaque accumulation at the gingival margin; interdental space filled with plaque	

56   Interdental Hygiene Index (HYG)

This index records plaque-*free* surfaces as a percentage. It is thus similar to the Approximal Plaque Index (API) of *Lange* (1981), which records percent plaque accumulation.

After staining, a simple yes/no decision is made with regard to whether or not stained plaque is present (+) on the approximal surfaces or not (–).

The HYG is usually scored within a quadrant *from only one aspect,* i.e., from the facial or from the oral. This is also the case with the Papilla Bleeding Index (PBI, p. 30).

The HYG score is calculated as:

$$HYG = \frac{\text{number of plaque-free areas } (-)}{\text{number of examined areas}} \times 100$$

The HYG is a sensitive index because small plaque quantity is also measured and because the index is scored in the interdental areas, which are in most cases not particularly well cleaned.

The HYG is well suited for recordings in *individual patients,* but less so for epidemiological studies.

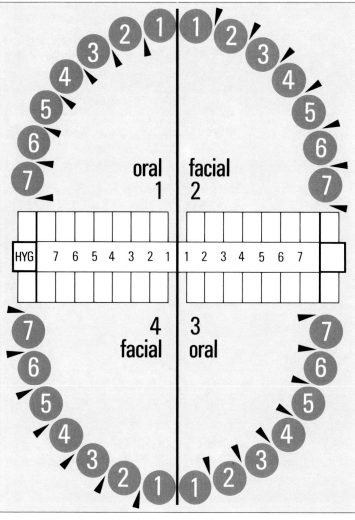

57   Hygiene Index (HI) – Recording plaque accumulation on all tooth surfaces

This most precise index involves measurement of plaque accumulation on *all four tooth surfaces* (facial, oral, mesial, distal).

With a simple yes/no decision the examiner can enter the presence (+) or absence (–) of plaque into a simple chart and in doing so precisely ascertain the cleanliness of a dentition and express it as a percentage. For this index, plaque is stained with a disclosing agent.

The HI was developed solely for use in *individual patients.*

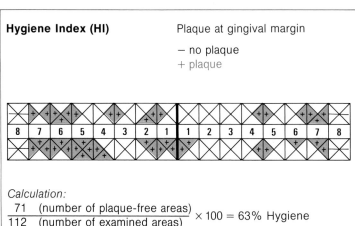

Hygiene Index (HI)   Plaque at gingival margin

– no plaque
+ plaque

Calculation:

$$\frac{71 \quad \text{(number of plaque-free areas)}}{112 \quad \text{(number of examined areas)}} \times 100 = 63\% \text{ Hygiene}$$

Gingival Indices

Many indices have been developed for the evaluation and quantitation of gingivitis (King 1945; Massler & Schour 1949; Mühlemann & Mazor 1958; Löe and Silness 1963; Mühlemann & Son 1971; Carter & Barnes 1974; Saxer & Mühlemann 1975; Ainamo & Bay 1975; Lindhe 1983).

The following indices will be described here:

– *Sulcus Bleeding Index* (SBI, Mühlemann & Son 1971)
– *Gingival Index* (GI, Löe & Silness 1963)

– *Gingival Index Simplified* (GI-S, Lindhe 1983) and *Gingival Bleeding Index* (GBI, Ainamo 1975)
– *Papilla Bleeding Index* (PBI, Saxer & Mühlemann 1975)

All of these indices share a common feature: In addition to other symptoms, they all recognize *bleeding* as an important symptom of inflammation. In this regard, the most sensitive and consistent of all these indices is the PBI, which utilizes exclusively the various manifestations of gingival hemorrhage.

Grade	
0	normal gingiva, no bleeding on probing
1	bleeding on probing, no changes in color or contour
2	bleeding on probing, erythema
3	bleeding on probing, erythema, mild edema
4	bleeding on probing, erythema, severe edema
5	bleeding on probing/spontaneous hemorrhage, severe edema with or without ulceration

58 Sulcus Bleeding Index (SBI)
The SB-Index considers bleeding from the sulcus after probing, as well as erythema, swelling and edema. It is generally scored separately on both the papilla (P) and gingival margin (M).

The SBI has been used in various clinical studies but is also applicable to individual patients in a private practice setting.

From the SBI, the Papilla Bleeding Index (p. 30) evolved, which considers bleeding as its only criterion.

Grade	
0	normal gingiva, no inflammation, no discoloration, no bleeding
1	mild inflammation, slight color change, mild alteration of gingival surface, no bleeding
2	moderate inflammation, erythema, swelling, bleeding on probing or when pressure applied
3	severe inflammation, severe erythema and swelling, tendency toward spontaneous hemorrhage, some ulceration

59 Gingival Index (GI)
This index is used worldwide in epidemiological studies and scientific investigations. The GI scores gingival inflammation on the facial, lingual and mesial surfaces of all teeth. The symptom of bleeding comprises a score of 2.

The GI is recommended for epidemiological studies. It is less applicable for individual patients because the differences between the scoring levels are too gross.

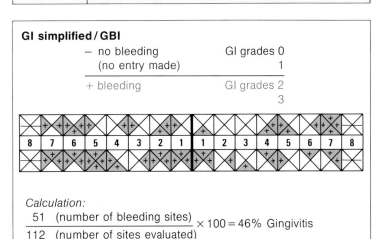

GI simplified / GBI

– no bleeding (no entry made)	GI grades 0 / 1
+ bleeding	GI grades 2 / 3

Calculation:

$$\frac{51 \ \text{(number of bleeding sites)}}{112 \ \text{(number of sites evaluated)}} \times 100 = 46\% \ \text{Gingivitis}$$

60 Gingival Index Simplified (GI-S, Lindhe 1981) and Gingival Bleeding Index (GBI, Ainamo 1975)
Similar to the HI (Fig. 57), all four tooth surfaces are scored as + or − for bleeding on probing. Negative observations are not entered into the chart. Gingivitis incidence is calculated as a percentage of affected (bleeding) units.

Because over 100 individual sites must be evaluated in both the GI-S and the GBI, these indices are suited only for individual practice application on a routine basis.

Papilla Bleeding Index (PBI)

The PBI was not developed for epidemiological studies. It is a *sensitive indicator* of gingival inflammation in individual patients and is therefore well suited for use by the practicing dentist or periodontist.

The PBI has proven to be particularly useful for gauging success or failure during a course of periodontal therapy. While the patient watches in a mirror, the practitioner can score the intensity of papillary inflammation. In this way, the PBI can also serve as an excellent method for motivating the patient toward good oral hygiene (see Motivation, p. 108). The patient can see when the gingival tissue bleeds, which helps him to realize where the diseased sites in his mouth are located.

Throughout therapy, repetitions of the PBI indicate any decrease in inflammation to the patient.

Grades   1   2   3   4

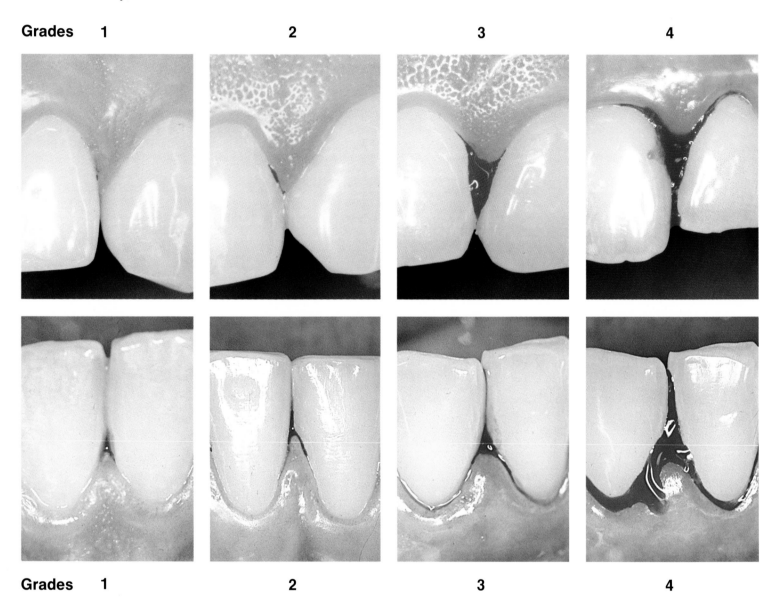

Grades   1   2   3   4

61   Grade 1 – Point
20–30 seconds after probing the mesial and distal sulci with a periodontal probe, a *single bleeding point* is observed.

62   Grade 2 – Line / Point
A fine line of blood or several bleeding points become visible at the gingival margin.

63   Grade 3 – Triangle
The interdental triangle becomes more or less filled with blood.

64   Grade 4 – Drops
Profuse bleeding. Immediately after probing, blood flows into the interdental area to cover portions of the tooth or gingiva.

Clinical procedure for the PBI

Using a blunt periodontal probe under light finger pressure, bleeding is provoked by sweeping the sulcus from the base of the papilla to its tip along the tooth's distal and mesial aspects. *After 20–30 seconds,* when a quadrant has been completely probed, the intensity of bleeding is scored in four grades (p.30) and recorded on the chart. Bleeding on probing indicates that the probe tip penetrated the pocket epithelium (or the disintegrating junctional epithelium) and achieved the highly vascular subepithelial connective tissue.

It is not necessary to score each interdental area from both facial and oral aspects in order to ascertain the gingival condition of the entire oral cavity. The dentist simply probes one quadrant from the facial and the next quadrant from the oral aspect.

The sum of the recorded scores gives the "bleeding number"; the PBI is calculated by dividing the bleeding number by the total number of papilla examined.

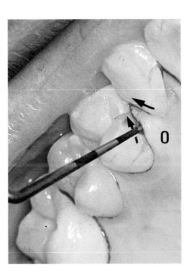

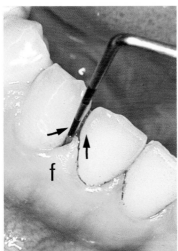

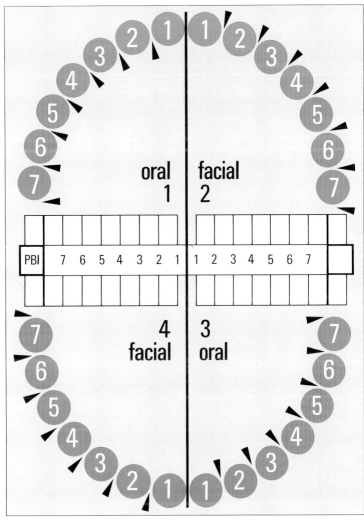

65 Probing to provoke bleeding (left)
Facially (in quadrants 2 and 4) and orally (in quadrants 1 and 3), the probe is inserted into the sulcus halfway between the papilla tip and most apical portion of the gingival margin, and moved coronally to the tip of the papilla. The same procedure is performed on mesial and distal aspects of each papilla (arrows).
   If periodontal pockets are present, the same movement is performed with the probe inserted only to a depth of about 3–4 mm.

66 Chart for recording the PBI (right)
The areas to be scored are indicated by black triangles in each of the four quadrants. The boxes in the middle of the chart are for recording the numerical score for each papilla examined.
   A single scoring sheet for inclusion in the patient's permanent records may contain several such PBI charts, side by side or one above the other, so that PBI recordings over an extended period of time be readily compared. A decrease in PBI score can be taken as evidence of improving gingival health. This can be readily comprehended by the patient as well.

Periodontal Indices

The determination of the severity of periodontitis through use of an index is difficult. Not only the degree of inflammation but also the degree of destruction of periodontal supporting structure (attachment loss) must be evaluated.

The *Periodontal Disease Index* (PDI) of Ramfjord (1959) is the most useful index for epidemiological studies.

For individual patients, the PDI cannot be used because it does not evaluate all 28 teeth; rather, six teeth

("Ramfjord teeth") are scored as representative of the entire dental arch: Teeth 16, 21, 24, 36, 41 and 44. If one of these teeth is missing, its distal neighbor (17, 11, 25, 37, 42 or 45, respectively) may be substituted (Marthaler et al. 1971).

The PDI evaluates these selected teeth for both gingivitis and attachment loss, with three gradations for each (see below).

67   Ramfjord teeth
Ramfjord demonstrated that for epidemiological purposes six teeth (red) could be taken as representative of the entire dentition. The substitutes for these six are shown on the chart in gray.

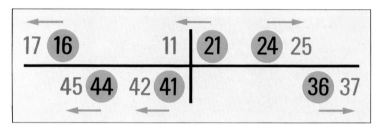

68   Periodontal Disease Index (PDI)
The PDI contains a *gingivitis index* in scores 1, 2 and 3, and a measure of *attachment loss* independent of gingivitis, in scores 4, 5 and 6.
     The PDI is designed for use in epidemiological studies, not for clinical practice.

Score	
0	No inflammation, no alterations in the gingiva
	Gingiva
1	Mild to moderate gingivitis at some locations on the gingival margin
2	Mild to moderate gingivitis of the entire gingival margin surrounding the tooth
3	Advanced gingivitis with severe erythema, hemorrhage, ulceration
	Periodontium
4	Up to 3 mm of attachment loss, measured from the cementoenamel junction
5	3–6 mm of attachment loss
6	More than 6 mm of attachment loss

Indices versus Clinical Findings

The indices described are useful in epidemiological studies or in the evaluation of individual symptoms in daily practice. Indices can never be a substitute for a complete examination of the oral cavity including charting of the following observations on *all* teeth:

- Probing or pocket depths
- Recession
- Attachment loss
- Tooth mobility
- Radiographic survey

Other specific observations and symptoms are discussed under "Diseases of the Periodontium" (p. 33) and "Charting – Diagnosis – Prognosis" (p. 87).

Other than the bleeding tendency, none of the indices provide definitive information about specific *etiology*, lesion *activity*, or the *prospective course* of an existent periodontitis. In the future, examination of the subgingival flora for the presence of pathogenic microorganisms, and detection of peculiarities in the host response mechanisms will assume greater prominence in patient evaluation.

Diseases of the Periodontium

The term "periodontal diseases" refers to inflammatory as well as recessive alterations of the gingiva and periodontium.

Gingivitis is an inflammatory process limited to the gingivae (no loss of attachment). In addition to the almost ubiquitous form of gingivitis elicited by plaque, gingival changes may also be detected during periods of hormonal imbalance and systemic diseases, or as medicinal side effects.

If the supporting alveolar bone is also affected by inflammatory processes in the periodontium, one speaks of *periodontitis.*

The term *recession* or *gingival recession* refers to the apical retreat of gingiva and alveolar bone, which usually occurs on the labial aspect in a clinically inflammation-free dentition.

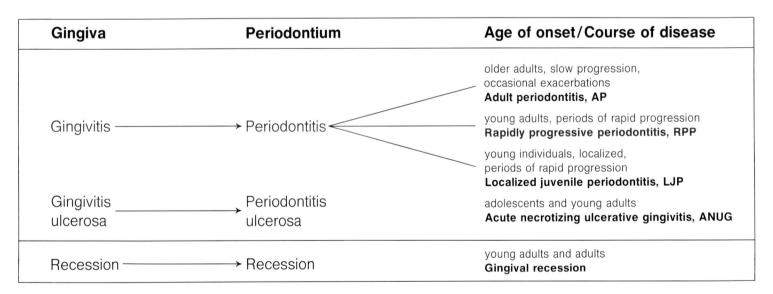

Gingiva	Periodontium	Age of onset/Course of disease
Gingivitis ⟶	Periodontitis ⟨	older adults, slow progression, occasional exacerbations **Adult periodontitis, AP** young adults, periods of rapid progression **Rapidly progressive periodontitis, RPP** young individuals, localized, periods of rapid progression **Localized juvenile periodontitis, LJP**
Gingivitis ulcerosa ⟶	Periodontitis ulcerosa	adolescents and young adults **Acute necrotizing ulcerative gingivitis, ANUG**
Recession ⟶	Recession	young adults and adults **Gingival recession**

Gingival and Periodontal Diseases, Local Etiology without Systemic Involvement

Gingivitis and periodontitis are *local* opportunistic infections of bacterial origin that may occur in an otherwise healthy individual. The progression of gingivitis to periodontitis, and the rapidity of attachment loss may be explained by the varying pathogenicity of plaque microorganisms. Some specific bacteria possess the capability to invade the periodontal tissues and cause acute inflammatory episodes (micronecrosis, abscess).

Host response to the bacterial insult, which varies from individual to individual, can dramatically alter the course of the disease process.

The etiology of noninflammatory gingival recession has not been completely clarified (see Recession, p.81).

Gingival and Periodontal Diseases, Etiology Partially Local but with Systemic Involvement

The clinical course of gingival and periodontal diseases can be accentuated, enhanced or caused in part by hormonal disturbances, side effects of drugs, autoimmune diseases, anomalies of keratinization, dermatological disorders, specific infections, injuries, allergies, poisons, metabolic disturbances, inadequate nutrition, blood dyscrasias and severe genetically-determined general syndromes.

It is not possible to draw sharp demarcations between diseases of the gingiva and those of the mucosa (see also Pindborg, in Lindhe 1983).

Those disorders printed below in *italics* are presented subsequently in clinical photographs.

Primarily gingival changes

- *Hormonal complications:*
  - *Pregnancy gingivitis*
  - *"Pill" gingivitis* (contraceptives)
  - Puberty gingivitis
  - Gingivitis menstrualis and intermenstrualis
  - Gingivitis climacterica

- *Side effects of drugs; gingival enlargement:*
  - *Phenytoin-induced overgrowth*
  - *Cyclosporine-A induced overgrowth*
  - *Idiopathic fibrosis*
  - *Epulis*
  - *Neoplasm (tumors)*

- *Autoimmune diseases, desquamative and bullous gingival alterations, keratinopathies, dermatological diseases:*
  - *Pemphigoid* (benign mucous membrane pemphigoid, chronic desquamative gingivitis)
  - *Pemphigus vulgaris*
  - Epidermolysis bullosa
  - Erythema multiforme
  - *Lichen planus*
  - Parakeratotic lesions
  - Premalignant lesions
  - Dermatomyositis, scleroderma, psoriasis etc.

- *Specific infections:*
  - *Aphthae*
  - *Herpes*
  - Toxoplasmosis
  - Actinomycosis
  - Candidiasis
  - Gonorrhea, syphilis etc.

- *Injuries/burns:*
  - mechanical, chemical, thermal, actinic

- *Allergies:*
  - to medicines, metals, plastics etc.

- *Poisons* (e.g., lead poisoning)

Gingival and periodontal changes

- *Metabolic disturbances:*
  - Diabetes
  - Acatalasemia

- *Blood cell dyscrasia:*
  - Panmyelopathia
  - Leukemias
  - Erythroblastic anemia
  - Cyclic neutropenia

- *Inadequate nutrition:*
  - Scurvy (ascorbic acid deficiency)
  - Kwashiorkor (protein deficiency)

- *Genetically-related general syndromes:*
  - Down's syndrome
  - *Papillon-Lefèvre syndrome* (see pp. 78–80)
  - Chediak-Higashi syndrome
  - Hypophosphatasia (Rathburn syndrome)

These general syndromes may be associated with periodontitis in the *deciduous dentition* and in *prepubescent* children.

In the case of Chediak-Higashi syndrome, PMN defects have been reported. This may also represent one etiologic factor in periodontitis accompanied by systemic diseases.

Gingivitis

Plaque-induced gingivitis

Gingivitis is ubiquitous. It is a bacterially-elicited inflammation of the marginal gingiva (Löe et al. 1965). In the chapter on "Etiology and Pathogenesis" (p.9), the development and progression of gingivitis from *healthy* tissue to an *initial* lesion, then an *early* lesion and on to *established* gingivitis was described (Page & Schroeder 1976).

The only form of gingivitis observed clinically in adults is the established lesion, which can manifest in varying degrees of severity. The amount of plaque accumulation, the types of microorganisms (virulence) and the resistance of the host (immune status) determine the intensity of the inflammatory reaction.

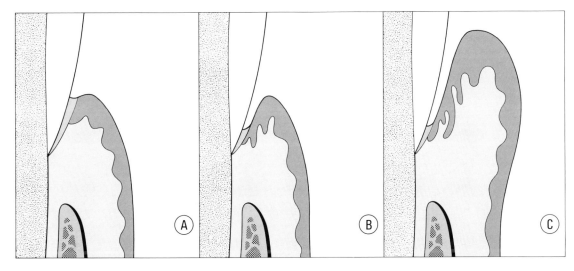

69 Sulcus and gingival pockets

A. Sulcus
Histologic sulcus in health = 0−0.5 mm, but probing depth = 2−3 mm as probe tip penetrates junctional epithelium (see p. 88).

B. Gingival pocket
Created when coronal junctional epithelium detaches from tooth in gingivitis; no connective tissue loss.

C. Pseudopocket
Created by gingival enlargement.

The fine line between healthy gingiva and gingivitis is difficult to discern. Even gingiva that appears healthy clinically will almost always exhibit histologically a small inflammatory infiltrate. With increasing clinical and histological inflammation, the basal cells of the junctional epithelium proliferate laterally. The junctional epithelium becomes detached from the tooth, which permits apical movement of bacteria between the tooth and the epithelium, forming a *gingival pocket*.

If gingivitis is severe, edema of the tissues occurs and *pseudopockets* may develop.

Gingival pockets and pseudopockets are *not* true periodontal pockets by definition, because no true apical proliferation of the junctional epithelium or loss of connective tissue attachment has occurred.

With treatment, gingivitis is reversible. Untreated, the condition can persist over many years with small variations in intensity, or it can develop into periodontitis.

Histopathology

The clinical and histopathological pictures of gingivitis are well correlated (Engelberger et al. 1983). The earliest mild infiltration of PMNs that occurs even in clinically healthy gingiva may be explained as a host response to the tiny amount of plaque that is present even in a clean oral cavity. Such plaque is composed of nonpathogenic or mildly pathogenic microorganisms, such as gram-positive cocci and rods.

As plaque accumulation increases, so does the severity of clinically detectable inflammation, as evidenced by the quantity of inflammatory infiltrate. It consists primarily of differentiated B-lymphocytes, with a smaller number of other types of leukocytes.

With increasing inflammation, more and more polymorphonuclear granulocytes (PMNs) transmigrate the junctional epithelium. If the inflammatory process is not stopped, the junctional epithelium will take on the character of a pocket epithelium (see p. 62; Müller-Glauser & Schroeder 1982).

70   Healthy gingiva (left)
Even in clinically healthy gingiva (GI = 0, PBI = 0), one can observe an initial, very discrete subepithelial round cell infiltrate. Scattered PMNs transmigrate the junctional epithelium, which remains for the most part intact (H & E, × 10).

71   Mild gingivitis (right)
As clinical inflammation increases (GI = 1, PBI = 1), the amount of inflammatory infiltrate increases (Masson stain, × 10).

72   Moderate gingivitis (left)
When gingivitis is clinically apparent (GI = 2, PBI = 2), the infiltrate becomes heavier and more widespread. The junctional epithelium proliferates laterally, creating a gingival pocket (Masson stain, × 10). P, subgingival plaque.

73   Severe gingivitis (right)
Pronounced edematous swelling (GI = 3, PBI = 3–4). The inflammatory infiltrate is expansive. The junctional epithelium has been transformed into a pocket epithelium (gingival pocket). Only in the apicalmost area are any remnants of intact junctional epithelium observed. The connective tissue attachment is intact (no loss of attachment; H & E, × 10).

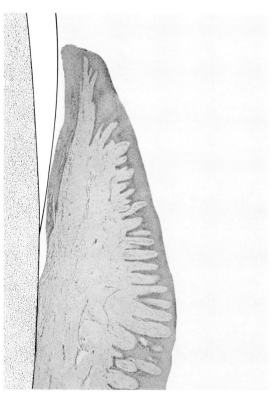

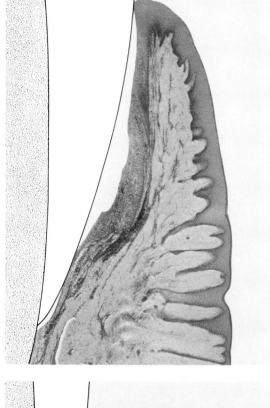

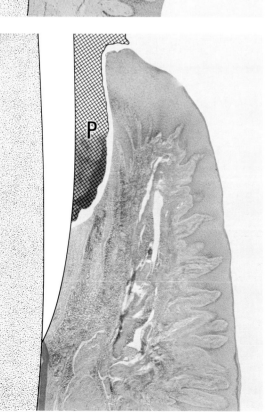

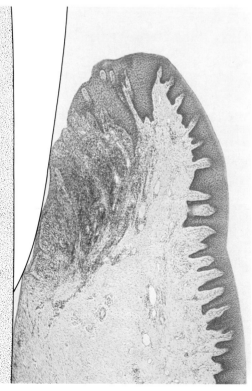

Clinical Symptoms

The first significant clinical symptom of an established lesion is bleeding subsequent to careful probing. This hemorrhage is elicited by the penetration of a blunt probe through the disintegrating junctional epithelium and into the vascular subepithelial connective tissue. At this stage of the inflammatory process (PBI = 1), no gingival erythema may be visible clinically.

Symptoms of advanced gingivitis include profuse bleeding after sulcus probing, obvious erythema and simultaneous edematous swelling. In the most severe cases, spontaneous bleeding and eventually ulceration may occur. Pronounced edematous enlargement of the gingivae leads to the formation of pseudopockets (Fig. 69), which are ideal sites for the accumulation of yet more plaque.

Even severe gingivitis need not progress to periodontitis. With proper treatment, gingivitis is reversible.

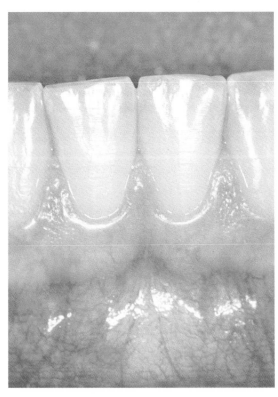
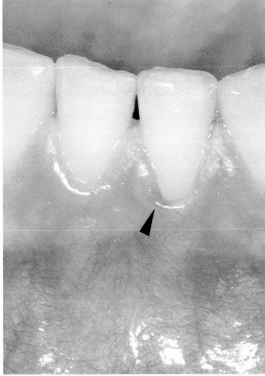

74 Healthy gingiva (left)
The gingiva is pale salmon pink in color and may be stippled. The narrow free gingival margin is clearly distinguishable from the attached gingiva. After gentle probing with a blunt periodontal probe, no bleeding occurs.

75 Mild gingivitis (right)
Localized mild erythema and slight edema. Some of the former stippling is lost. Minimal bleeding after probing.

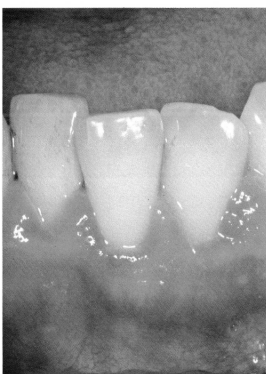
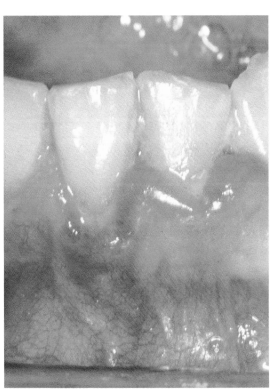

76 Moderate gingivitis (left)
Obvious erythema and edema. No stippling apparent; hemorrhage following probing of the sulcus.

77 Severe gingivitis (right)
Fiery redness, edematous and hyperplastic swelling; complete absence of any stippling; interdental ulceration, spontaneous bleeding.

Mild Gingivitis

A 23-year-old female came to the dentist for a routine check-up. She had no complaints and was not aware of any gingival problems, although in her medical history she indicated that her gingiva bleeds occasionally during toothbrushing. Her oral hygiene was relatively good. She had received toothbrushing instruction by a dentist once, but no subsequent instruction.

Findings:

HYG, Hygiene Index	70%
PBI, Papilla Bleeding Index	1.5
TM, Tooth Mobility	0
PD, Probing Depth,	1.5 mm in maxilla
interproximal	3 mm in mandible

Diagnosis: Gingivitis in initial stage
Therapy: Motivation, plaque and calculus removal
Prognosis: Very good

78   Mild gingivitis in anterior area
In the maxilla, one observes no overt signs of gingivitis, except for a very mild erythema.

In the mandible, especially in the papillary area, slight edematous swelling and erythema can be detected (arrows).

Radiograph: There is no evidence of loss of supporting structure in the interdental bony septa. The maxillary incisors exhibit short roots.

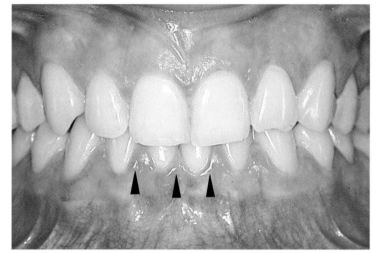 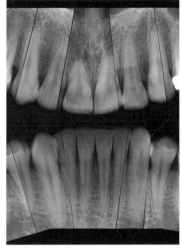

79   Papilla bleeding (PBI)
After gentle probing of the papillary sulci with a blunt periodontal probe, hemorrhages of grades 1 and 2 occur. This is a cardinal sign of gingivitis.

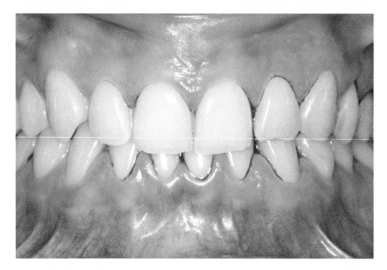

80   Stained plaque
Around the necks of the teeth and in interdental areas, small plaque accumulations are visible.

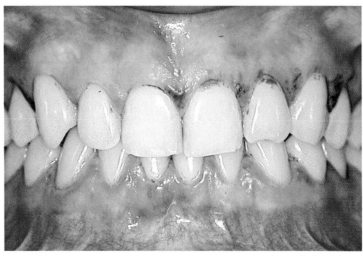

Moderate Gingivitis

A 28-year-old female presented with a chief complaint of gingival bleeding. She "brushes her teeth," but has never received any oral hygiene instruction from a dentist or hygienist. Generalized crowding of the teeth in both arches is evident, combined with an anterior open bite. These anomalies lessen any self cleansing effects and make oral hygiene difficult. They may also increase the severity of gingivitis.

Findings:

HYG	50%	TM	0 in maxilla;
PBI	2.6 in maxilla		1 in mandible
	3.4 in mandible	PD	3 mm in maxilla
			4 mm in mandible

Diagnosis: Maxilla, moderate gingivitis; mandibular anterior region, severe gingivitis (pseudopockets)

Therapy: Motivation, oral hygiene, plaque and calculus removal. After re-evaluation, possible gingivoplasty.

Prognosis: With patient cooperation, very good.

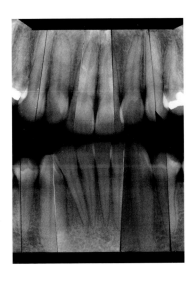 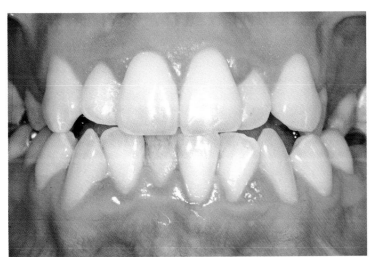

81 Moderate gingivitis in anterior segments
Erythema and enlargement of the gingiva. Symptoms are more pronounced in mandible than in maxilla.

Radiograph: There is no evidence of destruction of the interdental bony septa.

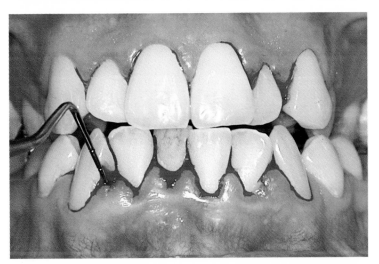

82 Papilla bleeding (PBI)
The pronounced gingivitis that is particularly obvious in the mandibular anterior area is corroborated by the PBI. Bleeding scores of 3 and 4 are recorded.

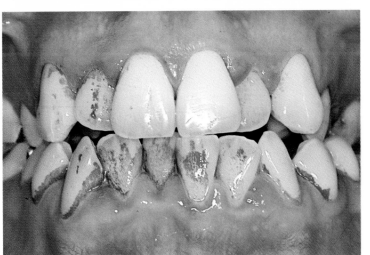

83 Stained plaque
Moderate plaque accumulation in the maxilla. In the mandible, heavier plaque, especially at the gingival margins.

Severe Gingivitis

This 17-year-old male had not been to the dentist "for years," and practiced no oral hygiene. He presented with a chief complaint of unsightly gingiva but also complained of gingival bleeding while eating, as well as spontaneous hemorrhage. He and his parents had refused the orthodontic treatment recommended several years ago (see same case in "Gingivectomy/Gingivoplasty," p. 163).

Findings:

HYG	0%	TM	0–1
PBI	3.5	PD	to 6 mm in interproximal areas (pseudopockets)

Diagnosis: Severe gingivitis with pronounced hyperplasia, tooth positional anomalies, mouth breathing.

Therapy: Motivation, plaque and calculus removal, gingivectomy (see p. 163); orthodontic treatment.

Prognosis: With intensive therapy and cooperation by the patient, good.

84 Severe gingivitis
Erythema and pronounced gingival hyperplasia. Abundant accumulations of plaque and calculus.

Radiograph: Despite the extreme hyperplastic inflammation, there is no evidence of destruction of interdental bony septa.

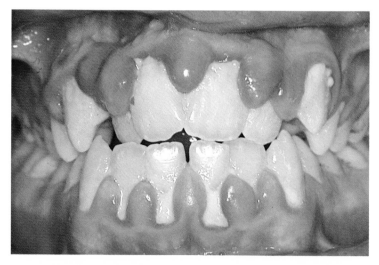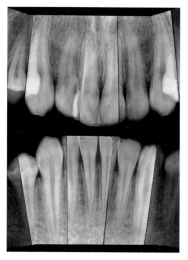

85 Mouth breathing
Weak lip muscle tone. Despite clear nasal passages, the patient constantly breathes through the mouth, also at night. In addition to plaque, the tooth position anomalies and mouth breathing (dehydration) also contribute to the clinical picture of gingivitis and hyperplasia.

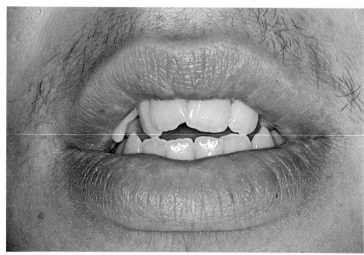

86 Stained plaque
Extremely heavy plaque accumulation results from complete lack of oral hygiene. Use of the toothbrush in the anterior area frightened the patient because of the severe bleeding it provoked.

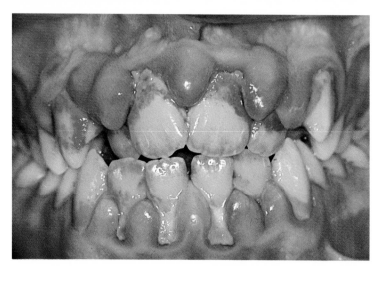

Acute Necrotizing Ulcerative Gingivitis

ANUG, Gingivitis ulcerosa, Vincent's infection, trench mouth

Acute necrotizing ulcerative gingivitis (ANUG) is an acute, painful, necrotizing, rapidly progressive inflammation of the gingiva, which may enter a subacute or chronic stage. The disease seldom occurs as a generalized process throughout the entire dentition, nor are its clinical manifestations of identical severity. It may be quite advanced in individual anterior teeth, while the adjacent premolars or molars are not affected at all or only mildly so. The reverse may also be the case. There is no all-encompassing reason for this irregular appearance, but poor oral hygiene, locally predominating pathogenic bacteria and the presence of plaque retentive areas are likely participants. Without treatment, ANUG may progress to Periodontitis ulcerosa (pp. 76–77).

In ANUG patients probing depths are usually small because gingiva propria is lost to necrosis as attachment loss proceeds. Secondary ulceration of other oral mucosal surfaces is rarely observed, even in severe cases of ANUG.

Next to Gingivitis simplex, ANUG is one of the most common diseases of the gingiva. Incidence figures ranging from 0.1–10% of the adolescent population have been reported.

The *etiology* of ANUG is not completely unterstood. In addition to plaque and a previously existing gingivitis, the following factors are suspected:

Local factors
  – Poor oral hygiene
  – Predominance of Spirochetes, Bacteroides and fusiform bacteria in plaque
  – Plaque-retentive areas (crowded teeth, overhanging restorations etc.)
  – Smoking (local irritation from tar substances)

Systemic factors
  – Poor general health
  – Fatigue or psychic stress
  – Smoking (*nicotine* as a sympatheticomimetic and chemotaxin; Totti et al. 1984)
  – Age
  – Season of the year (September/October and December/January; Škach et al. 1970)

Patients with ANUG are often young, heavy smokers, who exercise poor oral hygiene and are indifferent to their oral disease, becoming interested in treatment only during painful exacerbations.

The clinical course is acute, with destruction of affected papillae within days. Even without treatment the acute phase may enter a chronic stage. Increased host resistance or self-treatment such as rinsing with a disinfecting mouthwash may be benefical in shortening the acute episode. Without professional treatment ANUG usually recurs, and may develop into Periodontitis ulcerosa accompanied by attachment loss, especially in interdental areas.

Initial therapy should include debridement (Cavitron), thorough cleansing with hydrogen peroxide, oral hygiene instruction and motivation. A recall appointment several days later is advisable for follow-up on the patient's oral hygiene.

For advanced or intractable cases, initial therapy can be supplemented with chlorhexidine rinses and topical application of cortisone/antibiotic ointments. In severe cases of Gingivoperiodontitis ulcerosa, which may manifest fever or enlarged cervical lymph nodes, systemic penicillin, metronidazole (Flagyl) or ornidazole (Tiberal) may be used as adjunct therapy (see Medicaments, p. 263).

Histopathology

The clinical and histopathological pictures in ANUG are correlated. The histopathology of ANUG is significantly different from that of simple gingivitis.

As a consequence of the acute reaction, an enormous number of PMNs transmigrate the junctional epithelium in the direction of the sulcus and the col. In contrast to the situation in simple gingivitis, PMNs also migrate toward the oral epithelium and the tips of papillae, which undergo necrotic destruction. The ulcerated wound is covered by a clinically visible whitish pseudo-

membrane that consists of bacteria, dead leukocytes and epithelial cells, as well as fibrin. The tissue subjacent to the ulcerated areas is edematous, hyperemic and heavily infiltrated by PMNs. *Spirochetes and other bacteria often penetrate into the tissue* (Listgarten 1965; Listgarten & Lewis 1967). An inflammatory infiltrate is observed in deeper tissue zones. Plasma cells dominate the histologic picture of long-standing ANUG.

87 Papilla biopsy
Affected papilla excised from a patient with mild ANUG resembling the clinical situation in Figure 90. The tip of the papilla and the tissue approaching the col have been destroyed by ulceration (U). The oral epithelium (OE, stained yellow) remains essentially intact. In the deeper layers of the biopsy one observes the red-stained intact collagen, while beneath the decimated papilla tip the collagen is largely obliterated (van Gieson, × 10).

The arrow indicates the section that is enlarged in Figure 88.

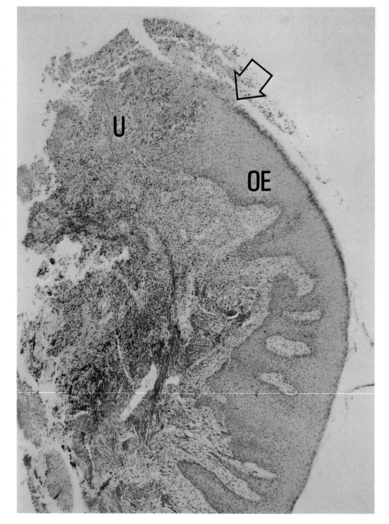

88 Surface of the disintegrated tissue
The upper portion of the figure exhibits thickly packed fusiform bacteria (FUS). Spirochetes present in this section are not visible with this staining technique, but the numerous PMNs are obvious. The brownish structures with weakly staining nuclei are dead epithelial cells (van Gieson, × 1000).

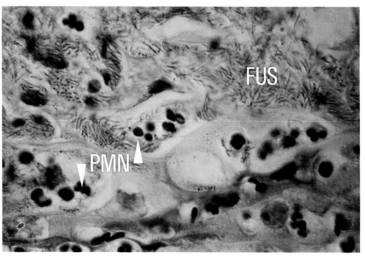

Clinical Symptoms

The first clinical symptom of ANUG is pain. Necrotic deterioration of papilla tips begins in the col tissues in the interdental area, followed by destruction of the entire papilla and even portions of the marginal gingiva. It is not clear whether the gingival destruction is caused by vascular infarction or by invasion (infiltration) of bacteria into the tissue. Without treatment, the osseous portion of the periodontal supporting apparatus can also become involved. The patient with ANUG is characterized by a typical, insipid, sweetish halitosis. In only a few cases are the depressed lesions on the cheeks, lips or tongue observed. Generalized ANUG may be accompanied by fever and malaise; it can be differentiated from acute herpetic gingivostomatitis by the vesicular pattern (see p. 54).

The diagnosis of ANUG can be supported by examination of a stained smear of the pseudomembrane with its characteristic composition (Fig. 89).

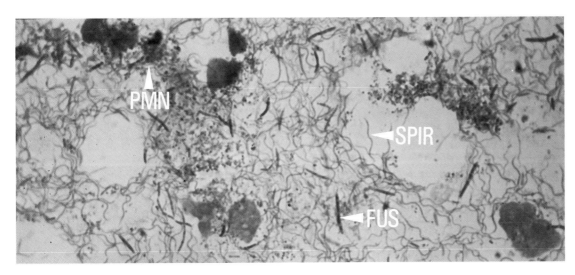

89   Smear of ANUG pseudomembrane
In addition to dead cells, PMNs and fusiform bacteria (FUS), innumerable spirochetes (SPIR) are visible (Giemsa, × 1000).

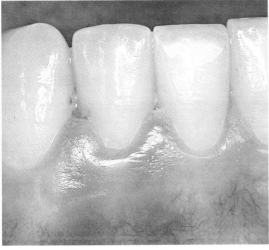
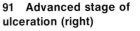

90   Earliest symptom of ANUG (left)
The most coronal portion of the papilla tip is necrotically destroyed from the col outward. The defects are coated with a typical whitish pseudomembrane. The first pain may be experienced even before any ulcerations become visible clinically. ANUG should be diagnosed and treated in this early, reversible stage.

91   Advanced stage of ulceration (right)

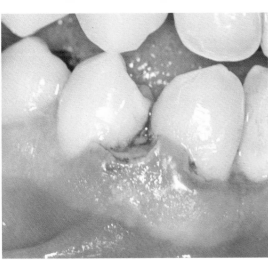
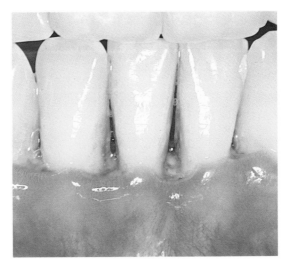

92   Complete destruction of the papilla (left)
Uneven involvement: Between the premolars there is no visible lesion, but areas of early necrosis can be seen on mesial and marginal aspects of the cuspid. Note the complete destruction of the papilla between cuspid and first bicuspid.

93   Acute recurrence (right)
The papillae are completely destroyed. The course of the gingival margin appears *inverse*. Beginning osseous destruction: Gingivoperiodontitis ulcerosa.

Mild ANUG (Gingivitis ulcerosa)

A 19-year-old female experienced gingival pain and bleeding for 3 days.

Findings:

HYG	60%
PBI	3.2 in anterior segments
	2.6 in bicuspid and molar areas
TM	0–1
PD	2–3 mm in interproximal areas

Diagnosis: Acute necrotizing ulcerative gingivitis, localized, early stage.

Therapy: During the first appointment, careful debridement (ultrasonic), hydrogen peroxide rinses, oral hygiene instruction and motivation. The patient may be instructed to rinse at home with chlorhexidine. At subsequent appointments, repeated motivation and home care instruction are provided, plaque and calculus are thoroughly removed by the dentist or hygienist. No systemic medications are indicated at this stage. Frequent recall!

Prognosis: With treatment and *good patient cooperation,* good.

94   Initial stage
Initial acute ulcerative destruction of several papilla tips (arrows). Other papillae exhibit signs of mild inflammation, but no destruction.

In the radiograph one observes no evidence of resorption of interdental septal bone.

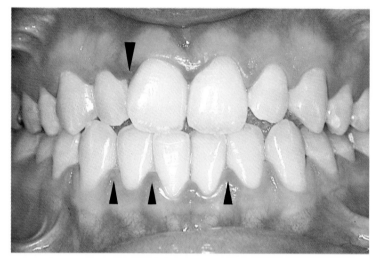
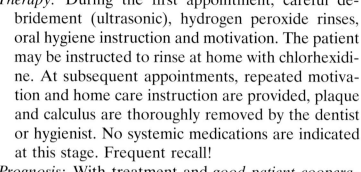
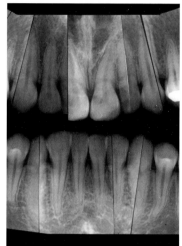

95   Destruction of papilla tips in the maxilla
Necrosis of the papilla between central and lateral incisor is apparent. Note simultaneous erythema and swelling, especially at the base of the papilla.
  Between the lateral incisor and the cuspid one observes the earliest signs of necrosis.
  Erythema of the papilla is noted between the two central incisors, but no clinically visible destruction. If the patient experiences pain when this area is probed gently, it is evidence that the necrotic process has already begun in the col area.

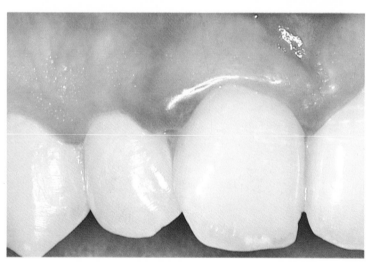

96   Destruction of papilla tips in the mandible
Each papilla exhibits signs of beginning ulceration, and each is already covered by a pseudomembrane consisting of fibrin, dead tissue cells, leukocytes and bacteria.

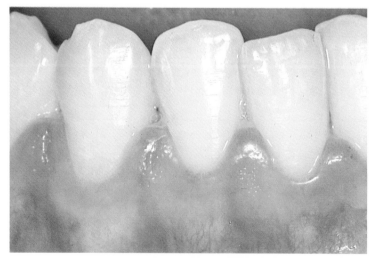

Severe ANUG

A 16-year-old female presented with a chief complaint of severe pain, inflammation and bleeding of the gingiva. Identical symptoms had been experienced twice before, at intervals of about 3 months. She treated the first acute episode herself with hydrogen peroxide rinses. She did not contact a dentist until this third incident.

Findings:

HYG	10%	TM	1
PBI	3.8	PD	maximum 3 mm interproximally

Diagnosis: Severe ANUG, generalized, 3rd exacerbation.

Therapy: 1. Careful debridement (ultrasonic), plaque and calculus removal, and topical application of antibiotic/cortisone ointment. Oral hygiene instruction and patient motivation. Re-evaluation, repeated oral hygiene instruction and patient motivation
2. Gingivoplasty as appropriate
3. Recall at short intervals!

Prognosis: Good, but only with excellent patient cooperation. There is a danger of recurrence.

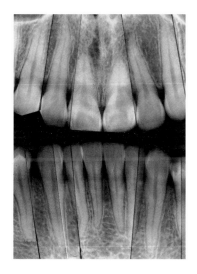
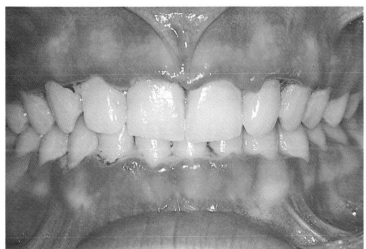

97 Acute exacerbation of advanced, generalized ANUG
Almost all interdental papillae are destroyed to a greater or lesser degree. The ulceration has already spread to the facial marginal gingiva. The gingivae are fiery red and bleed spontaneously or at the slightest touch.

The radiograph does not reveal any attack on the interdental bony septa.

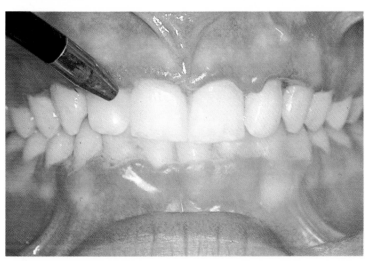

98 Spraying away loose debris and the pseudomembrane
Superficially located debris and the pseudomembrane can be easily removed from both teeth and gingiva by means of a water jet. Use of a spray or rinsing with chlorhexidine (CHX) will dramatically reduce the quantity of bacteria in the oral cavity.
   The operator should wear eye protection when using a water spray for this purpose.

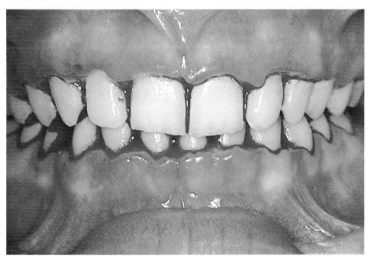

99 Hemorrhage after spraying
Heavy bleeding is provoked from the necrotic-ulcerated gingiva by the water spray.
   At this stage, the patient cannot be expected to perform efficient plaque control.

Gingivitis Modulated by Hormones

Alterations and dysregulation in the body's hormonal balance generally do not cause gingival inflammation, but can increase the severity of an already present gingivitis. In addition to insulin deficiency in Diabetes mellitus, it is primarily the female sex hormones that are associated with the progression of plaque-elicited gingivitis. One may distinguish:

- Puberty gingivitis
- Pregnancy gingivitis
- Gingivitis from the "pill"
- Gingivitis menstrualis and intermenstrualis
- Gingivitis climacterica.

Puberty gingivitis is the exception rather than the rule in a developing adolescent. However, epidemiological studies have demonstrated that Gingivitis simplex is somewhat more pronounced during puberty than before or after (Mühlemann & Mazor 1958; Curilović et al. 1977; Koivuniemi et al. 1980). If oral hygiene is poor and/or if the adolescent is a mouth breather, a typical gingival hyperplasia may ensue, especially in the maxillary anterior area (see Figs. 84–86).

Therapy: Plaque and calculus removal, oral hygiene instruction and gingivectomy/gingivoplasty. Mouth breathing may require consultation with an appropriate medical specialist.

Pregnancy gingivitis is not observed in every pregnant woman. Even if oral hygiene is good, however, the gingivae will exhibit an elevated tendency to bleed after toothbrushing or sulcus probing (Silness & Löe 1964).

Therapy: Oral hygiene; recall every one to two months until breast feeding is discontinued.

"Pill" gingivitis usually becomes evident only after regular long-term use of oral contraceptives (Lindhe & Björn 1967; Knight & Wade 1974; Pankhurst et al. 1981). The symptoms include gingival hemorrhage, mild erythema and edema.

Therapy: Oral hygiene and possibly a switch to a different brand of oral contraceptive.

Gingivitis menstrualis is exceedingly rare. Research has demonstrated that the desquamation of gingival epithelium changes over the course of the 28-day menstrual cycle, similar to the vaginal epithelium. In exceptional cases the desquamative cycle can be so pronounced that a diagnosis of "discrete" Gingivitis menstrualis may be made (Mühlemann 1952), or even less frequently Gingivitis intermenstrualis.

Therapy: Good oral hygiene to prevent secondary plaque-associated gingivitis. Some practitioners have advocated topical vitamin A preparations and dentifrices.

Gingivitis climacterica is also rare. The pathological alterations are observed less on the marginal gingiva than on the attached gingiva and oral mucosa. These appear dry and smooth, with salmon-pink spots. Stippling disappears and keratinization is lost. The patients complain of xerostomia and a burning sensation. The differential diagnosis should include desquamative gingivitis (p.52).

Therapy: Careful oral hygiene is necessary but may be painful. The patient should be instructed to use a soft-bristle toothbrush. Benzocaine in orabase may be beneficial as well as topical vitamin A ointments or dentifrices. In severe cases, systemic estrogen therapy may be prescribed by a gynecologist.

Mild Pregnancy Gingivitis

A 28-year-old female appeared for a dental check-up in her 7th month of pregnancy. She complained of occasional gingival bleeding during toothbrushing. The patient is quite motivated and performs home care rigorously.

Findings:
HYG 85%
PBI 1.8 in maxillary and mandibular
      anterior segments
      3.2 in all bicuspid and molar segments

TM   1–2
PD   2.5 mm in maxillary and mandibular
      anterior interproximal areas
      4–5 mm in bicuspid and molar areas
      (pseudopockets)

Diagnosis: Mild pregnancy gingivitis, localized.
Therapy: Removal of restoration overhangs; scaling; emphasize interdental hygiene.
Prognosis: After the pregnancy, very good.

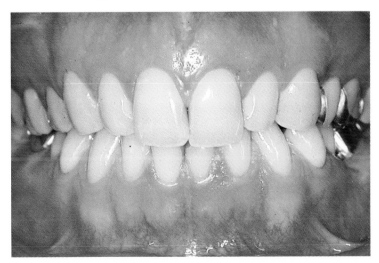

100 Healthy appearing gingiva
At first glance, one notices no signs of inflammation in the anterior area. In the posterior segments, however, mild to moderate gingivitis is obvious clinically.

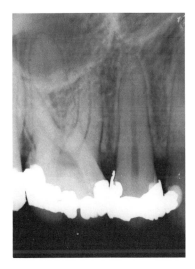
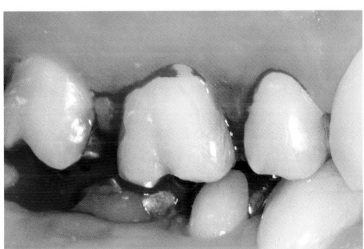

101 Localized inflammation
Adjacent to inadequate restorations that enhance plaque accumulation, the inflammation is particularly pronounced. Interdental papillae are edematous and probing of the sulcus elicits copious hemorrhage.

The radiograph reveals overhanging restorations, especially on the second bicuspid.

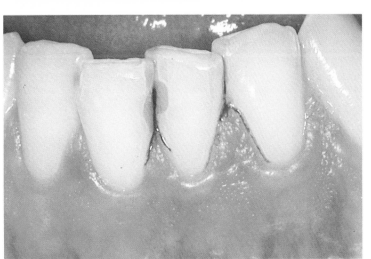

102 Bleeding on probing
The healthy-appearing mandibular anterior gingiva yields a score of 2 in the PBI test. The increased tendency to bleeding is characteristic during the second and third trimesters of pregnancy. The very high level of circulating hormones during this time may elicit these symptoms even when the teeth appear clean clinically.

Severe Pregnancy Gingivitis, Gravid Epulis

This 24-year-old woman was 8-months pregnant. She presented complaining that she "bites the swollen gums" on the left side of her mouth. Clinical examination reveals a severe generalized gingivitis as well as the gravid epulis ("pregnancy tumor").

Diagnosis: Severe generalized pregnancy gingivitis with large pyogenic granuloma near 34–35.

Therapy: ...

During the pregnancy: Motivation, repeated oral hygiene instruction, plaque and calculus removal, gingivoplasty around 34 and 35 using electrosurgery.

After breast feeding is terminated: Re-evaluation, further treatment planning.

Prognosis: With treatment, good.

Findings:

HYG	40%	PD	7 mm around teeth 34 & 35,
PBI	3.2		otherwise generally 4 mm
TM	0–1		(pseudopockets)

103 Severe pregnancy gingivitis
With poor oral hygiene, a pronounced gingivitis has developed during the last half of the pregnancy. A large epulis is observed buccally and lingually around the mandibular second bicuspid.

The histological section (of gingiva, not the epulis; see black line) exhibits normal oral epithelium, a relatively mild inflammatory infiltrate and widely dilated vessels (H & E, × 40).

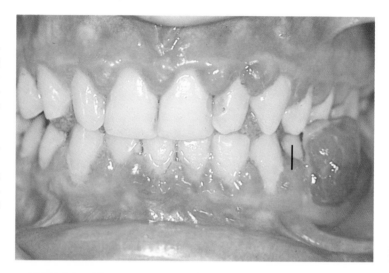 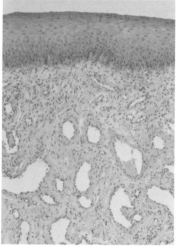

104 Gravid epulis
The surface of the epulis is ulcerated because the patient's maxillary teeth bite into the tissue during mastication. For this reason, the redundant tissue must be removed while the patient is still pregnant. Heavy hemorrhaging may be expected during the surgery; therefore, electrosurgery is the treatment of choice.

The radiograph depicts some horizontal bone loss.

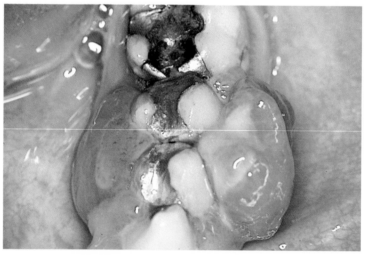 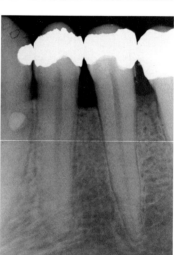

105 3 months after gingivoplasty; 2 months post-partum
Definitive periodontal therapy and treatment planning for restorative work that is sorely needed should begin at this time.

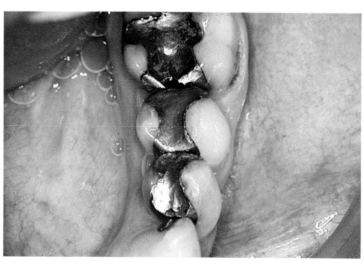

Gingival Overgrowth, Tumors

Swelling ("Tumor") is one of the classical signs of inflammation. In conjunction with hemorrhage and erythema, swelling caused by edema and hyperplasia is a common symptom of Gingivitis simplex, puberty gingivitis, pregnancy gingivitis and other forms of inflammatory changes in the gingiva. There are other types of gingival enlargement, especially papillary enlargement, whose etiologies are not solely plaque-related. Specific infections and hormonal imbalances may be prime etiological factors. Pindborg (1974, 1983) classified gingival enlargements as:

- Idiopathic fibrosis (Fibromatosis gingivae)
- Overgrowth elicited by drugs
  (e.g., phenytoin & cyclosporine-A)
- Epulis
- Benign and malignant tumors.

Idiopathic fibrosis is a firm, fibrous thickening of the gingiva. It is often observed as a localized lesion on the maxillary tuberosity and on the palatal aspect of posterior segments; it may also manifest as a generalized gingival enlargement. The cause is unknown but genetic factors cannot be ruled out (Emerson 1965).
Therapy: Gingivectomy, gingivoplasty.

Phenytoin (hydantoin)-induced gingival enlargement is a fibrous thickening of the gingiva that may be involved with secondary inflammation. The lesions occur in about half of all persons who ingest the antiepileptic drug phenytoin on a chronic regimen. A pharmacogenetic factor has been suggested (Hassell 1981). The lesions develop via selection of fibroblast subpopulations characterized by elevated synthesis of connective tissue macromolecules. Plaque may play a role in both incidence and severity of the enlargement (secondary inflammation).
Therapy: Motivation, oral hygiene, scaling, gingivectomy/gingivoplasty.

Cyclosporine-A (CS-A), a relatively new immunosuppressant drug, may also elicit gingival *enlargement and overgrowth.* The drug is used primarily in organ transplant patients to prevent rejection of the allograft and to prevent graft-versus-host reaction. It is also being tested clinically in the treatment of arthritis, psoriasis, type I Diabetes mellitus and several autoimmune diseases. The CS-A induced lesions manifest clinically as cauliflower-like protuberances that begin in the interdental area. Lesion severity appears to be related to daily drug dose. Inflammatory symptoms may appear secondarily as oral hygiene becomes difficult due to the excess tissue.
Therapy: Motivation, oral hygiene instruction, scaling and gingivectomy with antibiotic coverage (Rateitschak-Plüss et al. 1983a, b).

Epulis is a benign, tumor-like thickening of interdental papillae. It is possible to distinguish granulomatous, giant cell and fibrotic epulis histologically.
Therapy: Scaling, flap surgery to remove the excess tissue, osseous curettage. Recurrence is not uncommon.

Malignant tumors (carcinoma, sarcoma) of the gingivae are quite rare. Figure 113 depicts a rhabdomyosarcoma.
Therapy: Radical operation by oral surgeon; chemotherapy and/or irradiation to prevent metastasis.

106 Idiopathic fibrosis (Fibromatosis gingivae)

The etiology of this generalized gingival enlargement, present for years in this patient, is unknown. This 14-year-old female is not taking any medication (e.g., phenytoin).

Subsequent to gingivectomy, the redundant tissue returned slowly. Thirteen years later, surgical intervention to resect the recurrent fibrosis was again required.

The radiograph reveals no bone loss.

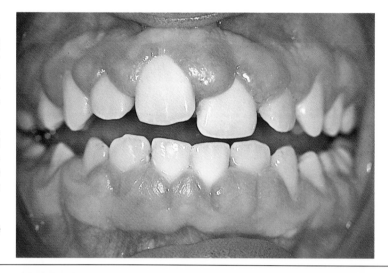
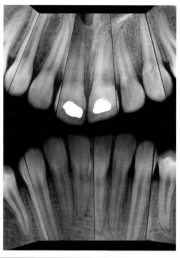

107 Mild phenytoin-induced gingival overgrowth

Fibrous-type gingival overgrowth in a 19-year-old female epileptic treated with a chronic regimen of phenytoin. With proper oral hygiene, the severity of the lesion can be markedly reduced, and secondary inflammatory sequelae can be avoided.

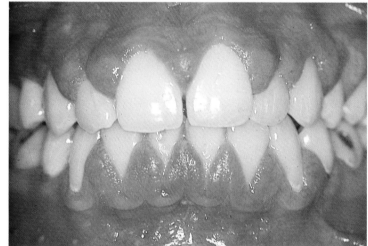

108 Severe phenytoin-induced gingival overgrowth with secondary inflammation

This 44-year-old female had taken phenytoin since a neurosurgical operation six years previously. She was slightly debilitated and unable to perform effective oral hygiene.

In the radiograph, resorption of the alveolar septa is obvious.

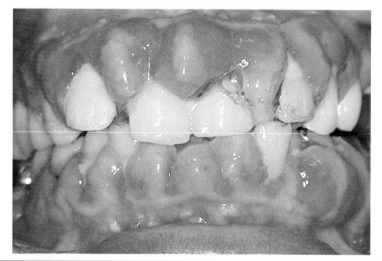
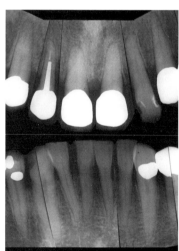

109 Gingival enlargement elicited by cyclosporine-A

A kidney transplant was performed in this 51-year-old female six years ago. The gingival lesions depicted here developed after cyclosporine-A was added to her immunosuppressant regimen.

A high power histological view reveals plasma cells and numerous PMNs in the subepithelial connective tissue. This is nothing more than host response to microbial plaque on the teeth, not a medicament-related phenomenon (H & E, × 400).

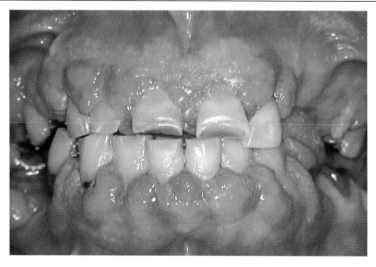
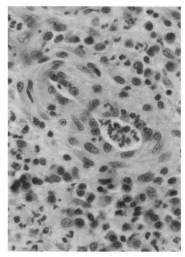

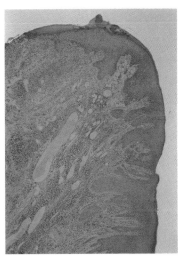
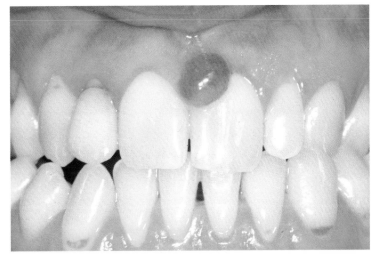

110 Granulomatous epulis, pyogenic granuloma

Localized, tumor-like, bright red, soft mass on the labial gingival margin in a 34-year-old woman. Such an epulis usually emantes from the interdental papillae. When probed, the lesion exudes a copious mixture of blood and pus.

The histological view exhibits a loose granulation tissue filled with blood (H & E, × 40).

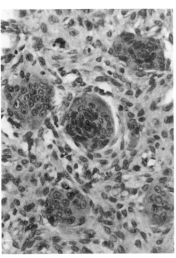
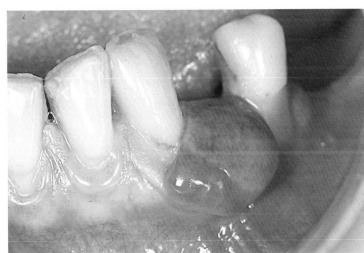

111 Giant cell epulis

Resembling clinically the granulomatous epulis, the giant cell epulis can only be diagnosed histologically. These lesions can become very large and, as in this 50-year-old patient, can cause migration of adjacent teeth. The etiology is unknown, but may be due to local irritants.

The histological section reveals an inflammatory infiltrate and multinucleated giant cells in the subepithelial connective tissue (H & E, × 400).

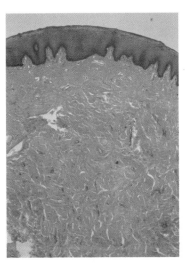
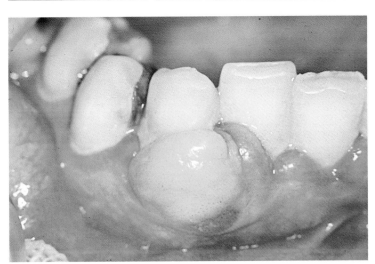

112 Epulis fibromatosa (fibroma)

Localized, fibrous, pale, firm, tumor-like mass on the gingiva of a 56-year-old female. Local marginal irritating factors can play an etiologic role.

Histologically one observes an accumulation of fibrous connective tissue that may also exhibit an inflammatory infiltrate if the mass become secondarily inflamed (Masson, × 40).

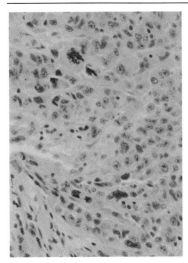
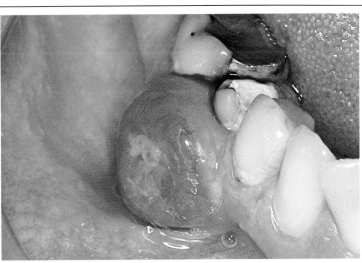

113 Malignant tumor, rhabdomyosarcoma

Very rare malignant tumor in a 38-year-old female. Displays invasive growth into the alveolar bone. Metastasizes rapidly throughout the skeletal system.

A high power (× 400) *histologic view* reveals growth of "strands" of the malignant tissue. Dramatic number of mitotic figures (H & E).

Courtesy of *B. Maeglin*

Autoimmune Diseases
Anomalies of Keratinization
Viral Infections

Autoimmune diseases such as desquamative and bullous alterations of the mucosa, anomalies of keratinization, and viral infections are often localized on the gingivae. These lesions have essentially nothing to do with plaque-induced gingivitis and must be differentiated from it. Patients who suffer from these diseases often have difficulty performing adequate oral hygiene because of pain and ease of gingival injury. The result of this situation is often the superimposition of a plaque-induced gingivitis. We shall describe several of these types of lesions:

- Desquamative gingivitis (gingivosis)
- Pemphigoid
- Pemphigus vulgaris
- Lichen planus
- Herpetic gingivostomatitis.

Gingivosis (Gingivitis desquamativa) is observed more frequently in women than in men. The initial stage is characterized by the appearance of reddish spots on the gingiva, followed by desquamation of the epithelium. In more severe cases blisters may be observed; at this stage it is difficult to differentiate the lesions from those of pemphigoid. Gingivosis is an autoimmune disease in which the host produces antibodies against its own epithelial basement membrane.

Therapy: It is not possible to treat the cause. Dental treatment is polypragmatic and symptomatic. Vitamin A or cortisone preparations may be employed in severe cases.

Pemphigoid is most common in women past middle age, with lesions developing on the oral mucosa and gingiva. The conjunctiva are often affected, and sometimes the skin as well. There is gingival erythema and vessicle formation. When vessicles rupture, an erosion covered with fibrin develops, which heals with mild scarring. Pemphigoid is also an autoimmune disease.

Therapy: Immunosuppressants and systemic corticosteroids. The painful lesions may be treated topically with cortisone ointment.

Pemphigus vulgaris is a disease of the elderly, affecting females somewhat more often than males. Before corticosteroid medication became available, the disease led to death. Affected sites include mucosal surfaces throughout the body, the skin, as well as oral mucosa and gingiva.

Intraepithelial vessicles develop, which burst easily and leave behind painful erosions. Epithelial desquamation occurs.

Therapy: Immunosuppressants and systemic corticosteroids prescribed by the dermatologist or internist.

Lichen planus is experienced by those over the age of 30, with males and females equally affected. It is a skin disease that can also affect the gingiva and oral mucosa. The symptoms include milky-whitish, spoon-shaped, hyperkeratotic effluorescences and/or a spiderweb-like network referred to as Wickham's striae. The etiology is unknown, possibly psychosomatic.

Therapy: None. Periodic re-examination only. In *erosive forms,* therapy consisting of vitamin A preparations, sometimes combined with systemic administration of corticosteroids may be instituted. The lesions may be facultatively premalignant.

Herpetic gingivostomatitis see p. 54.

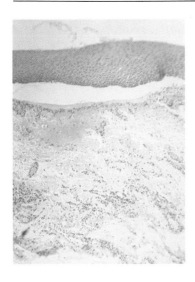

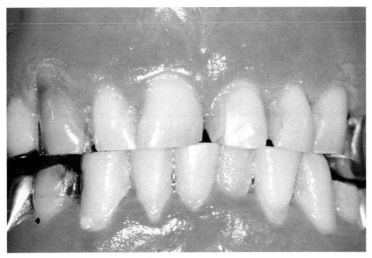

114 Desquamative gingivitis (gingivosis)

Severe erythema of the entire attached gingiva in this 62-year-old female. The epithelium can be easily separated from the subepithelial tissues. A secondary gingivitis elicited by plaque accumulation is also observed.

The histological section exhibits a thin oral epithelium that is devoid of rete ridges and not keratinized. The epithelium has separated from the underlying connective tissue (carbol fuchsin stain, × 100).

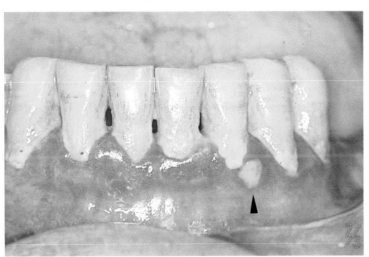

115 Pemphigoid

There are no strict criteria for clinical differentiation between gingivosis and pemphigoid. In this 54-year-old female, one observes a severely reddened gingiva, with vessicles that burst and form erosions (arrow). There is also a secondary, plaque-induced gingivitis.

The histological picture is essentially identical to that of gingivosis.

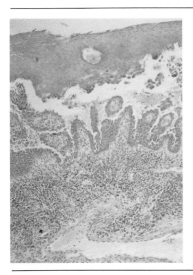

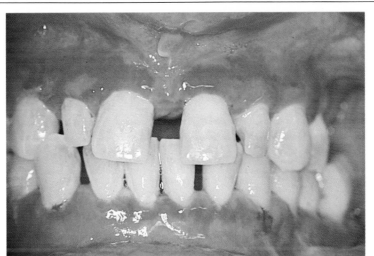

116 Pemphigus vulgaris

Fiery red gingiva with secondary effluorescences (burst vessicles). This 50-year-old female also manifested pronounced symptoms on her skin.

In the histological view, it is clear that vessicle formation and sloughing of the superficial layer of gingiva occurs intra-epithelially. The basal cell layer remains attached to the connective tissue component (H & E, × 250).

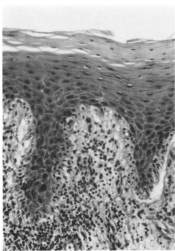

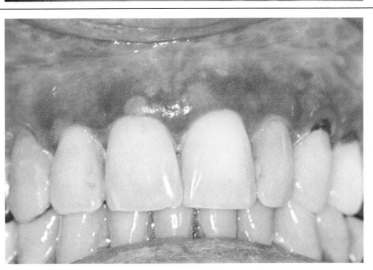

117 Lichen planus

A 42-year-old male presented with a whitish, hyperkeratotic net-like coating (Wickham's striae) on the gingiva and oral mucosa.

Histologically the epithelium exhibits rete ridges and hyperkeratosis. An inflammatory infiltrate is visible subepithelially (H & E, × 400).

Courtesy of *B. Maeglin*

Gingivostomatitis Herpetica

This viral infection is most commonly detected in children and in young adults between the ages of 20 and 25 (Herrmann 1972). Once primary infection has occurred, the patient experiences *fever* and painful swelling of the lymph nodes. Intraoral examination reveals an acute, painful gingivitis with blister-like aphthae, erosive lesions on the attached gingiva and not infrequently on the oral mucosa and lips as well. The differential diagnosis must include Gingivitis ulcerosa (ANUG) and common recurrent aphthous ulcer. The etiology is clear: Infection with *Herpes simplex virus*. Predisposing factors include mechanical trauma, sun exposure, inadequate diet, hormonal disturbance and psychic trauma. The lesions generally disappear spontaneously within 1–2 weeks, without any therapy.

Therapy: Topical application of palliative ointments, and perhaps a plaque-inhibitory agent (chlorhexidine) to prevent a bacterial superinfection. *Systemic* protection against the viral infection is not yet feasible, nor is there any specific medicament available. In severe cases antibiotics may be used to combat the bacterial superinfection.

118 Mild herpetic gingivostomatitis
Whitish patches and erosive alterations, especially on the attached gingiva. This female patient exhibited good oral hygiene, very little plaque accumulation and hardly any signs of marginal inflammation. The possibility that the herpes infection occurred secondary to a toothbrush injury cannot be ruled out.

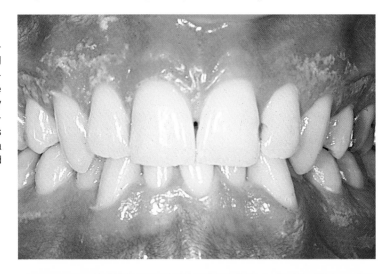

119 Herpetic gingivostomatitis
The patient's lack of oral hygiene coupled with the plaque retention fostered by orthodontic bands and wires led to gingivitis, which became superinfected with Herpes.

Right: Solitary aphthous ulcer
Whitish ulcer surrounded by fiery red mucosal tissue; often recurrent. Etiology is unknown. Differential diagnosis should include herpetic gingivostomatitis.

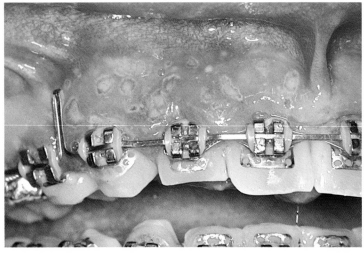
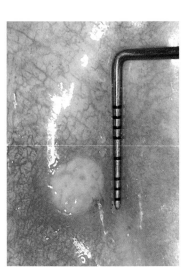

120 Severe herpetic gingivostomatitis
This 20-year-old male experienced fever and swollen cervical lymph nodes. A severe gingivitis was present even before the Herpes infection. This acute clinical picture is reminiscent of ulcerative gingivitis, which should be included in the differential diagnosis.

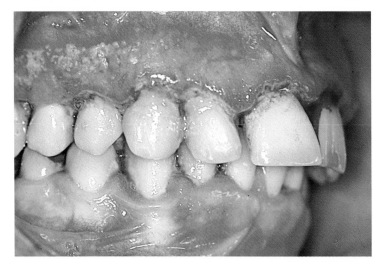

Periodontitis

Periodontitis in its various forms is one of the most widespread diseases of mankind, along with dental caries. The most important symptoms of periodontitis include inflammation, pocket formation and bone resorption (attachment loss).

In general, periodontitis develops from a previously existing gingivitis. On the other hand, not every case of gingivitis will progress to periodontitis. The quantity and virulence of the plaque microorganisms (pathogens), as well as host resistance factors (immune status) will determine the inflammatory activity and progression of periodontal destruction. With proper oral hygiene (plaque and calculus removal) periodontitis can almost always be prevented.

In the permanent dentition three different forms of progression of periodontitis are acknowledged, among which there exist ill-defined borders (Page & Schroeder 1982; Page et al. 1983).

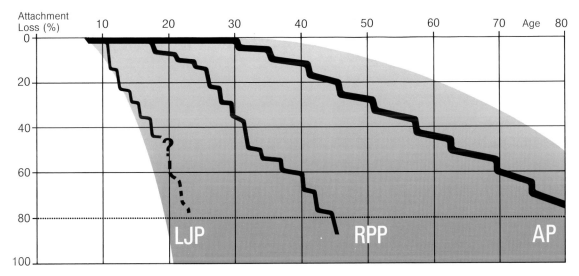

121 Forms of periodontitis
The stepwise loss of periodontal support (attachment loss) is shown schematically in relation to average subject age.

1. Slowly progressing periodontitis in adults; "adult periodontitis" (**AP**).

2. Rapidly progressive periodontitis in young adults (**RPP**).

3. Localized, rapidly progressing periodontitis in young persons ("localized juvenile periodontitis," **LJP**).

Adult periodontitis (AP) progresses slowly and is the most frequently encountered form of the disease. Approximately 95 % of all cases of periodontitis are AP. *Rapidly progressive periodontitis (RPP)* in young adults accounts for but 5 % of all cases. *Juvenile periodontitis (LJP = localized juvenile periodontitis)* has an incidence of less than 0.1 % in Caucasians. The figure for LJP is apparently higher in India and Africa (see review by Saxén 1980). From an epidemiological point of view, RPP and LJP are not of particular public health significance. But it is precisely these cases of RPP and LJP that give the clinical periodontist his greatest problems. Loss of attachment in all 3 forms of periodontitis in the permanent dentition does not proceed at a regular pace, as was previously assumed. The course of the disease is actually one of acute exacerbations that occur in the depth of the pocket, alternating with periods of quiescence or remission. The acute phases usually occur around individual teeth or groups of teeth, or on a single root surface, and not generalized in the entire dentition (Socransky et al. 1984). This explains the usually observed clinical situation in which the distribution of attachment loss is irregular (see Single Tooth Diagnosis, Single Tooth Prognosis, pp. 97–98).

Slowly Progressing Adult Periodontitis (AP)

This most common form of periodontitis develops between the ages of 30 and 40, with a gradual development, generally from a pre-existing gingivitis. The entire dentition may be equally affected. More often, however, the distribution of the disease is irregular, with more severe destruction primarily in molar areas but also in anterior segments. In beginning stages, bone loss progresses horizontally for the most part (suprabony pockets); vertical bone loss may ensue subsequently. The gingivae exhibit various degrees of inflammation, with recession in some areas and fibrotic manifestations elsewhere. As was the case with beginning gingivitis, the plaque is composed primarily of gram-positive rods and cocci. This plaque provides the matrix for those organisms responsible for progression of AP and also for subgingival calculus.

Exacerbations of AP occur at rather lengthy intervals. The disease leads to tooth loss only in much later years, or not at all.

Therapy: With professional mechanical treatment, AP can be successfully controlled even if the patient's cooperation with home care is not optimal.

Rapidly Progressive Periodontitis of Young Adults (RPP)

This relatively rare disease can begin immediately after puberty but is usually diagnosed initially between ages 20 and 30. Females are more frequently affected than males. In contrast to localized juvenile periodontitis (LJP), from which it is often difficult to differentiate, in RPP all teeth may be affected. Some authors have referred to RPP as *postjuvenile periodontitis.* Severity and degree of attachment loss vary considerably, but in advanced cases the bone loss picture is mainly vertical.

Acute exacerbations are followed by periods of relative quiescence or chronicity, with no bone loss. The etiology of these acute stages is to be found in the specific microorganisms (gram-negative anaerobes) which may to some degree actually invade the ulcerated pocket epithelium (infection). Specific serum antibodies have been identified against *Bacteroides gingivalis* and *Actinobacillus actinomycetemcomitans.* In addition, PMN and monocyte defects have been detected in RPP patients.

Clinical symptoms of an acute exacerbation include increased gingival inflammation with bleeding upon probing, as well as exudation and suppuration from the pockets. Without treatment, RPP progresses rapidly and tooth loss may result. With treatment, the symptoms of disease activity can be eliminated. Clinically, the gingivae may be rendered free of inflammation.

Therapy: With intensive local treatment including scaling and root planing, the progress of RPP can be halted. Supportive therapy with *systemic* medications such as *metronidazole* or *ornidazole,* in combination with chlorhexidine rinses, is indicated for aggressive treatment of this severe form of periodontitis (see Side Effects – Contraindications, p. 265).

Localized Juvenile Periodontitis (LJP)

This rare disorder attacks the permanent dentition. LJP begins in puberty but is usually not diagnosed until several years later, often when lesions are discovered serendipitously on bitewing radiographs. In the initial stages, incisors and first molars are affected in both maxilla and mandible. Later, other teeth may also be included in the disease process. The radiographic picture is primarily one of vertical bone loss. Hereditary factors likely play a role. Girls are affected four times more often than boys. The boundary between late LJP and RPP is often indistinct.

In its earliest stages, LJP seldom manifests as gingival inflammation. Patients exhibit normal appearing gingiva and very little supragingival plaque. The pocket harbors a nonadherent gram-negative anaerobic bacterial flora. In virtually every instance, one observes *Actinobacillus actinomycetemcomitans* (Aa) and *Capnocytophaga ochracea* (Zambon et al. 1983). The patient's serum contains high antibody titers to a bacterial leukotoxin, which has the ability to injure PMNs. Defects in PMNs and monocytes have been demonstrated in LJP patients. Without treatment, the disease progresses very rapidly on incisors and first molars.

Therapy: With prompt diagnosis and therapy consisting of vigorous mechanical debridement and systemic administration of *tetracycline* (see Medicaments p. 263), the destructive process can be halted. Osseous defects may eventually regenerate.

Pockets, Loss of Attachment

Pocket formation without any loss of (connective tissue) *attachment* is seen in gingivitis in the form of the *gingival pocket.* Additional edema may create a *pseudopocket.*

True pockets with loss of attachment are symptomatic of periodontitis. One may differentiate between:
- *Suprabony pockets*
  resulting from horizontal loss of bone
- *Infrabony pockets*
  resulting from vertical, angular bone loss.

A true pocket will exhibit apical migration of the junctional epithelium down the root surface and transformation of the junctional epithelium (JE) into a pocket epithelium (Müller-Glauser & Schroeder 1982). If the most apical extent of the pocket is coronal to the alveolar crest, one speaks of a suprabony pocket. If the base of the pocket is apical to the alveolar crest, an infrabony pocket is present.

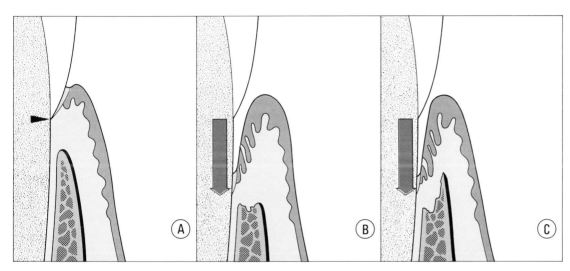

122   Types of pockets

A. Normal sulcus
Apical termination of the JE is at the cementoenamel junction (arrow).

B. Suprabony pocket
Proliferating pocket epithelium. A remnant of junctional epithelium persists (pink).

C. Infrabony pocket
Extends beyond alveolar crest.

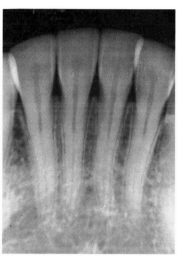
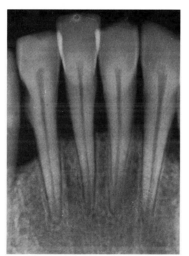
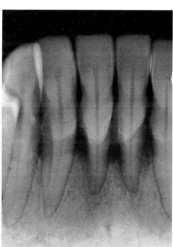

123   No attachment loss, normal alveolar septa (left)
Lamina dura remains intact.

124   Horizontal bone loss (middle)
Up to 50% loss of interdental septal bone.

125   Severe horizontal bone loss (right)
Up to 80% bone loss. Heavy calculus accumulation.

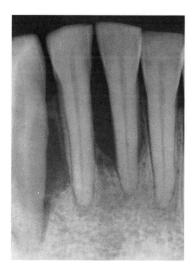
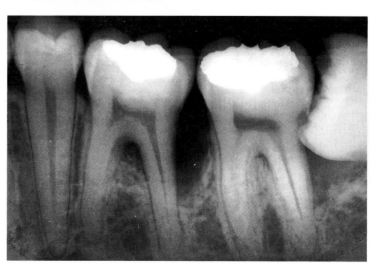

126   Vertical bone loss – Craters (left)
Irregular pattern of destruction of alveolar septa. Mesial to the cuspid, evidence of undermining or cyst formation.

127   Vertical bone loss – Furcation involvement (right)
Severe bone loss distal to the first molar. On the same tooth the interradicular bone (furcation) is also involved in the destruction.

Infrabony Pockets

Vertical bone loss (infrabony pocketing) may exhibit various forms in relation to the affected tooth (Goldman & Cohen 1980). Osseous defects are classified as follows:

3-wall bony pockets are bordered by one tooth surface and three osseous surfaces.

2-wall bony pockets (interdental crater) are bordered by two tooth surfaces and two osseous surfaces (one facial and one oral).

1-wall bony pockets are bordered by two tooth surfaces, one osseous surface (facial or oral) and a soft tissue border.

Crater ("cup") *defects* are a combined form of pocket, bordered by several surfaces of a tooth and several of bone. The defect surrounds the tooth.

The causes for this wide variation in pocket morphology and resorption of bone are myriad and cannot always be wholly elucidated in each individual case. In the early

128   Schematic representation of pocket morphology
The walls of each pocket are shown in red.

A. 3-wall bony defect

B. 2-wall bony defect

C. 1-wall bony defect

D. Combined bony pocket, crater-like resorption ("cup").

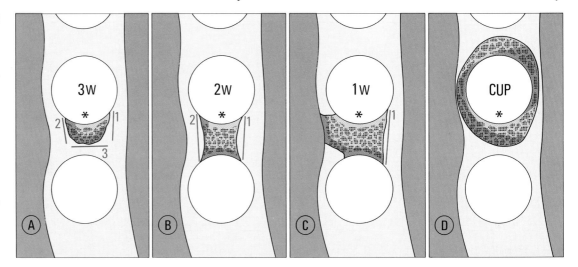

129   Small 3-wall defect
Early pocket formation on the mesial aspect of the second bicuspid. The color-coded probe (CP 12) measures a depth of ca. 3 mm. If gingiva were present, the total probing depth would be ca. 5 mm.

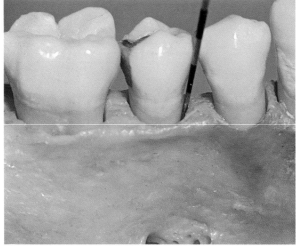
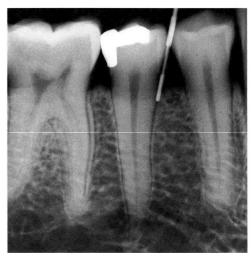

130   Deep 3-wall bony pocket
The periodontal probe descends almost 6 mm (measured from the alveolar crest) to the base of this 3-wall defect.

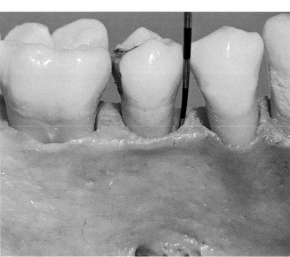
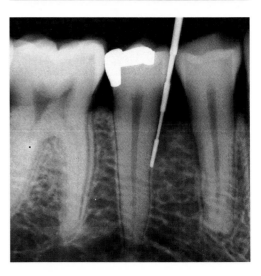

stages of periodontitis, especially in the slowly progressing form (AP), bone loss is mostly in a horizontal direction. If infrabony pockets then develop as the disease process advances, the following factors *may* account for the morphology of the resulting pocket:
– Local inadequate oral hygiene
– Local acute exacerbation elicited by specific bacteria in the pocket
– Crowding and tipping of teeth (plaque-retentive areas)
– Tooth morphology (root irregularities, furcations)

– Osseous morphology
– Improper loading due to functional disturbances.

The morphology of the bony pocket is of importance in both prognosis and treatment planning. The amount of bone remaining will effect the chances of osseous regeneration after treatment.

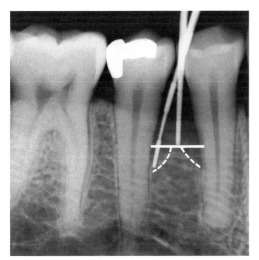 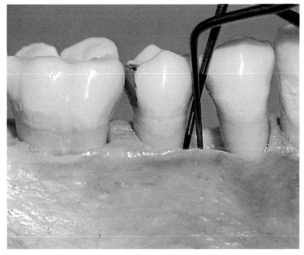

131 2-wall bony pocket, interdental crater
The coronal portion of this defect is bordered by only two bony walls (and two tooth surfaces). In the apical areas the 2-wall defect actually becomes *two* 3-wall defects (see probe tip left of interdental septum in radiograph, left).

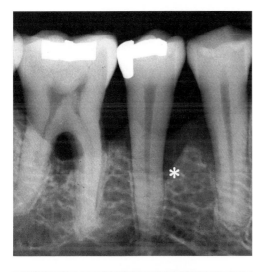 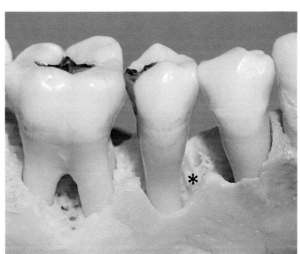

132 1-wall bony pocket on the mesial of tooth 45
Advanced bone loss in bicuspid/molar area. On tooth 45 the facial wall of bone is reduced almost to the level of the depth of the mesial pocket (∗). A portion of the lingual plate of bone (one wall) remains intact.

The facial root surface and the interdental spaces could be covered with soft tissue to the cementoenamel junction, masking the defect clinically.

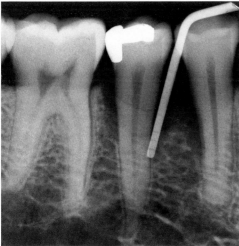 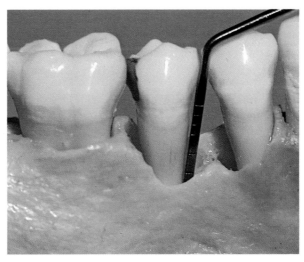

133 Combined pocket, crater defect
In the region of tooth 45, the apical portion of the osseous defect courses around the tooth, creating a "moat" or "cup" (Goldman probe in situ). The bony pocket is therefore bordered by several osseous and tooth surface walls.

Furcation Involvement

Periodontal bone loss in multirooted teeth presents a special problem when bi- or trifurcations are involved. Partially or completely open furcations tend to accumulate plaque. Exacerbations, abscesses, progressive loss of attachment and rapid deepening of periodontal pockets occur frequently, especially with through-and-through furcation involvement. In addition, open furcations are particularly susceptible to caries.

Hamp et al. (1975) presented three degrees of furcation involvement (F1–F3), and Ramfjord and Ash (1970) similarly classified furcation involvement into three degrees of severity, both *measuring horizontally*.

In this *Atlas,* furcation involvement will be referred to according to horizontal measurements, as follows:

Class 1: The furcation can be probed to a depth of 3 mm with the periodontal probe (F1).

Class 2: The furcation can be probed to a depth of more than 3 mm, but is not through-and-through (F2).

Class 3: The furcation is through-and-through and can be probed completely (F3).

134 Classification of furcation involvement

A. F0: Pocket, but without furcation involvement.

B. F1: Furcation can be probed 3 mm in horizontal direction.

C. F2: Furcation can be probed deeper than 3 mm.

D. F3: Through-and-through furcation involvement.

Furcation involvement often occurs in conjunction with an infrabony defect.

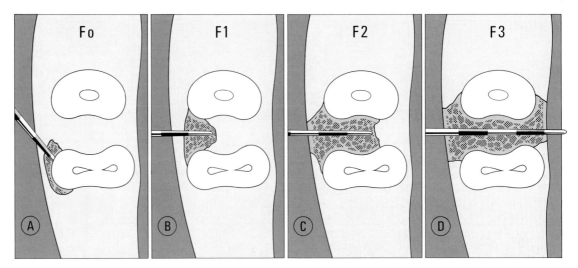

135 No furcation involvement – F0
In this situation one could detect a ca. 5 mm deep suprabony pocket in the area of the buccal furcation.

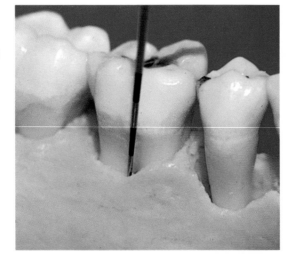
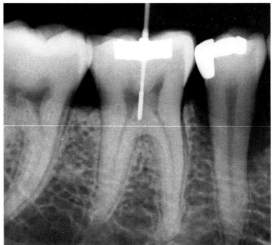

136 Furcation involvement – F1
Using a curved explorer the buccal furcation can be probed to a depth of less than 3 mm. Probing is performed from both buccal and lingual aspects during clinical examination.

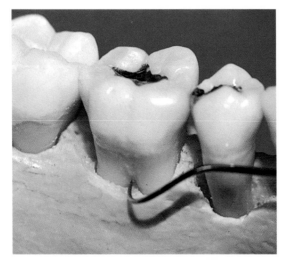
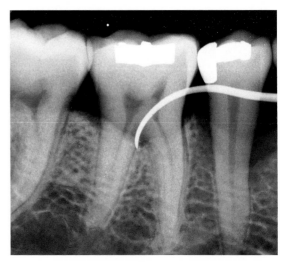

This classification of furcation involvement is applicable both in the mandible and in the maxilla, where it can rarely be diagnosed radiographically. In such cases it is necessary to ascertain whether, in class F 3 involvement, a through-and-through situation exists among all three roots of the maxillary molar or whether bone or attachment is still present on any two roots, e.g., the mesiobuccal and the palatal root. In order to ascertain furcation involvement in the maxillary molars, the probing must be performed from buccal, distobuccal and mesiopalatal aspects.

The *vertical bone loss* in an open furcation can also be classified (subclasses A – C, Tarnow & Fletcher 1983); it is measured from the roof of the furcation. *Therapy:* Class F 1 and F 2 furcation involvement may be successfully treated by root planing alone or by flap procedures (Ramfjord technique). A narrow furcation may be extended by odontoplasty.

The class F 3 involvement carries a less favorable prognosis, but can be treated the same as 1 and 2. Hemisection and resection of one root offer additional possibilities (pp. 221–227).

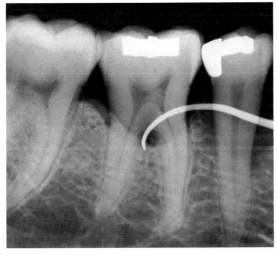
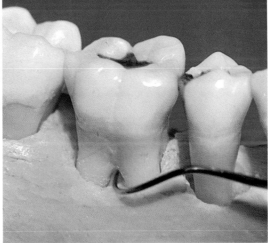

137 Furcation involvement – F 2
The explorer can probe more than 3 mm into a furcation, which is not yet through-and-through.

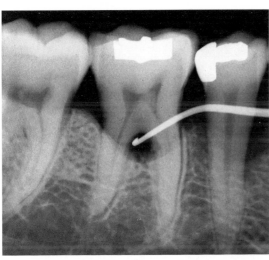
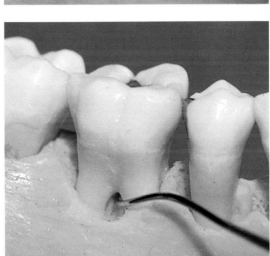

138 Furcation involvement – F 3, mild (subclass A)
Narrow, through-and-through bifurcation in the face of relatively minor bone loss (Nabers 2 explorer). Vertical interradicular bone loss is less than 3 mm.

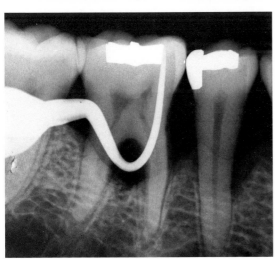
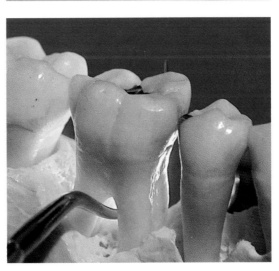

139 Furcation involvement – F 3, severe (subclass C)
Wide through-and-through bifurcation involvement in a case exhibiting severe horizontal and vertical bone loss (cowhorn explorer). Vertical interradicular bone loss greater than 6 mm.

Histopathology

The primary symptoms of periodontitis are attachment loss and pocket formation. *Pocket epithelium* has the following features (modified from Müller-Glauser & Schroeder 1982):

1. Irregular boundary with subjacent connective tissue, exhibiting rete pegs; toward the periodontal pocket, epithelium often very thin and partially ulcerated.
2. In the apicalmost region, the pocket epithelium becomes a very narrow junctional epithelium.

3. Transmigration of PMNs through the pocket epithelium.
4. Defective basal lamina complex on the connective tissue aspect.

A heavy inflammatory infiltrate and collagen loss occur within the connective tissue compartment. In acute stages, pus formation and microabscesses occur. Bone is resorbed, and deeper osseous marrow is transformed into fibrous connective tissue.

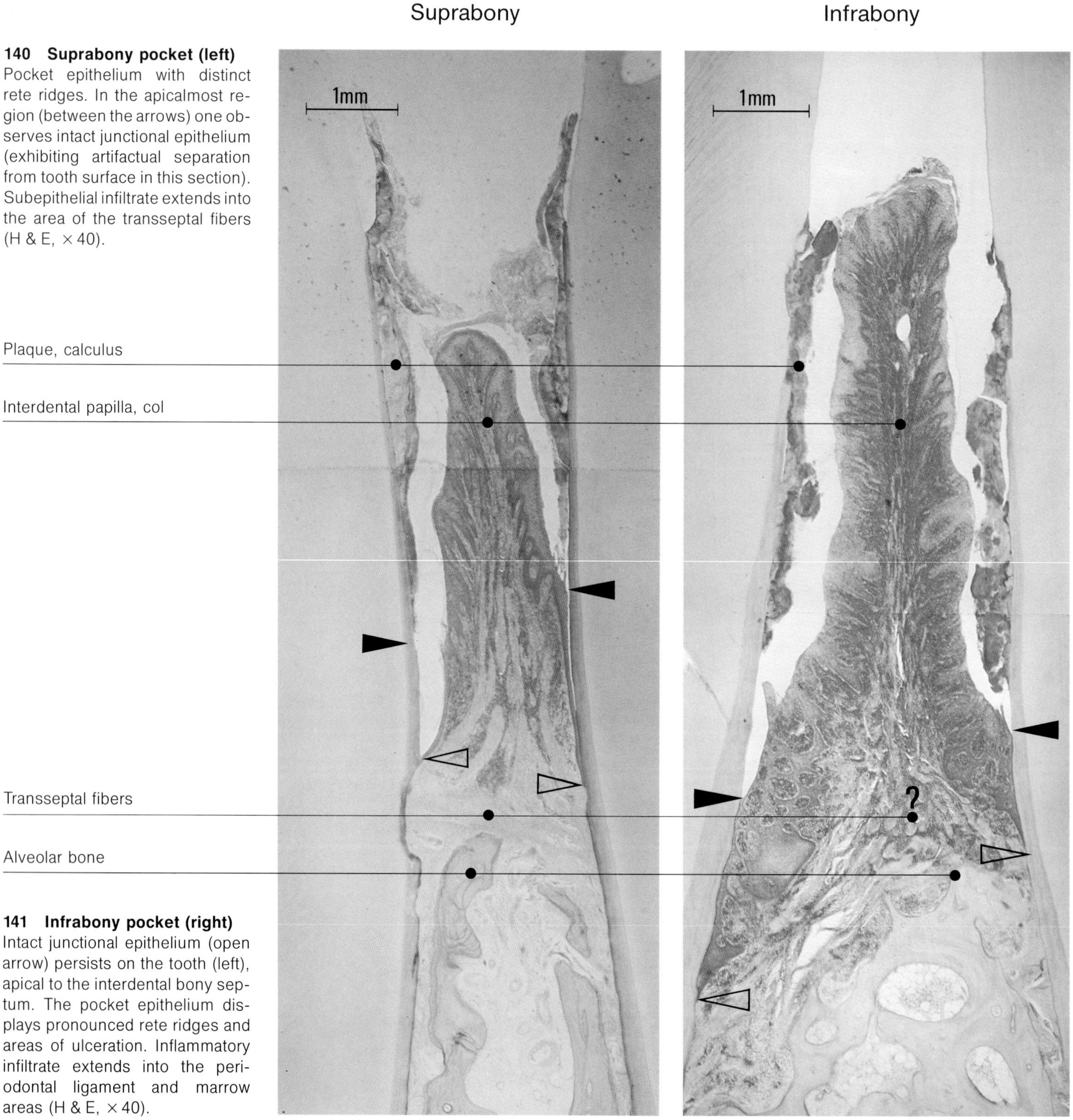

Suprabony

Infrabony

140   Suprabony pocket (left)
Pocket epithelium with distinct rete ridges. In the apicalmost region (between the arrows) one observes intact junctional epithelium (exhibiting artifactual separation from tooth surface in this section). Subepithelial infiltrate extends into the area of the transseptal fibers (H & E, × 40).

Plaque, calculus

Interdental papilla, col

Transseptal fibers

Alveolar bone

141   Infrabony pocket (right)
Intact junctional epithelium (open arrow) persists on the tooth (left), apical to the interdental bony septum. The pocket epithelium displays pronounced rete ridges and areas of ulceration. Inflammatory infiltrate extends into the periodontal ligament and marrow areas (H & E, × 40).

Clinical Symptoms

The main clinical symptoms of periodontitis are *inflammation, bone loss (attachment loss) and the true periodontal pocket*. These can occur in varying degrees of severity and in differing forms. They may be complicated or modified by other pathological processes:

- Activity of the pocket
  (bleeding, exudate, suppuration)
- Gingival swelling
- Gingival recession (retraction)
- Pocket abscess, furcation abscess
- Fistula
- Tooth movement, tipping, extrusion
- Tooth loosening.

The measurement of *pocket depth (probing depth)* is not a measure of *attachment loss* (see Charting – Diagnosis – Prognosis, p. 87). Only when the marginal gingiva is at its normal level vis-à-vis the cementoenamel junction does pocket probing correspond approximately to the loss of tooth supportive attachment.

The activity of a pocket is of more importance than pocket depth, especially with regard to treatment planning and prognosis. Bleeding on probing, presence of exudate, and suppuration after application of finger pressure are the signs of an active pocket. This is often observed in rapidly progressive periodontitis in young adults (RPP), and in juvenile periodontitis (LJP) in particular.

If the gingiva is *edematous or hyperplastically* enlarged beyond the cementoenamel junction, attachment loss and true pocket depth will be overestimated by the degree of swelling.

If periodontitis persists untreated for an extended period of time (years), gingival *shrinkage* may occur. This is particularly true in AP. Gingival shrinkage can also occur after spontaneous transition of an acute exacerbation into a chronic, quiescent stage, or following comprehensive periodontal therapy, or after opening of abscesses. Gingival shrinkage, whatever the cause, leads to exposure of root surfaces. This sort of gingival shrinkage must not be confused with true gingival *recession*, which can occur in the *abscence* of clinical inflammation. True recession occurs without the formation of periodontal pockets. If, as a result of shrinkage, the gingival margin is located apical to the cementoenamel junction, clinical probing of any true pockets will underestimate the actual loss of attachment. True attachment loss must be measured from the cementoenamel junction to the base of the pocket.

An additional symptom of active periodontitis is the *pocket abscess*. This develops during an acute exacerbation if necrotic tissue cannot be either resorbed or expelled. This can occur in furcations, e.g., if the coronal gingiva closes off the pocket. An abscess may also be the consequence of injury, for example biting upon hard, sharp foodstuffs, improper oral hygiene efforts (a broken toothpick), or iatrogenic trauma. In rare instances a periodontal abscess can develop into a submucosal abscess (parulis). An abscess is one of the few manifestations of periodontitis that may elicit *pain.* If an abscess is expansive, extending to the apical region, the tooth may become sensitive to percussion. A painful abscess must be opened on an emergency basis, either by way of the pocket itself or via incision through the lateral wall. An abscess may also release spontaneously through a fistulous tract or at the gingival margin.

Fistulae often create a patent connection between the suppurating periodontal pocket and the intraoral orifice. If clinical treatment is improper, such a fistula may persist for an extended period of time without any pain.

In advanced periodontitis additional clinical symptoms including *migration* and *tipping* of teeth may occur. The result of such tooth movements is the creation of diastemata, which can be an esthetic problem depending upon the size and location. There are many factors that could be responsible for tooth migration and it is not possible in every case to determine the specific cause. Missing antagonists, functional occlusal disturbances, oral parafunctions (lip biting, tongue thrust etc.) and oral habits (e. g., pipe smoking) may cause tooth migration. There is also speculation that a tooth exhibiting a deep pocket on one side and essentially intact periodontal fiber structure on the other side may migrate not so much as a result of pressure exerted by granulation tissue in the pocket as by forces deriving from the yet intact collagenous supracrestal fiber bundles in the healthy tissues. The fact that migrated teeth usually exhibit their unilateral pocket on the side opposite the direction of wandering would appear to support this theory.

Pathologically *increasing tooth mobility* is a symptom of severe, advanced periodontitis. However, this symptom must be interpreted carefully because it can be influenced by numerous factors. In a healthy periodontium the teeth exhibit physiological differences in mobility de-

pending on number of roots, root morphology and root length. Occlusal trauma can lead to increased tooth mobility even when the periodontal supporting structures are intact. In moderate to severe periodontitis, it is the quantitative loss of bone that is the primary determinant of tooth mobility.

However, inflammation and the edematous condition within the soft tissue may also enhance tooth

142 Active pocket (left):
Suppuration
Pus exudes from a pocket on tooth 11 after finger pressure is applied.

143 Pocket (right):
The probing depth corresponds to the attachment loss (AL)
The measurement (8 mm) is made from the gingival margin, which in this case is still in its normal position at the cementoenamel junction (see also Fig. 220, p. 89).

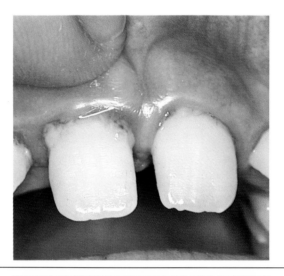

144 Pocket (left):
Overestimation of attachment loss (AL)
The measurement (7 mm) is made from the gingival margin, but the hyperplastic gingivae extend beyond the CEJ, creating a pseudo-pocket. The true AL is 3 mm less than the probing depth.

145 Pocket (right):
Underestimation of attachment loss (AL)
The measurement (7 mm) is made from the gingival margin, but the true AL is 10 mm.

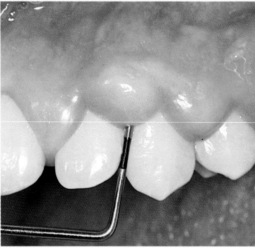
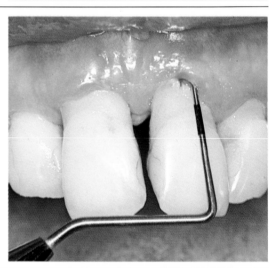

146 Periodontal abscess
Originating from a 12 mm pocket on the mesial aspect of the tipped molar 47, the abscess is just about to drain spontaneously (fistula).

Radiograph: Severe vertical bony defect on mesial of 47. Probing revealed a 1-wall bony pocket (open lingually).

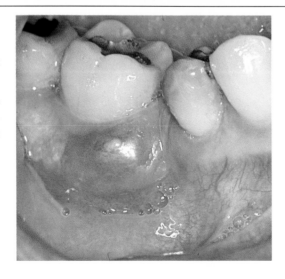
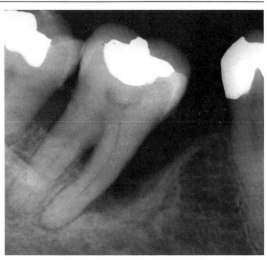

mobility somewhat in periodontitis. Occlusal trauma in a periodontally compromised dentition can increase tooth mobility still further. If tooth mobility continues to increase over time, the prognosis for the tooth is not favorable. A tooth may appear less firm in its alveolus after periodontal therapy, but this does not necessarily effect the prognosis adversely.

The primary symptoms of periodontitis are inflammation, attachment loss and the formation of pockets. However, when charting the patient's oral condition the dentist must not neglect the secondary symptoms described here. These may modify the diagnosis, the prognosis and the treatment plan.

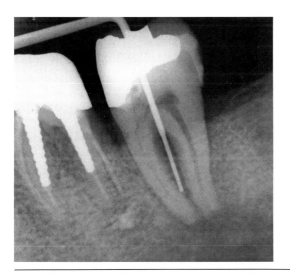
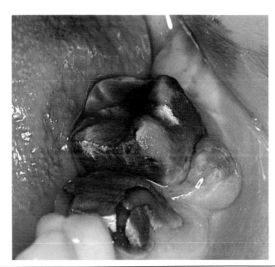

147 Furcation abscess
The abscess originates from a 9 mm pocket on the buccal of tooth 37, which has an open furcation.

The radiograph depicts the probe (CP 12) in situ. The probe penetrates to a depth of 9 mm before encountering intact bone; the soft tissue at the base of the pocket is easily traversed by the probe tip.

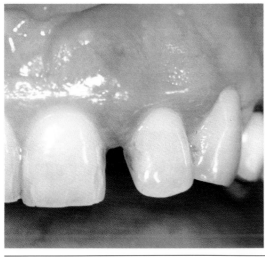
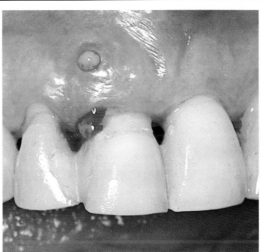

148 Tooth migration (left)
Creation of a diastema between teeth 21 and 22. The osseous septum between these teeth has been destroyed to the root apices. Granulation tissue, tension from intact periodontal fibers and oral parafunctions (e.g., tongue thrust) could have elicited the migration.

149 Periodontal fistula (right)
13 mm pocket on the distal of tooth 11, which is a candidate for extraction. After probing, pus escapes from both the fistulous tract and the gingival margin.

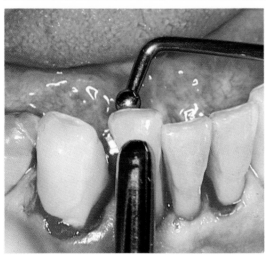
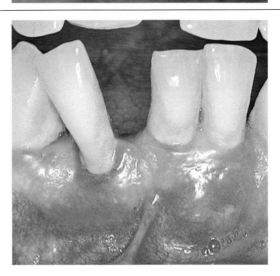
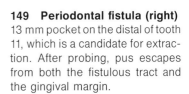

150 Tooth mobility (left)
Increased tooth mobility can be caused by functional disturbances and/or by periodontal attachment loss. Mobility is measured clinically by using 2 instruments or one instrument and the fingertip (see Diagnosis, p. 95).

151 Tooth migration and tipping (right)
Creation of a diastema by severe tipping of tooth 41 after loss of 42. Patient exhibits a heavy tongue thrust when swallowing.

Adult Periodontitis (AP)

This 51-year-old male had received restorative dental care at irregular intervals. The dentist had never performed any periodontal diagnostic procedures nor any therapy. The patient himself complained of occasional gingival bleeding and calculus that disturbed him. The patient was unaware of any periodontal disease and felt he was completely functional in mastication.

Findings: See chart and radiographic survey (p.67).
Diagnosis: Slowly progressing, mild to moderate adult periodontitis (AP).

Treatment planning: Motivation, oral hygiene instruction and follow-up; initial therapy.
After *re-evaluation,* modified Widman procedure and full flap reflection at several sites. No systemic therapy. Possible bridges in mandibular posterior areas.
Recall every 4–6 months.
Prognosis: Even if the patient's cooperation is only average, the prognosis is good. In cases such as this, the dentist or periodontist is always "very successful."

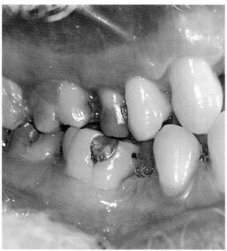
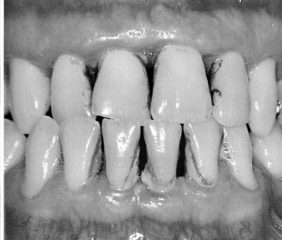
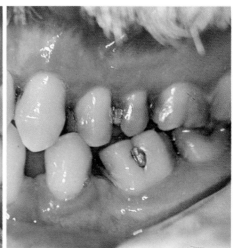

152   Clinical picture (above)
A cursory inspection reveals only mild gingivitis. The interdental papillae have shrunk. The mandibular first molars were extracted 30 years ago, with resultant slow tooth migration, mesial tipping and the formation of diastemata. Recently, the migration seems to have stabilized.

153   Plaque disclosure, oral hygiene (right)
The labial surfaces exhibit almost no plaque accumulation, while the interproximal areas are filled with plaque and calculus.

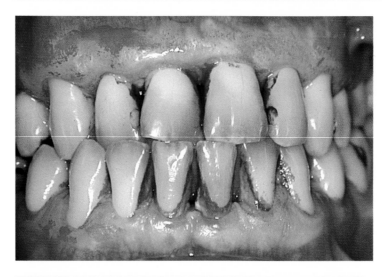

154   Mandible during the flap procedure
The facial crest of bone is bulbous but shows no signs of active destruction. Interdental 3 mm craters were detected. Treatment consisted solely of root planing, minor recontouring of the bulbous bony margin (osteoplasty) and repositioning of the flaps.

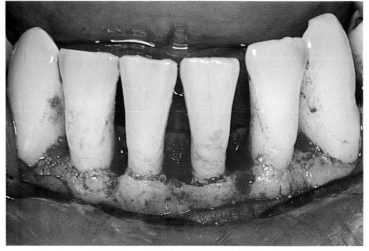

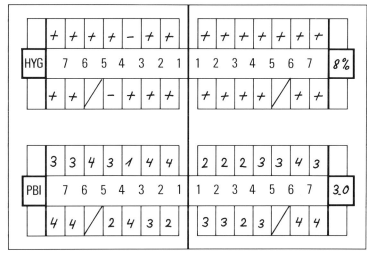

155 Hygiene Index (HYG) and Papilla Bleeding Index (PBI)

The HYG (plaque in interdental areas) and the PBI (severity of bleeding after probing) were scored on *oral* surfaces in quadrants 1 and 3, and on *facial* surfaces in quadrants 2 and 4.

Interdental hygiene is very poor. Copious hemorrhaging (score 3–4) indicates severe gingivitis.

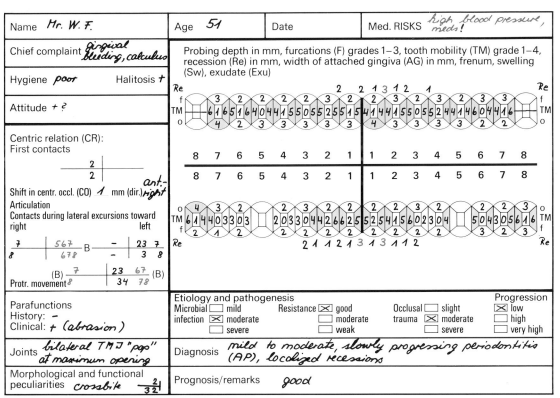

156 Periodontal charting

Probing depths are uniform throughout, especially in the interdental areas. For an assessment of true attachment loss, the mm measurements entered by "Re" (recession) must be considered; these indicate the amount of gingival shrinkage.

Tooth mobility (TM) is low (grade 0–2). Functional analysis reveals premature contact between the upper and lower right lateral incisors (crossbite, increased mobility). Disturbances in lateral excursion as well as in protrusion are also noted. A slight "popping" in the TMJ does not cause the patient any pain or discomfort.

Complete information concerning the periodontal chart and its use is presented on page 97 (Fig. 244).

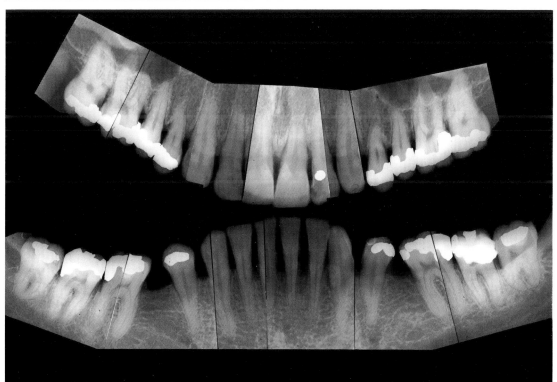

157 Radiographic survey

The radiographs confirm the clinical observations: Localized, mild to moderate horizontal bone loss. Some of the restorative work is inadequate.

(*Author's note:* This is not a "panorama radiograph" in the usual sense of the term. Rather, this survey was prepared by cutting and fitting the individual periapical radiographs into a unified whole. This practice, common in Switzerland and elsewhere, provides a more detailed overview of each individual segment of the dentition than any available panoramic x-ray device.)

Rapidly Progressive Periodontitis (RPP)

This 45-year-old female complained of loose teeth, especially in the maxilla, as well as pain in tooth 37 during mastication. Oral hygiene was good on all facial surfaces and gingival bleeding occurred only seldom.

Findings: See chart and radiographic survey (p. 69).
Diagnosis: Localized, rapidly progressive periodontitis.
Therapy: Immediate extraction of 37; oral hygiene instruction to modify the patient's oral hygiene methods; initial therapy, possibly supported by systemic administration of Metronidazole or Ornidazole (see Medicaments, p. 263).
After re-evaluation: Extraction of any hopeless remaining maxillary teeth with *simultaneous* surgical revision of periodontal structures adjacent to them; temporary partial denture; definitive reconstruction (see Periodontal Surgery, p. 206).
Recall every 3 months.
Prognosis: With optimal oral hygiene, good.

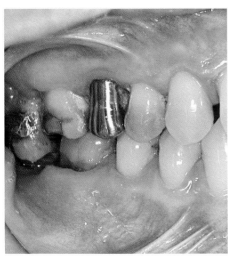 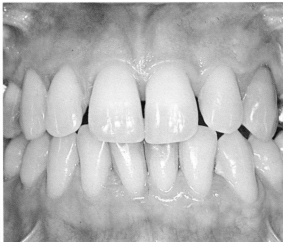 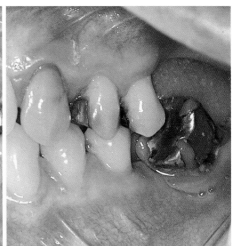

158   Clinical picture (above)
Anterior gingiva appears almost healthy! The severe attachment loss is not obvious.

In the posterior segments one notes missing teeth (upper left, lower right), tipping of 37 and supereruption of 17.

159   Palatal view of maxillary anterior segment (right)
Inflammation of the gingiva; active pockets up to 9 mm depth.

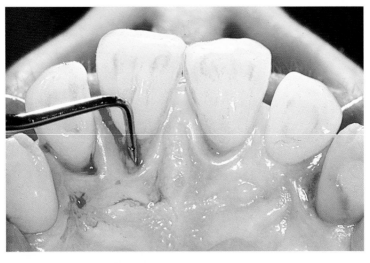

160   Mandibular anterior segment, lingual surface, after disclosing solution
Gingivitis, plaque and calculus, brown-gray discolorations, but no deep pockets.

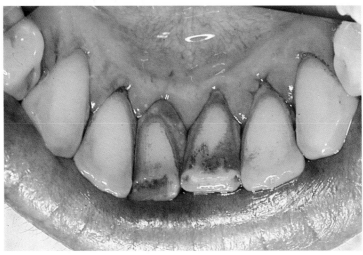

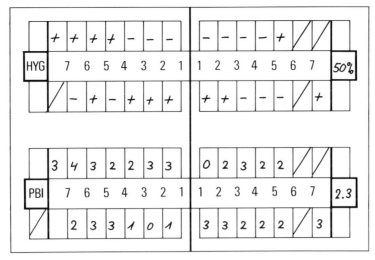

HYG															
+	+	+	+	–	–	–		–	–	–	–	+	/	/	
7	6	5	4	3	2	1		1	2	3	4	5	6	7	50%
/	–	+	–	+	+	+		+	+	–	–	/	+		

PBI															
3	4	3	2	2	3	3		0	2	3	2	2	/	/	
7	6	5	4	3	2	1		1	2	3	4	5	6	7	2.3
/	2	3	3	1	0	1		3	3	2	2	2	/	3	

161 HYG and PBI

The upper anterior region is plaque free, but deposits are present in the interproximal areas of almost all other segments of the dentition.

Despite several areas that do not manifest clinical signs of gingivitis, the PBI is relatively high.

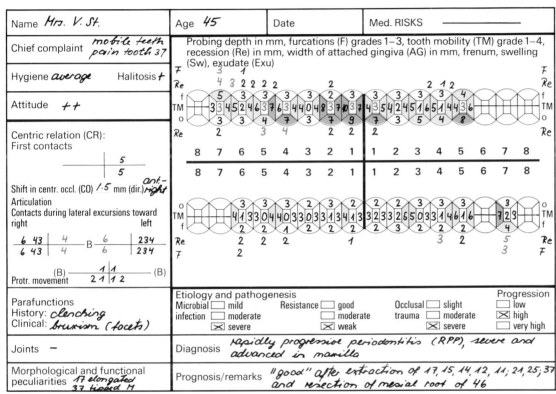

Name *Mrs. V. St.*	Age **45**	Date	Med. RISKS ————
Chief complaint *mobile teeth pain tooth 37*			
Hygiene *average* Halitosis +			
Attitude *+ +*			

Centric relation (CR):
First contacts
$\frac{5}{5}$
Shift in centr. occl. (CO) *1.5* mm (dir.) *ant.- right*
Articulation
Contacts during lateral excursions toward
right   left

6 43	4	B	6	234
6 43	4		6	234

Protr. movement (B) $\frac{1|1}{2\ 1|1\ 2}$ (B)

Parafunctions
History: *clenching*
Clinical: *bruxism (facets)*

Joints —

Morphological and functional peculiarities *17 elongated 37 tipped M*

Probing depth in mm, furcations (F) grades 1–3, tooth mobility (TM) grade 1–4, recession (Re) in mm, width of attached gingiva (AG) in mm, frenum, swelling (Sw), exudate (Exu)

8	7	6	5	4	3	2	1	1	2	3	4	5	6	7	8
8	7	6	5	4	3	2	1	1	2	3	4	5	6	7	8

Etiology and pathogenesis

				Progression
Microbial infection	☐ mild ☐ moderate ☒ severe	Resistance ☐ good ☐ moderate ☒ weak	Occlusal trauma ☐ slight ☐ moderate ☒ severe	☐ low ☒ high ☐ very high

Diagnosis *rapidly progressive periodontitis (RPP), severe and advanced in maxilla*

Prognosis/remarks *"good" after extraction of 17, 15, 14, 12, 11; 21, 25; 37 and resection of mesial root of 46*

162 Periodontal charting

Probing reveals some very deep pockets that one would not have expected upon first clinical inspection. Compare the clinical picture of the maxillary anterior region (Fig. 158, middle) and the periodontal destruction indicated in the chart and on the radiographs.

On several teeth, gingival recession (Re) is noted. All furcations are involved to some degree.

Those teeth exhibiting pronounced attachment loss are also highly mobile.

A functional analysis shows premature contact between the upper and lower left second bicuspids in centric relation, as well as a balancing side interference during lateral excursion (red numbers, left).

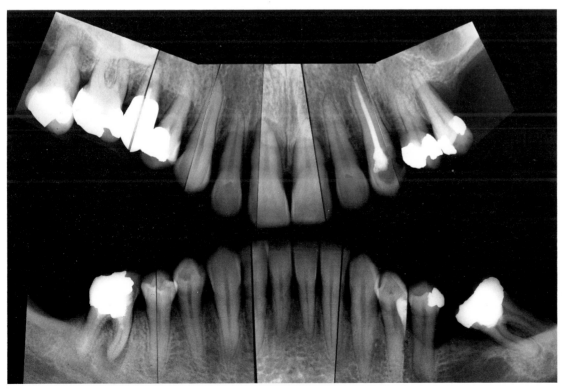

163 Radiographic survey

The radiographs confirm the clinical observations. Severe periodontal destruction is obvious at teeth 17, 15, 14, 12, 11; 21, 25 and 37.

Note the pronounced apical lesion on mesial root of 47.

Rapidly Progressive Periodontitis (RPP) – Acute Phase

This 35-year-old female complained of heavy gingival bleeding and noticeable loosening of her upper front teeth on the right side. She presented seeking information about the possibility of periodontal treatment. The patient had never been instructed in oral hygiene procedures. Until this time, she had seldom been to the dentist.

Findings: See charting and radiographs (p.71).
Diagnosis: Localized, advanced, rapidly progressive periodontitis in an acute phase.

Therapy: Motivation; repeated oral hygiene instruction and re-evaluation; initial local therapy with systemic support (metronidazole, ornidazole). Extraction of 12 and 11, and insertion of a temporary bridge; re-evaluation, then flap procedure; extraction of 17, 27, 47 and 48; definitive bridgework in maxillary anterior and mandibular left segments.
Prognosis: Good only if patient cooperation is excellent and recall interval is short (3 months).

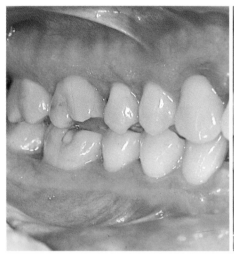
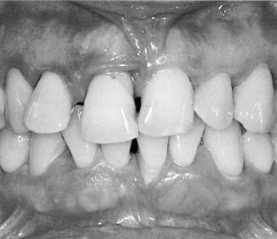
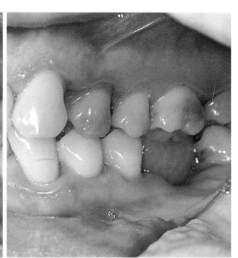

164   Clinical picture (above)
Severe gingival inflammation is obvious. Tooth migration and supereruption in the maxillary right anterior area have occurred within the past 2 years.

Tooth 36 was recently extracted on an emergency basis due to a periodontal abscess.

165 Maxilla, palatal view (right)
Very pronounced gingival inflammation. Spontaneous hemorrhage in the anterior area.

Inadequate composite resin restorations in bicuspids and molar.

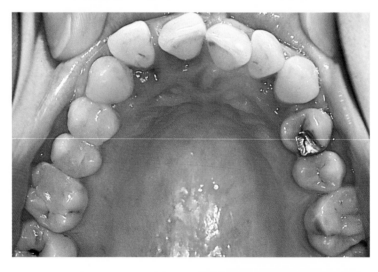

166   Active pocket
Suppuration is noted at the gingival margin of tooth 11 when finger pressure is applied to the labial surface. This is a typical sign of an active pocket in RPP.

A subsequent microscopic assessment of the exudate (p.92) revealed large quantities of motile bacteria including Spirochetes.

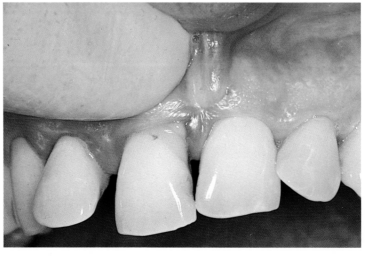

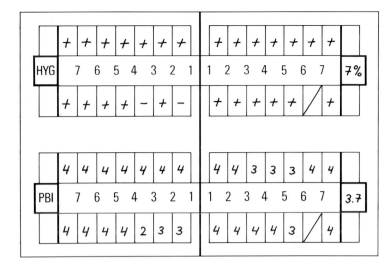

167 HYG and PBI
Almost every interdental space harbors deposits.

The PBI is correspondingly high.

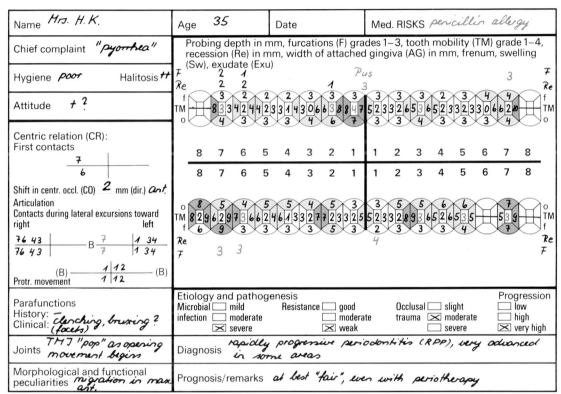

168 Periodontal charting
Probing reveals especially deep pockets at 17, 12, 11, 27, 37, 33, 47 and 48. These teeth are also mobile. Furcations are involved to some degree in most molars. Only slight gingival recession (Re) is noted.

Premature contacts exist in centric relation between 17 and 46, and a balancing side interference between 17 and 47 (see functional analysis, left).

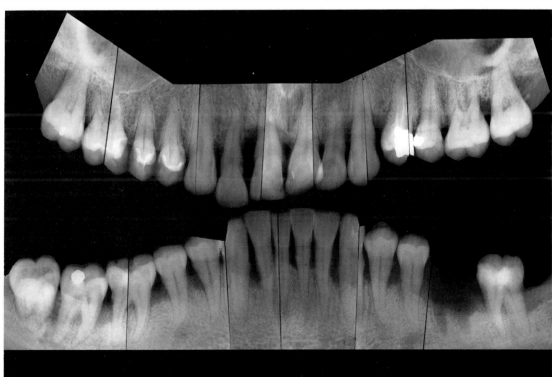

169 Radiographic survey
The radiographs generally confirm the clinical observations. Note the irregular distribution of bone loss, including vertical defects (infrabony pockets) and open furcations.

Some of the restorations are inadequate, exhibiting overhangs. Use of composite materials in posterior teeth is contraindicated.

Juvenile Periodontitis (LJP) – Initial Stage

This 14-year-old female was referred to the periodontist because of severe gingivitis. She practiced virtually no oral hygiene. Her chief complaint was the malpositioned upper left cuspid, which was destined for orthodontic treatment at a later time (see p. 290).

Findings: See charting and radiographs (p. 73).
Diagnosis: Juvenile periodontitis (incisor/molar type) in an early stage, with initial attachment loss mesial of

mandibular first molar and on several anterior teeth. Superimposed severe hyperplastic gingivitis.
Therapy: "Introduction" to oral hygiene procedures; repeated oral hygiene instruction. Initial therapy without use of systemic drugs; subsequent re-evaluation for possible gingivectomy / gingivoplasty; orthodontic treatment; *initial short-interval recall* (2–3 months).
Prognosis: Good after overcoming the patient's neglect of hygiene.

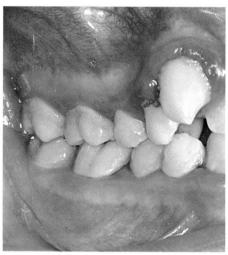 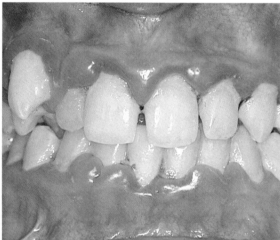 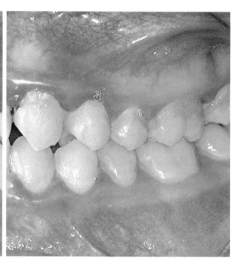

170   Clinical picture (above)
Very heavy plaque accumulation and severe gingivitis. Pronounced gingival hyperplasia in maxillary and mandibular anterior segments. Crowding, cuspid malposition.

171   Plaque disclosure (right)
Heavy plaque accumulation, especially in interdental areas and at the gingival margin.

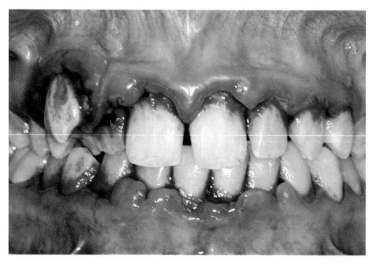

172   Special observations: LJP
A 5 mm pocket can be probed mesial of 46, indicating early loss of attachment.

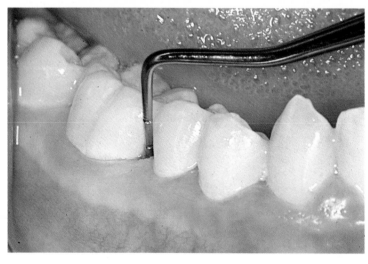

173 HYG and PBI
The patient does not practice any oral hygiene. The HYG score is 0%. The PBI achieves almost the maximum average score of 4.

	+	+	+	+	+	+	+		+	+	+	+	+	+	+	
HYG	7	6	5	4	3	2	1		1	2	3	4	5	6	7	0%
	+	+	+	+	+	+	+		+	+	+	+	+	+	+	

	4	4	4	3	4	4	4		4	4	4	4	4	4	4	
PBI	7	6	5	4	3	2	1		1	2	3	4	5	6	7	3.9
	4	4	4	3	4	4	4		4	4	4	4	3	4	4	

174 Periodontal charting
The probing depths recorded in the anterior area can be partially explained by the pronounced inflammatory gingival hyperplasia in this area (pseudopockets). Nevertheless, beginning attachment loss has occurred. On the lower first molars, attachment loss of 5–6 mm is recorded. This destruction is more severe than that in the anterior region.

Functional dysharmonies are evident, with premature contacts in centric relation, and a pronounced shift of 3 mm after initial contact. Balancing side interferences exist (left, red entries).

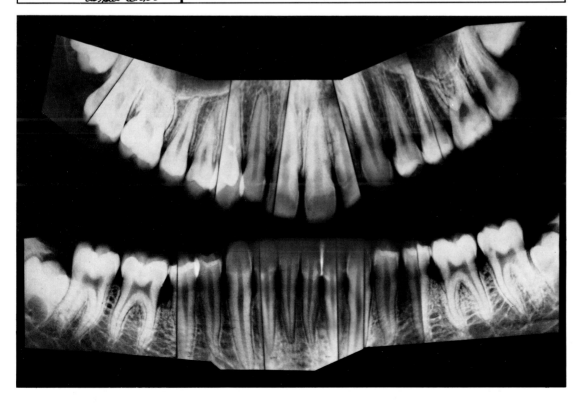

| Name | Miss S.S. | Age | 14 | Date | | Med. RISKS | ———— |

Chief complaint *none!* (referral)

Hygiene *very poor* Halitosis +

Attitude — ?

Centric relation (CR):
First contacts
$\frac{5}{5}$

Shift in centr. occl. (CO) 3 mm (dir.) *ant.-left*
Articulation
Contacts during lateral excursions toward
right   left

$\frac{654\ 2}{65432}$ | $\frac{67}{67}$ B $\frac{7}{7}$ | $\frac{23456}{23456}$

(B) $\frac{2\ 1|1}{3\ 2\ 1|1}$ (B)
Protr. movement

Parafunctions
History: *bruxism*
Clinical: *bruxing (abrasion)*

Joints —

Morphological and functional peculiarities *max. right cuspid ectopic*

Probing depth in mm, furcations (F) grades 1–3, tooth mobility (TM) grade 1–4, recession (Re) in mm, width of attached gingiva (AG) in mm, frenum, swelling (Sw), exudate (Exu)

Etiology and pathogenesis

				Progression
Microbial infection	☐ mild ☐ moderate ☒ severe	Resistance	☐ good ☐ moderate ☒ weak	Occlusal trauma ☐ slight ☒ moderate ☐ severe	☐ low ☒ high ☐ very high

Diagnosis *juvenile periodontitis (LJP), initial stage, severe gingivitis*

Prognosis/remarks *good*

175 Radiographic survey
A cursory inspection of the radiographs reveals no dramatic evidence of bone resorption. But a careful tooth-by-tooth examination of the films shows beginning periodontal destruction at those sites typical of juvenile periodontitis: Mesial of teeth 46 and 36.

Juvenile Periodontitis (LJP) – Advanced Stage

A 21-year-old Black female student was referred to an oral surgeon for surgical extraction of an impacted third molar (38). The diagnosis of LJP was a serendipitous finding after radiographs were prepared. The patient had relatively good oral hygiene and little evidence of gingivitis.

Findings: See charting and radiographs (p.75).
Diagnosis: Juvenile periodontitis with deep pockets on *typical* teeth (maxillary incisors and first molars).

Therapy: Oral hygiene instruction; initial therapy including systemic administration of *tetracycline;* flap procedure including thorough root planing with direct vision; second *tetracycline regimen;* extraction of 28 and 38; *recall* every 3 months.
Prognosis: For the severely affected maxillary incisors, questionable. For all of the first year molars, poor (due also to furcation involvements). All remaining teeth have a good prognosis for retention.

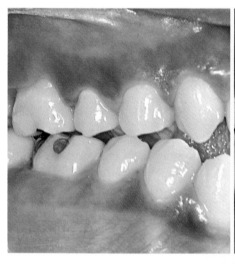 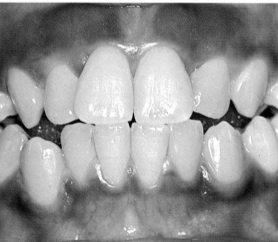 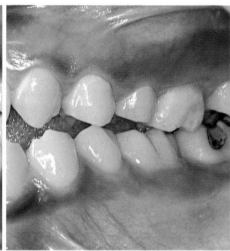

176   Clinical picture (above)
Pigmented gingiva. Very mild gingivitis in anterior area and posterior segments.
 The type and severity of the disease process cannot be ascertained by a "quick look."
 An open bite is obvious in cuspid and bicuspid areas.

177   Maxillary anterior area during flap procedure (right)
9 mm of attachment loss can be seen in those areas typical for LJP, teeth 21 and 22.

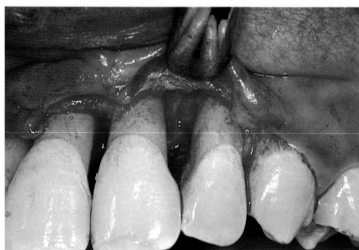

178   Maxillary molars 26 and 27 during flap surgery and on radiograph
The buccal roots of the first molar have practically no bone support. Note the crater defects and open trifurcation (class F 3).

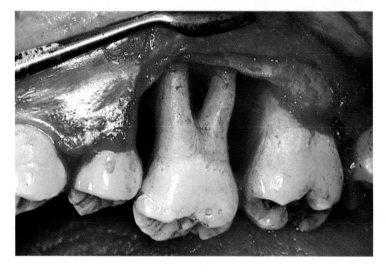 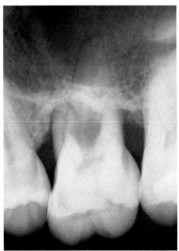

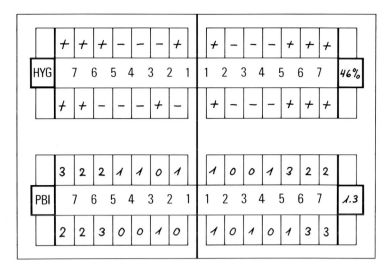

HYG

	7	6	5	4	3	2	1	1	2	3	4	5	6	7	
	+	+	+	–	–	–	+	+	–	–	–	+	+	+	
	+	+	–	–	–	+	–	+	–	–	–	+	+	+	46%

PBI

	7	6	5	4	3	2	1	1	2	3	4	5	6	7	
	3	2	2	1	1	0	1	1	0	0	1	3	2	2	
	2	2	3	0	0	1	0	1	0	1	0	1	3	3	1.3

179 HYG and PBI
In the anterior area and in cuspid and bicuspid regions, oral hygiene is quite good and the PBI is low.

In the molar segments, interdental plaque accumulation is evident, with a correspondingly higher PBI.

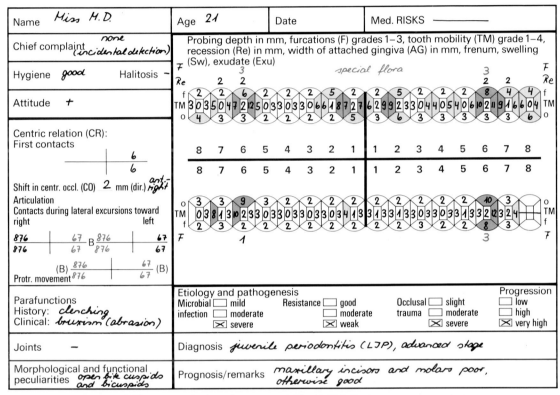

Name	Miss M.D.	Age	21	Date		Med. RISKS	———

Chief complaint *none (incidental detection)*

Hygiene *good*   Halitosis –

Attitude +

Centric relation (CR):
First contacts   6 / 6

Shift in centr. occl. (CO) 2 mm (dir.) *ant. right*

Articulation
Contacts during lateral excursions toward
right   left

| 876 | 67 | B | 876 | 67 |
| 876 | 67 | | 876 | 67 |

(B) 876 / 876   67 / 67 (B)
Protr. movement

Parafunctions
History: *clenching*
Clinical: *bruxism (abrasion)*

Joints –

Morphological and functional peculiarities *open bite cuspids and bicuspids*

Probing depth in mm, furcations (F) grades 1–3, tooth mobility (TM) grade 1–4, recession (Re) in mm, width of attached gingiva (AG) in mm, frenum, swelling (Sw), exudate (Exu)

special flora

8	7	6	5	4	3	2	1	1	2	3	4	5	6	7	8
8	7	6	5	4	3	2	1	1	2	3	4	5	6	7	8

Etiology and pathogenesis

				Progression
Microbial ☐ mild	Resistance ☐ good	Occlusal ☐ slight		☐ low
infection ☐ moderate	☐ moderate	trauma ☐ moderate		☐ high
☒ severe	☒ weak	☒ severe		☒ very high

Diagnosis *juvenile periodontitis (LJP), advanced stage*

Prognosis/remarks *maxillary incisors and molars poor, otherwise good*

180 Periodontal charting
Periodontal probing reveals the deep pockets in the maxillary anterior area and on the first permanent molars (LJP, incisor/molar type). The furcations are through-and-through on all first molars (class F3).

Poor functional relationships, with balancing contacts during lateral excursion and protrusive movement of the mandible are evident (red in functional analysis, left).

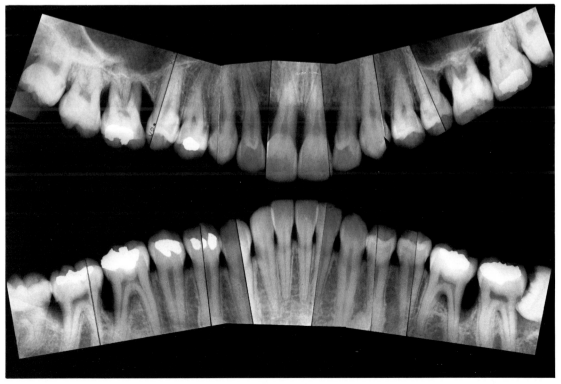

181 Radiographic survey
The radiographs corroborate the clinical observations and the diagnosis: Juvenile periodontitis with typical involvement of first permanent molars and maxillary anterior teeth. Note crater formation and vertical defects.

Periodontitis Ulcerosa – Symptoms

The epidemiology, etiology, histopathology, microbiology and clinical picture of ANUG, as well as the stress level and attitude of patients manifesting this disease were described on page 41. If ANUG recurs repeatedly, it may develop into a Periodontitis ulcerosa with rapid destruction of interdental bony septa. Because the gingival tissue is being destroyed by ulceration with simultaneous resorption of the osseous structure, it is not uncommon to find only shallow periodontal pockets upon clinical probing, despite dramatic loss of attachment. The interdental spaces are wide open and cratered due to loss of the papilla to necrosis, and thus represent plaque-retentive areas. Bone loss may vary in different segments of the dentition, and may progress with varying rapidity. Without treatment, Periodontitis ulcerosa eventually leads to tooth loss.

182   Localized Periodontitis ulcerosa, dormant stage
There is loss of attachment and gingival destruction between 22 and 23. The measured pocket is only 3 mm deep. The true attachment loss is 10 mm, measured from the CEJ (compare radiograph).

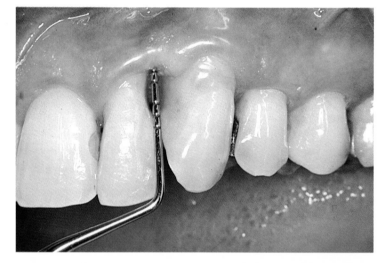 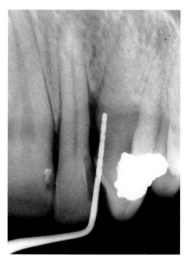

183   Localized Periodontitis ulcerosa, acute stage
Advanced destruction in the mandibular anterior area, beyond the mucogingival line and into the mobile oral mucosa. Note attachment of labial frenum.

The gingiva is bulbous and thickened. Plaque and calculus are present. Tooth 31 is highly mobile.

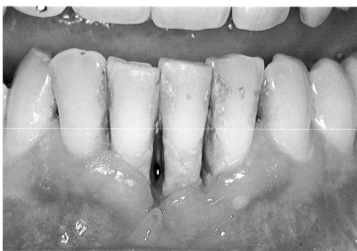

184   Detritus and ulcerated tissue around the erupting third molar (48)
The soft tissue pocket around the erupting tooth is a plaque-retentive area. The bacterial infection (Spirochetes, fusiforms) is accompanied by destruction of the soft tissues.

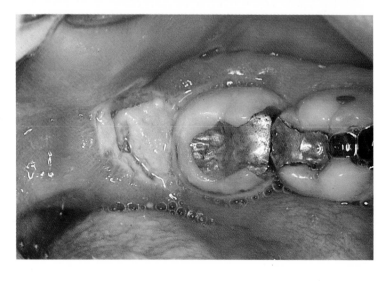

Periodontitis Ulcerosa – Acute Phase

A 30-year-old man complained that his gums were painful and receding. He stated that similar symptoms had occurred many times over the past several years. He had treated these former exacerbations himself with various "medicines" applied topically, but no definitive professional care had ever been rendered.

Findings:

HYG 10%   PBI 3.4

See periodontal chart below for probing depths, tooth mobility and gingival recession values.

Diagnosis: Generalized acute Periodontitis ulcerosa.

Therapy for acute phase: Topical chemotherapy including chlorhexidine rinses, cortisone ointment with antibiotics; gross debridement (Cavitron); oral hygiene instruction and motivation with frequent follow-up.

Subsequent therapy: Subgingival scaling, flap surgery, extraction of 48.

Prognosis: Fair (see Gingivitis ulcerosa – ANUG, p. 41). Too often, the patient's cooperation declines as the pain subsides.

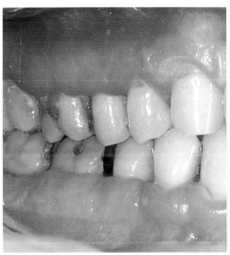 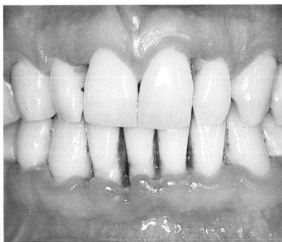 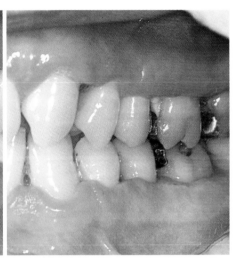

185 Clinical picture (above)
This is a typical presentation of generalized Periodontitis ulcerosa. As the interdental papilla deteriorate, an inversion of the gingival marginal architecture occurs.

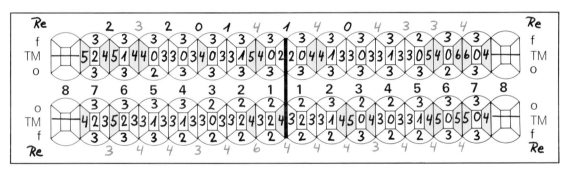

186 Probing depths, gingival recession and tooth mobility (left)
Probing depths (PD) are not great, but considerable attachment loss (AL) has occurred: AL = PD + Re (recession).

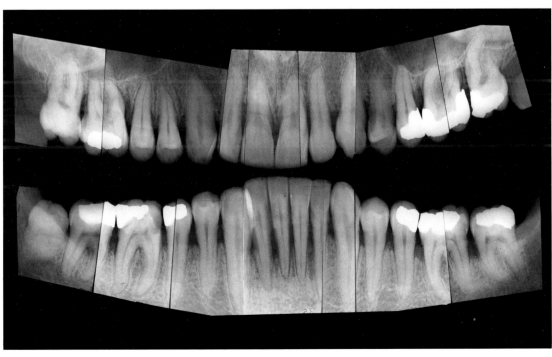

187 Radiographic survey
A generalized loss of attachment is observed. In some cases of Periodontitis ulcerosa, attachment loss is localized.

Unsatisfactory restorations create plaque-retentive areas that enhance the bacterial infection.

The pseudopocket around tooth 48 (see also clinical view, Fig. 184) is likewise a harbor for plaque accumulation.

Prepubertal Periodontitis with Systemic Disease
Papillon-Lefèvre Syndrome

Several systemic disorders (see also p. 34) can either accentuate, promote or be partially responsible for the initiation of gingivitis and/or periodontitis. An example presented here is the Papillon-Lefèvre syndrome, a rare disease that occurs in two persons per million in the population. The disorder appears to have a genetic basis. The obligate symptoms include severe periodontitis and hyperkeratoses, usually localized to palms, soles of the feet and other skin areas that commonly absorb minor trauma (elbows, knees). These patients routinely lose deciduous teeth prematurely. Permanent teeth exhibit periodontitis soon after eruption and are most often lost prematurely (Haneke 1979).

Case: A 9-year-old boy was referred by a pediatrician to the periodontist because of extreme halitosis and loose teeth. The boy's masticatory function was already impaired. No oral hygiene had been practiced, for fear that the loose teeth would be dislodged (Rateitschak-Plüss & Schroeder 1984).

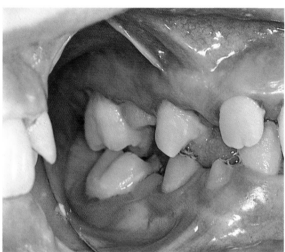
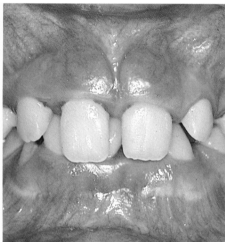
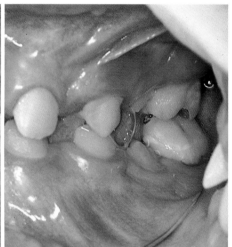

188 Clinical picture (above)
Severe gingivitis and periodontitis, plaque, spontaneous hemorrhage, exudate and suppuration. Abscess on the facial of 11 and 21. Poor occlusion, severe overbite.

189 Probing depths and tooth mobility (right)
All of the deep pockets exhibit advanced signs of activity (pus).

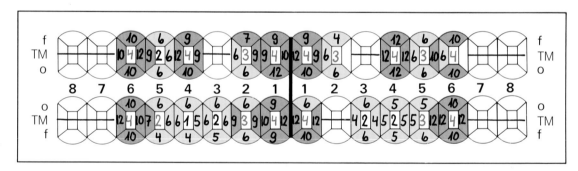

190 Radiographic survey
The indicated (✳) teeth 16, 14, 11; 21, 24, 26 and 36, 31; 41, 46 are in the process of being exfoliated.

Teeth 17, 13, 23, 27, 37 and 47 are erupting. The loss of alveolar bone has proceeded at an extremely rapid pace. Vertical defects (infrabony pockets) are most common. Class F3 furcation involvements are noted on most molars.

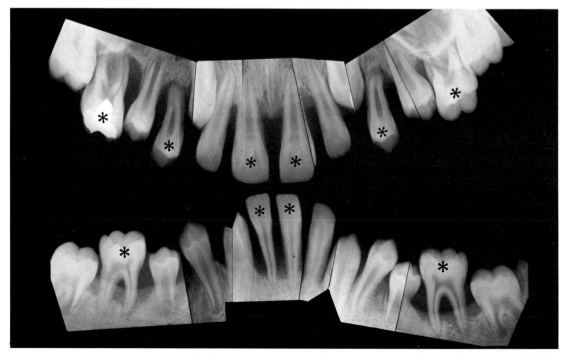

Findings:
HYG 0%   PBI 3.9
Pockets, radiographs, TM and skin lesions: See Figures 188, 191–193.

Other observations: PMN defect (decreased host response); specific pocket flora (Spirochetes). The appropriate medical specialist (dermatologist, internist) should be consulted.

Diagnosis: Acute, severe prepubertal periodontitis related to Papillon-Lefèvre syndrome.

Therapy: Very intensive professional treatment including plaque and calculus removal with simultaneous topical application of chlorhexidine and administration of systemic medication (metronidazole/tetracycline). A very short recall interval should be maintained. Removable partial denture to facilitate oral hygiene. Teeth that can be "saved" through puberty can sometimes be maintained (see next case).

Prognosis: Almost hopeless.

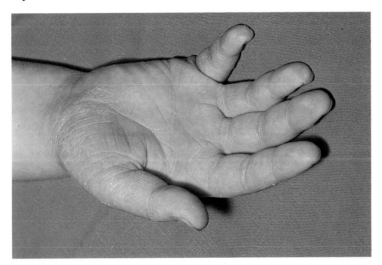

Papillon-Lefèvre syndrome

191 Hyperkeratosis on palm of hand
The hyperkeratotic area exhibits cracks and fissures, which are actually wounds that have occurred during normal function. These heal slowly and poorly. The patient suffers most from these palmar lesions in winter.

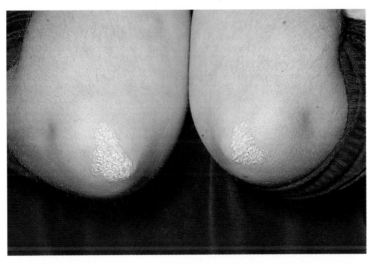

192 Hyperkeratosis on elbows

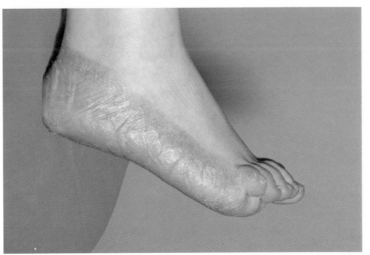

193 Hyperkeratosis on sole and lateral border of foot
The sharp line of demarcation between hyperkeratotic area and normal-appearing skin corresponds to the outline of the shoe worn by this patient.

Minor trauma to the skin elicits this type of severe hyperkeratotic response. Dermatologists, too, can only treat this disease symptomatically.

Papillon-Lefèvre Syndrome – "An exception for every rule"

A 7-year-old girl was referred to the dental clinic because of severe mobility of her recently erupted permanent incisors and first molars. The patient remained under dental care for 24 years thereafter.

Diagnosis: Acute, severe periodontitis associated with Papillon-Lefèvre syndrome.

Course of the disease: In this one exceptional case, it was possible to maintain 15 permanent teeth through puberty until the present. With intensive periodontal therapy, regular and frequent recall, teeth 18, 17, 15,

13; 23, 25, 28 and 38, 37, 35, 34; 44, 45, 47 and 48 were saved.

The patient is now wearing maxillary and mandibular fixed total reconstructions that are cemented temporarily. They are removed at recall appointments, cleaned, and recemented. The abutment teeth are cleaned professionally and checked at each recall. At age 18, a surgical procedure was performed to correct prognathism, and the chin was also remodeled (note osteosynthesis wires in radiographic survey, Fig. 196).

194   Radiographic survey (7-year-old female)
The first permanent molars are supererupted only one year after their appearance into the oral cavity. The mandibular anterior teeth exhibit severe periodontitis.

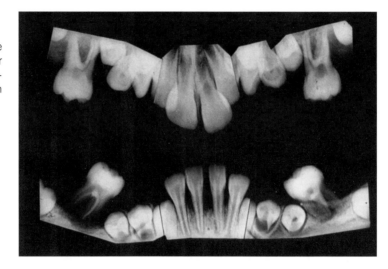

195   Same patient, age 31
The patient smiles with her own teeth, which were deemed "hopeless" due to her Papillon-Lefèvre syndrome when she was first examined 24 years previously. She displays advanced hyperkeratosis on both palms, and painful cracks through the hyperkeratotic area on her heel.

The skin on the backs of her hands is paper thin, hyperkeratotic, dry and visibly erythematous.

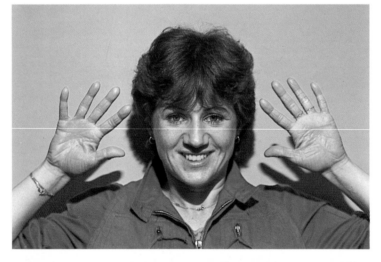
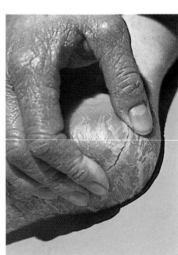

196   Radiographic survey (31-year-old female)
Destructive periodontitis came to a halt after the patient had traversed puberty. The remaining teeth in both arches were prepared as abutments to support fixed total reconstructions of porcelain-fused-to-metal. Both appliances are cemented temporarily with Temp-Bond.

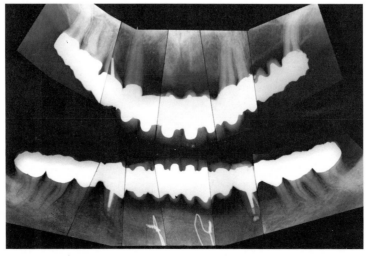

Recession

Gingival recession accounts for 5–10% of all attachment loss. Recession is defined as a seemingly inflammation-free clinical condition characterized by the retreat in an apical direction of the facial and less often of the oral (palatal, lingual) periodontium. Despite recession of the gingival margin, the interdental papillae usually fill the entire embrasure areas in younger patients. Recession is usually localized to one or several teeth; generalized gingival recession is seldom observed. Teeth exhibiting gingival recession do not display increased mobility. The periodontal supporting structures are generally of excellent quality.

Teeth are never lost due to gingival recession alone!

If the patient's oral hygiene is inadequate, or if the recession reaches the movable oral mucosa, secondary inflammation may ensue and eventually pocket formation (periodontitis) may occur.

Etiology: The causes of recession have not been completely elucidated. It is probable, however, that a primary factor is purely the morphology and anatomy of the situation. The facial plate of bone overlying the root is usually very thin. Not infrequently the root surface is completely denuded of alveolar bone or exhibits *fenestrations* in the thin osseous lamella. The total lack of bone over the facial root surface is referred to as a *dehiscence.* This situation is most frequently observed on cuspids and incisors, less often on premolars and seldom on molar teeth (except mesiobuccal root of 1st maxillary molars!). The situation is also frequently associated with tooth positional anomalies such as buccoversion, supereruption etc. Despite the lack of a buccal plate of bone over the root, the gingival margin may maintain its normal position just coronal to the CEJ. Some possible etiologic factors in gingival recession include:

- Improper, traumatic toothbrushing, e.g., horizontal scrubbing
- Mild chronic inflammation that may be only slightly visible clinically
- Frenum pulls, especially when fibers of the frenum attach near the gingival margin
- Orthodontic treatment (tooth movement labially; arch expansion).

Bernimoulin and Curilović (1977) were unable to demonstrate that functional disturbances (bruxism) can elicit gingival recession. As is the case in inflammatory diseases, recession appears to follow a nonlinear course as it becomes more severe; the pattern of development is step-wise.

Clinical picture and radiographic survey: In the following pages, recession is depicted schematically, on skull preparations and in clinical situations.

Pure recessions localized to the facial surfaces of teeth *cannot be diagnosed radiographically.*

Therapy: With good oral hygiene, recession can be brought to a halt without any further treatment. The vertical-rotatory brushing technique (modified Stillman) should be recommended.

Surgical treatment for severe recession is described in detail on page 228.

Fenestration and Dehiscence of the Alveolar Bone

In a healthy periodontium the facial margin of the alveolar bone lies approximately 1–2 mm apical to the gingival margin, which courses near to the cemento-enamel junction. The facial aspect of the alveolar bone covering the root is usually very thin. As revealed by a flap operation or on a skull preparation, the coronal portion of the root often is not covered by bone *(dehiscence)* or there is *fenestration* of facial osseous lamella. Towards the apex, the facial plate of bone becomes

thicker, and spongy bone fills the interval between facial and lingual cortical plates. In these thicker areas, recession generally stops spontaneously.

In older individuals, recession of facial periodontal tissues may appear in combination with horizontal bone loss in the interdental area. In such cases, the interdental papillae usually also recede. Nevertheless, no true periodontal pockets develop.

197 Normal periodontium and various manifestations of recession as viewed in orofacial section
The junctional epithelium is depicted in *pink* (no pockets), the mucogingival line is indicated (◄).

A. Normal gingiva and bone.
B. Parallel recession of bone *and* gingiva; *fenestration.*
C. *Bony dehiscence* more pronounced than the gingival recession.
D. Recession with formation of *McCall's festoons* (compare Fig. 205).

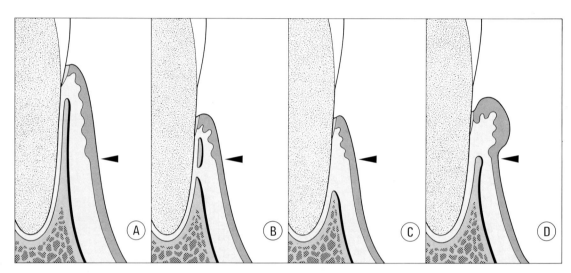

Skull observations

198 Fenestration (left)
Adjacent to the fenestration on the facial aspect of tooth 13 (circled), dehiscences and primarily horizontal bone loss in interdental area are visible.

199 Dehiscence (right)
A pronounced dehiscence that extends almost to the apex is observed on the facial of 13. The other teeth exhibit dehiscences of lesser severity. Generalized interdental bone loss is also observed.

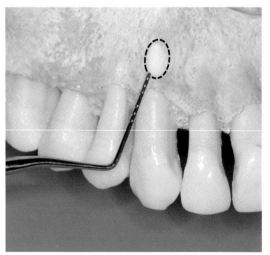
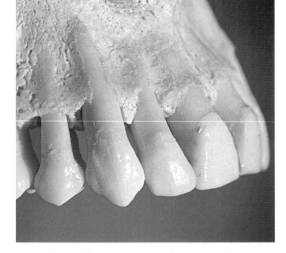

Clinical views

200 Multiple fenestration (left)
In the course of an Edlan operation, large fenestrations became visible after reflection of the periosteum on teeth 16, 15, 13 and 12.

201 Dehiscence on 13 (right)
During the first phase of an extension operation involving free gingival grafting, an unexpected osseous dehiscence was observed. This was not detectable with the periodontal probe before surgery. The dehiscence is more severe than the gingival recession.

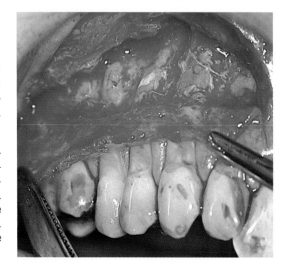
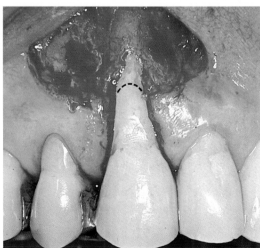

Clinical Symptoms

The clinical manifestations of recession are numerous. Gingival recession usually begins with a gradual apical migration of the entire *facial aspect* of the gingiva, revealing the CEJ. Less frequently the first sign of recession is the relatively rapid formation of a small groove in the gingiva, a so-called *Stillman's cleft*. This can expand into a pronounced recession. As a consequence of recession, the remaining attached gingiva may become somewhat thickened and rolled, a noninflammatory fibrotic response known as *McCall's festoons*.

If the recession proceeds as far as the mucogingival line, secondary inflammation of the marginal gingiva may ensue. Though rare, recession may also be observed on the palatal roots of maxillary molars and on the lingual aspect of mandibular incisors.

Esthetic considerations may prompt the patient to seek professional care if recession becomes pronounced in the maxillary anterior segment. As root surfaces are exposed, cervical sensitivity may also become a problem.

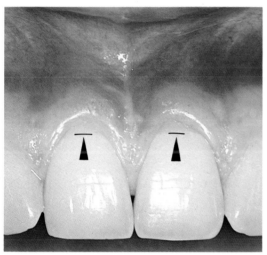

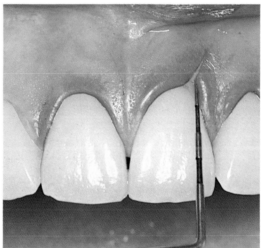

202   Initial recession (left)
The cementoenamel junction is marked in this view, to demonstrate early gingival recession.

203   Stillman's cleft (right)
The periodontal probe reveals the presence of a cleft, which may expand laterally and develop into general recession. The exposed root surface is often very sensitive, and is usually covered with plaque, which leads to secondary inflammation.

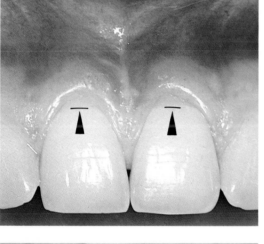

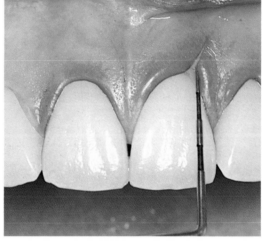

204   Palatal recession (left)
Due probably to tooth morphology and osseous anatomy, recession on the palatal or lingual surfaces is considerably less frequent than on facial surfaces.

205   McCall's festoons (right)
The attached gingiva in this case consists of nothing more than a collar-like, fibrous thickening. The arrow indicates the CEJ. This *may* be a tissue response to further recession beyond the mucogingival line. It is *not* an indication for mucogingival surgery!

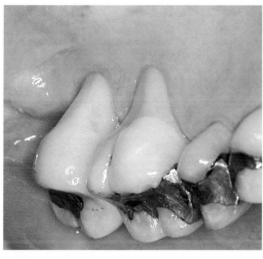

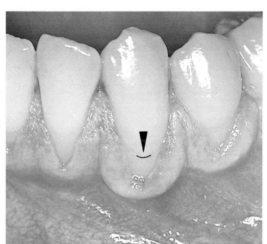

206   Dehiscence of alveolar process (left)
Orofacial section through an anterior tooth, as viewed in a radiograph. Remarkably little bone surrounds the tooth, both facially and lingually.

207   Deep localized recession (right)
The root of this tooth has been denuded all the way to the mucogingival line. The gingival margin is secondarily inflamed.
   Following initial therapy, a mucogingival surgical intervention *is* indicated in this case (see p. 228).

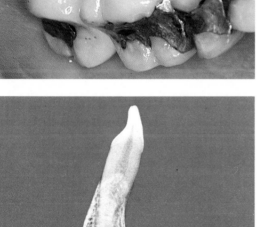

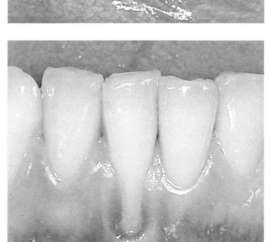

Recession – Localized

A 26-year-old male presented to the clinic with a chief complaint of recession on his maxillary cuspids. His oral hygiene was impeccable; he claimed to brush his teeth four times a day. Neither a dentist nor a dental hygienist had ever observed his toothbrushing technique.

Findings:

HYG 91%   PBI 0.8

Figure 209 depicts probing depths and tooth mobility.

Diagnosis: Pronounced facial recession on cuspids. Initial generalized gingival recession.

Therapy: Instruction in the vertical-rotatory toothbrushing method (modified Stillman) using a soft toothbrush; repeated evaluation for gingival trauma; study models to document progression of gingival recession, should it continue. Mucogingival surgery should be considered only if the recession continues unabated.

Recall interval: 6 months or less frequent.

Prognosis: Good.

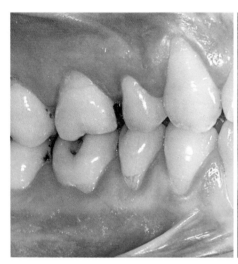
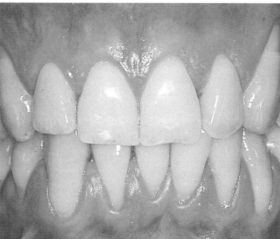
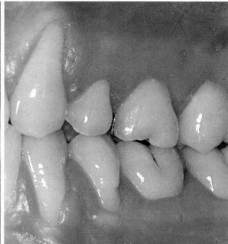

208 Clinical picture (above)
The recessions are of varying severity, with pronounced areas over the cuspids. The papillae still fill the interdental spaces. In the molar segments, mild marginal inflammation is noted. Tooth 35 exhibits a wedge-shaped defect.

209 Probing depths, recession, tooth mobility (TM)
The classical recession is associated with neither pathologically deepened pockets nor elevated tooth mobility. Attachment loss is restricted mainly to the facial surfaces.

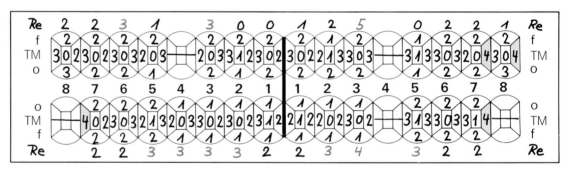

210 Radiographic survey
The facial osseous dehiscences are *not visible* on the radiograph. In young patients, no loss of interdental septal height is noted. Recession cannot be diagnosed using radiographs alone.

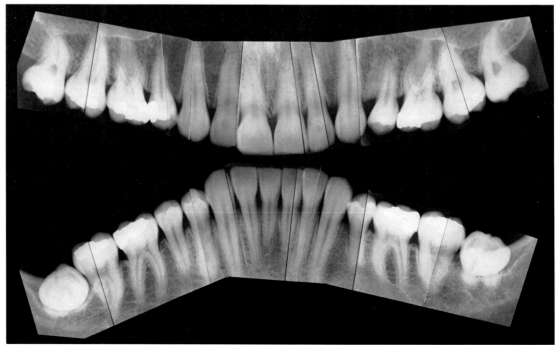

Recession – Generalized

This 43-year-old female was worried that her teeth kept getting longer, and she complained that her teeth were "sensitive at the gumline." She expressed the desire to have her "gum condition" treated if possible.

Findings:
HYG 80%   PBI 1.0
Probing depths, recession, TM: see Fig. 212

Diagnosis: Generalized, advanced facial recession. Mild loss of periodontal supporting structure in interdental areas, shallow pocket formation but no hemorrhage.

Therapy: Change home care technique to vertical-rotatory brushing, modified Stillman; fabricate study models; check-ups at regular interval of 3–6 months. If documented recession continues, then mucogingival surgery with free gingival graft in mandible (see p. 233).

Prognosis: Good, if secondary inflammation is avoided.

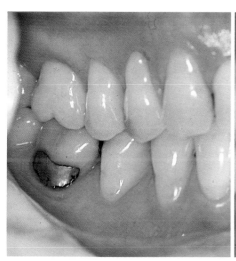 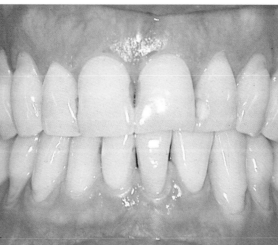 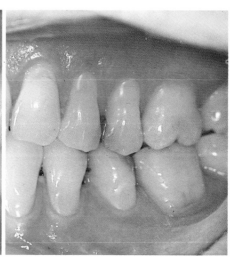

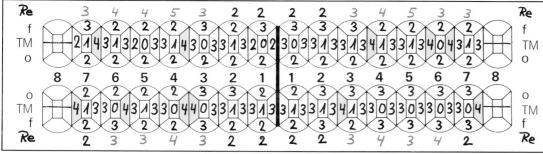

211 Clinical picture (above)
Generalized gingival recession is apparent in this middle-aged female. The interdental papillae have also receded slightly.

212 Probing depths, facial recession, tooth mobility (TM)
In the maxillary bicuspid area, the facial attached gingiva is almost completely absent due to the gingival recession. In this area, attachment loss continued slowly despite changing the patient's brushing technique.

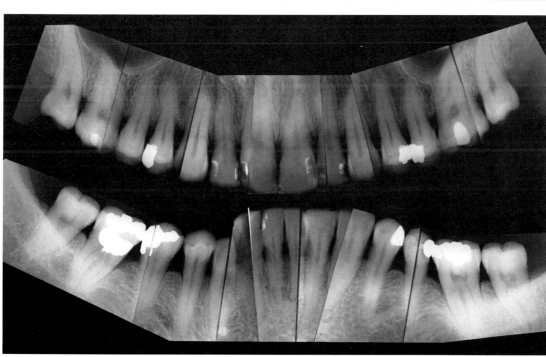

213 Radiographic survey
Mild generalized reduction of interdental septal height is noted. The more advanced bone loss on the facial surfaces is not visible radiographically.

"Destruction and Shrinkage" – Clinical Situations Resembling Recession

In addition to the classical recession, there are other forms of clinically observable attachment loss:

- *Recession of the entire periodontium in old persons.* This condition is *not* the rule. It may be caused by a mild chronic inflammation and shrinkage; it can be enhanced by improper toothbrushing technique or other iatrogenic irritation.
- *Recession with a superimposed secondary periodontitis.* This combination occurs seldom, because patients who practice proper oral hygiene usually exhibit neither plaque accumulation nor inflammation.

- *Destruction or shrinkage of the gingiva as a consequence of untreated periodontitis* (see also Symptoms of Periodontitis, pp. 64–65).
- *Status following periodontal therapy.* "Long teeth," open interdental spaces and cervical sensitivity are often the uncomfortable consequences of treatment for advanced periodontal disease.

214 Shrinkage in an elderly man
This 81-year-old man exhibited *no* periodontal pockets. The dentist had performed only restorative treatment.

The patient took care of the periodontal "treatment" by himself through vigorous brushing and a coarse diet (note wedge-shaped defects and abrasion).

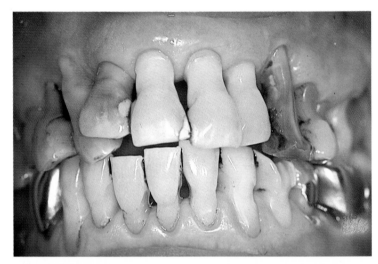

215 "Recession" (shrinkage) in a case of untreated periodontitis
This 32-year-old female with rapidly progressive periodontitis has 5–6 mm pockets in the interdental areas. In addition she exhibits 4–5 mm of gingival recession; thus, the true measure of *attachment loss* is 9–11 mm.

This uncommon degree of gingival recession appears to have been enhanced by improper toothbrushing technique (note wedge-shaped defects at cervical areas).

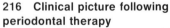
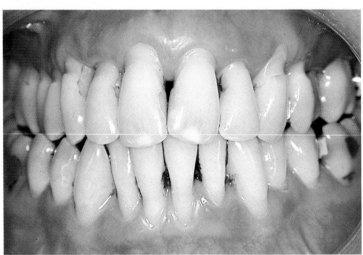

216 Clinical picture following periodontal therapy
In this 36-year-old female with advanced, rapidly progressive periodontitis (9 mm pockets), the esthetic consequences of radical surgical intervention for treatment of the disease process are severe. The appearance is similar to advanced gingival recession.

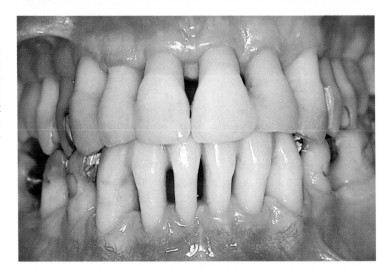

Charting – Diagnosis – Prognosis

Recognition, diagnosis and differential diagnosis of a periodontal disorder are only possible by means of an accurate history and a systematic oral examination. However, such information pertains only to the clinical situation at the time of the examination. The course of the disease and its progression up to that time remain a matter of speculation.

How the disease might progress in the future, i.e., the prognosis arrived at after thorough examination, is always tentative. During the initial phase of therapy, the reaction of the periodontal tissues to the therapist's efforts, and the intensity of the patient's cooperation in home care are unknowns. During active therapy and maintenance phase, the periodontal tissues must be examined regularly for any changes in the status of home care or rate of disease progression. Any such re-examination may lead to a modification of the original prognosis.

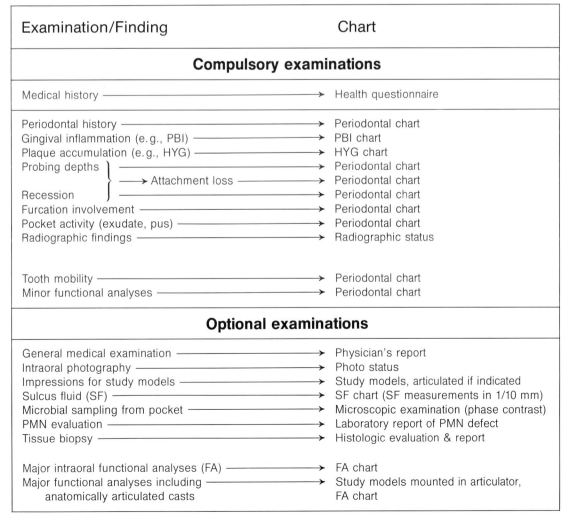

Examination/Finding	Chart
Compulsory examinations	
Medical history →	Health questionnaire
Periodontal history →	Periodontal chart
Gingival inflammation (e.g., PBI) →	PBI chart
Plaque accumulation (e.g., HYG) →	HYG chart
Probing depths ⎫ →	Periodontal chart
→ Attachment loss →	Periodontal chart
Recession ⎭ →	Periodontal chart
Furcation involvement →	Periodontal chart
Pocket activity (exudate, pus) →	Periodontal chart
Radiographic findings →	Radiographic status
Tooth mobility →	Periodontal chart
Minor functional analyses →	Periodontal chart
Optional examinations	
General medical examination →	Physician's report
Intraoral photography →	Photo status
Impressions for study models →	Study models, articulated if indicated
Sulcus fluid (SF) →	SF chart (SF measurements in 1/10 mm)
Microbial sampling from pocket →	Microscopic examination (phase contrast)
PMN evaluation →	Laboratory report of PMN defect
Tissue biopsy →	Histologic evaluation & report
Major intraoral functional analyses (FA) →	FA chart
Major functional analyses including anatomically articulated casts →	Study models mounted in articulator, FA chart

217 Checklist of compulsory and optional exams

Compulsory:
Periodontal charting cannot be performed properly using the dental charts commonly employed in general practice. A special periodontal charting page is required, often enhanced by additional charts for recording hygiene and gingival indices, functional analyses etc. Many such periodontal charting systems are commercially available. It is imperative that the *compulsory* examinations be systematically performed and recorded *for each tooth* in a logical and clearly arranged manner.

Optional:
In advanced cases, such as rapidly progressive periodontitis (RPP) and/or cases involving severe functional disturbances, it may also be necessary to record the optional findings as well (see chart, left). Which *optional exam is to be performed will be determined by the individual situation.*

The primary symptoms of periodontitis are the loss of tooth-supporting tissues ("attachment loss") and the formation of true gingival and bony pockets. Thus, the measurement of probing depths and loss of attachment are essential. The significance of these measurements is relative at best, and not completely congruent with the anatomical-histological relationships (Listgarten 1972, 1980; Armitage et al. 1977; Van der Velden 1979; Van der Velden & Vries 1980). The measurement of probing depths is nevertheless justified because "periodontal therapy" is often synonymous with "pocket therapy."

When a light force of 25 g is applied, the probe tip penetrates beyond the histological bottom of the sulcus or pocket. In healthy gingiva, the histological sulcus is about 0.5 mm deep, but the probe tip normally penetrates to a depth of 2.5 mm. If gingivitis or periodontitis is present, the tip of a periodontal probe may penetrate through the pocket epithelium, through infiltrated and highly vascular connective tissue (with attendant hemorrhage) until resistance is met at the first intact collagen fibers that insert into cementum. Therefore, it is clear that the "probing depth" is also dependent upon

218 Periodontal probes for measurement of pocket depth
The tip of the probe should be rounded and thin; the markings should be easy to read.

1. **CP 12:** 3, 6, 9, 12 mm
2. **Michigan-O:** 3, 6, 8 mm
3. **Williams:** 1, 2, 3, 5, 7, 8, 9, 10 mm
4. **Goldman:** 1, 2, 3, 5, 7, 8, 9, 10 mm
5. **Plast-O-Probe:** 3, 6, 9 mm

The cross sectional profiles of the five probes listed are shown in the diagram at right.

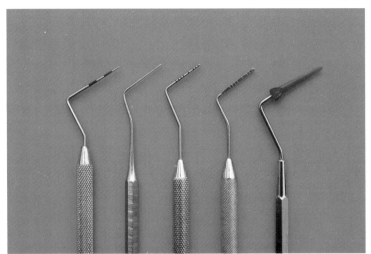

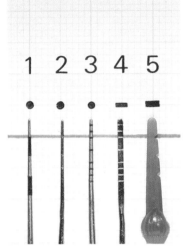

219 Probing depth versus pocket depth
This photomontage shows a periodontal probe (Michigan-O) in a shallow gingival pocket (compare also Fig. 221).

The pocket epithelium is perforated and the gingiva severely deflected. It is only the alveolar crest of bone or the healthy collagenous fiber bundles that stop the probe tip from further penetration. The white arrow indicates the histologic bottom of the sulcus/pocket. The blue arrow represents the probing depth, determined in fact by the counterforce exerted by intact dentogingival fibers (adapted from Armitage et al. 1977).

In diseased gingiva, the measurement error may be as much as 2 mm; in healthy tissues, less. This sort of error is not particularly important when performing the initial examination; however, for the "before and after" comparison, it may be of significance.

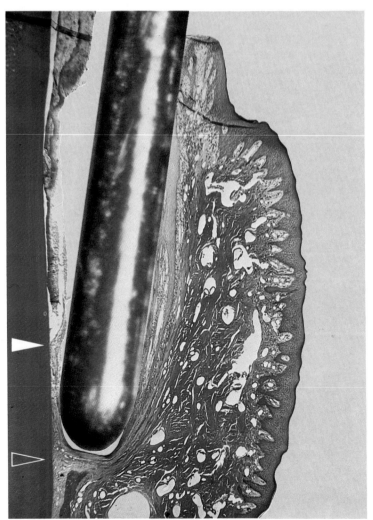

the degree of health or disease in the periodontal tissues. Probing depth will be 0.5–2 mm greater than the actual histological sulcus depth. It is for this reason that it is more correct to speak of *probing depth* and not of *pocket depth*.

The measurement of probing depths provides information about attachment loss only when the gingival margin is at its normal location at the cementoenamel junction. Attachment loss will be underestimated if gingival recession has occurred, and overestimated if gingival enlargement is present. Clearly, true attachment loss must be measured from the CEJ and not from the gingival margin.

More important than the effective attachment loss is the expanse of the *remaining* attachment. This is directly dependent upon the length and thickness of the root (which determines the *area* available for insertion of collagen fibers), and can therefore only be appropriately estimated by combining clinical and radiographic observations.

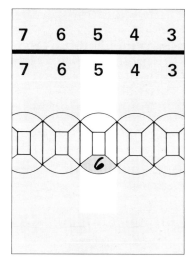

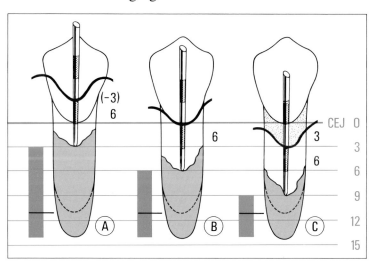

220 "Pocket depth 6 mm…"
This statement provides no information concerning attachment loss or how much attachment remains on a tooth (blue columns).

A. 6 mm pocket depth
−3 mm pseudopocket
=3 mm attachment loss

B. 6 mm pocket depth
=6 mm attachment loss

C. 3 mm gingival recession
+6 mm pocket depth
=9 mm attachment loss

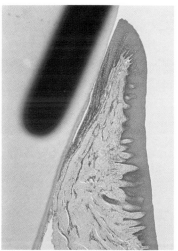

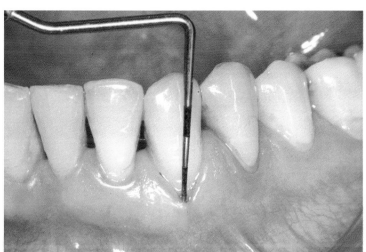

221 "3 mm gingival pocket"
During sulcus probing, the tip of the probe extends beyond the sulcus bottom, penetrates the junctional epithelium and splits it. The internal basal lamina and several JE cell layers always remain attached to the tooth. It is this splitting of the JE that results in a reading of 3 mm for a "normal" sulcus depth.

The cellular turnover rate in the JE repairs such a split within 4–6 days by means of cell proliferation in the Stratum basale (see Fig. 12).

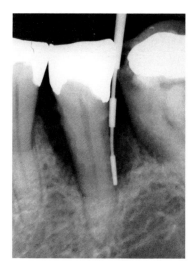

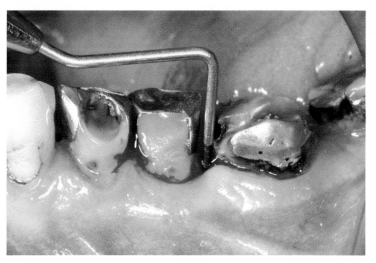

222 "10 mm bony pocket (active)"
In this severely abraded dentition, probing with very light pressure leads to probe tip penetration beyond the base of the soft tissue pocket, through the pocket epithelium, until contact is made with the bone. The radiograph reveals the vertical osseous defect.

Hemorrhage and purulence from the pocket are typical signs of an acute exacerbation of inflammatory periodontal disease. These symptoms of *current pocket activity* are more important than pocket depth.

Furcation Involvement – Root Irregularities

Treatment would be greatly facilitated if all tooth roots exhibited a round-oval profile! Very often, however, roots exhibit an hour-glass shape. In the case of multi-rooted teeth, the practitioner must ascertain to what degree the furcation is involved by attachment loss, and whether the individual roots are fused. Fusion or partial fusion often create deep, narrow grooves along the root. Enamel projections may occur at the furcation area (Fig. 35).

Ascertaining pocket depth and root morphology becomes even more difficult as severity of attachment loss increases and as root cross-sectional profile becomes more bizzare. In addition to naturally occurring irregularities, root surfaces may develop lacuna-like areas of resorption after exposure due to periodontitis. Such areas must also be recognized and recorded in the patient's chart (Schroeder & Rateitschak-Plüss 1983).

223 Special probes for diagnosis of furcations and root irregularities:

- **CH 3:** Fine and pointed, paired left and right, curved. For surfaces and narrow grooves.
- **Nabers 2:** Blunt, paired left and right, curved. For probing furcations.
- **CP 12 (right):** Periodontal probe for horizontal measurement of furcation involvement (Hu-Friedy).

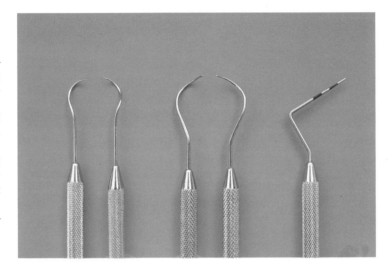

Classes of furcation involvement, horizontal measurement (p. 60)

F 0: —
F 1: Up to 3 mm
F 2: Over 3 mm
F 3: Through-and-through between two roots

Subclasses of F 3 furcation involvement, vertical measurement

A: Up to 3 mm
B: 3 to 6 mm
C: 7 or more mm

224 Section through maxilla
This view, with the cut root surfaces colored red, clearly depicts the enormous variations in root morphology. The narrow furcations, root fusions and hour-glass shape of some roots can also be observed. The interdental and interradicular osseous septa are also of varying dimension.

Maxillary molars (right)
These teeth were sectioned 3–5 mm apical to the furcation. The differences in morphology of the furcations are dramatic.

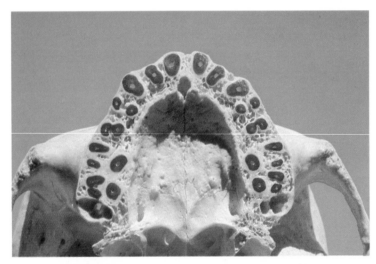

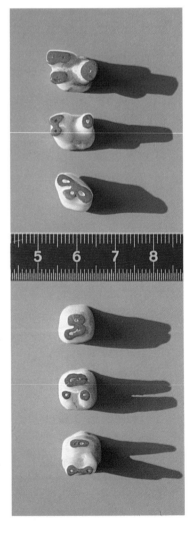

225 Section through mandible
Root morphology in the mandible is more uniform and less complicated than in the maxilla, but almost all of the roots exhibit some depressions labiolingually.

Mandibular molars (right)
These three teeth exhibit root fusion (top), narrow interradicular areas (middle) and widespaced roots (bottom). Over one-fourth of all molar roots (maxillary and mandibular) are fused to some degree!

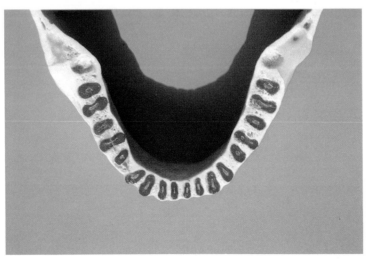

For practical purposes, diagnosis of morphologic and pathologic root variations cannot be performed using only a blunt, straight periodontal probe. Adjunct probes that are specially curved and/or pointed are required (Fig. 223).

It is important for the practitioner to ascertain the presence of root irregularities, because they represent potential plaque-retentive areas that must be dealt with during the course of periodontal therapy, for example during root planing. Furthermore, when a flap opera-

tion permits direct vision of the exposed root surfaces, the practitioner quickly realizes that Nature has even more morphological fantasy than perhaps was apparent at the initial examination.

The radiograph can often provide additional evidence of root peculiarities, but cannot portray exactly the variations in root morphology that occur from tooth to tooth. The radiograph cannot replace a meticulous tactile examination of each root surface using a fine probe.

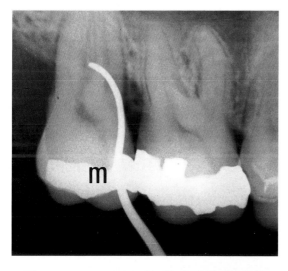
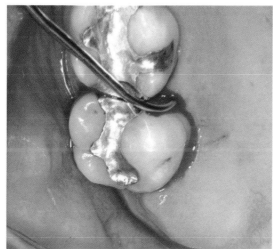

226 "Mesial" furcation – m
In the radiograph, no furcation involvement is visible. However, using a Nabers-2 probe, it is possible to probe the interradicular area of tooth 17 via the mesial furcation.

The mesial furcation can only be probed from a mesiopalatal approach.

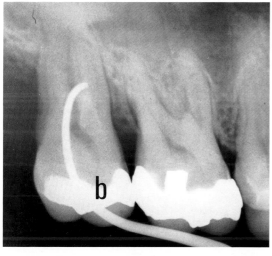
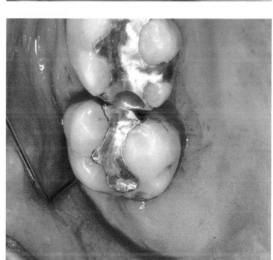

227 "Buccal" furcation – b
Through the narrow buccal furcation, between the mesiobuccal and distobuccal roots, the probe can also be guided into the interradicular area of the same tooth.

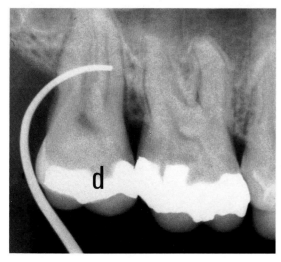
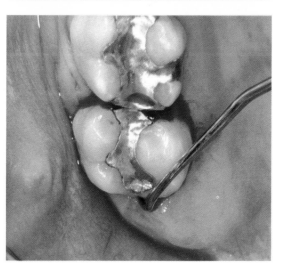

228 "Distal" furcation – d
When the second molar is the most posterior tooth in an arch, the distal furcation can be probed from either distobuccal or distopalatal approaches. As shown, the Nabers-2 probe achieves the interradicular area from the distal approach.

Thus, tooth 17 is shown to have a Class F3 furcation involvement regardless of the probing approach, mesial, distal or buccal.

Pocket Activity – Subgingival Flora

Based on the scientific discoveries of recent years, a complete periodontal examination must include not only clinical and radiographic findings but also a determination of the composition of subgingival flora (Keyes 1978a,b; Socransky 1977; Newman & Socransky 1977; Evian 1982; Singletary 1982). The former represent a summary of past disease, while the latter is a measure of potential future destruction.

Adding an examination of subgingival flora to the practice regimen will serve two purposes. First, it will demonstrate to the patient his own plaque microorganisms, living and moving in the phase contrast microscope or on a TV monitor. This can be a significant motivating influence. Second, the knowledge of the approximate percentage composition of subgingival plaque helps the dentist to determine if the disease is in an active or quiescent stage. Elevated numbers of motile rods and Spirochetes are an indication of an acute stage of periodontitis. This knowledge can also help in the diagnosis of RPP in younger patients.

229 Phase contrast microscope with TV camera and monitor
Pocket flora can be viewed immediately in smears, and the patient can see his "personal enemies," represented by the moving bacteria. This experience motivates the patient and will encourage his cooperation during the treatment phase.

A good laboratory microscope should be available for the actual percentage evaluation of the plaque composition.

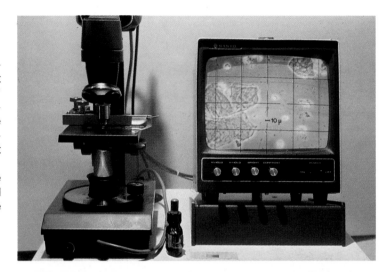

230 Filaments (left) and an amoeba (right)
The TV monitor attached to the microscope can be fitted with a measurement standard to permit size comparisons and morphological identification of the microorganisms.

The filaments were scraped from the root surface (adherent plaque), while the slowly moving amoeba came from the fluid contents of a periodontal pocket (non-adherent plaque).

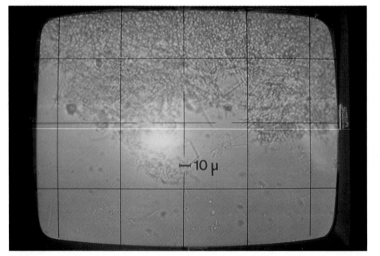

231 Spirochetes!
The monitor displays a smear from the depth of an active pocket. In addition to a few cocci and rods, the major component of this sample is made up of rapidly motile Spirochetes. The clear white spots are red blood cells with a constant diameter of 7–8 μm.

Spirochetes and motile rods are found in elevated numbers in active pockets, comprising over 2/3 of all organisms. In inactive or treated sites, these organisms are seldom encountered.

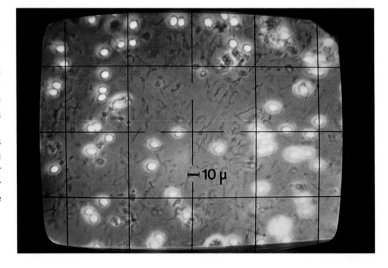

Morphological differentiation of motile and nonmotile microorganisms

- Spirochetes
- Motile rods

- Rods
- Fusiforms
- Cocci
- Filamentous organisms

Several fields from diluted pocket contents are examined and the listed bacterial forms are counted. The percentage composition is then calculated.

Gingival Recession

Recession of the gingiva may be the primary reason a patient seeks dental care. Recession is easy to recognize during an examination of the oral cavity, but a more objective assessment is required for recording recession in the patient's records. The extent of gingival recession is measured with the periodontal probe as the mm distance from the CEJ to the gingival margin. It also must be determined whether a normal sulcus or a pathological pocket is present at the recession site. The width of the remaining attached gingiva between the free gingival margin and the mucogingival line is of little consequence as long as no inflammation is present (Wennström 1982; Wennström & Lindhe 1983).

However, a recession site where *no* attached gingiva remains is a significant observation, particularly when the movable mucosa or frena extend directly into the gingival margin. The dentist also must clarify whether or not the recession is an esthetic problem for the patient.

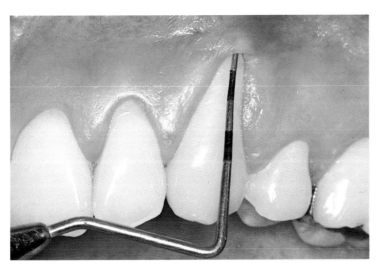

232 Attachment loss through recession
Recession on the facial surface of the cuspid is measured at 5 mm between the CEJ and the gingival margin. The probe extends an additional 2 mm into the gingival sulcus. It appears that there is absolutely no attached gingiva remaining in this area. Also absent is a McCall's festoon, which, if present, could be considered as a reparative attempt on the part of the host tissues to the minimal gingival width.

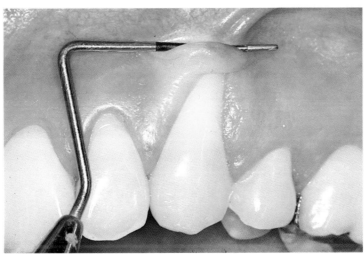

233 Roll test
Using a finger or a periodontal probe, the movable mucosa is pushed toward the recession site. This permits verification of presence or absence of attached gingiva, which will offer resistance. In this case, the movable mucosa extends directly to the gingival margin.

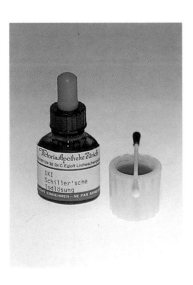
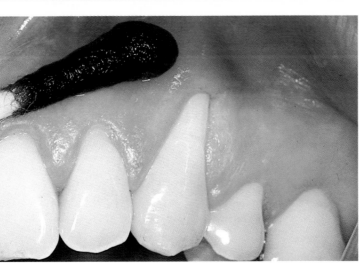

234 Iodine test
Gingva and oral mucosa are painted with Schiller or Lugol solution (a solution of iodine and potassium iodide). The mucosa takes on a brown color owing to its glycogen content, while the glycogen-free attached gingiva remains unstained. The iodine test depicted here reveals that no attached gingiva remains on the facial surface of tooth 23.

Radiography

A complete radiographic survey is necessary for an exact periodontal diagnosis. The survey shows what "is," i.e., the current status of the remaining interdental alveolar bone. The radiograph provides another diagnostic dimension along with clinical probing depth measurement and determination of attachment loss, but it is not a substitute.

Probing depths and radiographically visible bone loss may often disagree (Schweizer & Rateitschak 1972). The periodontal probe may catch on root irregularities, subgingival calculus etc., which leads to an inaccurate measurement of the pocket.

Early periodontal alterations such as triangulation resulting from occlusal trauma can be detected radiographically but are often not visible clinically. On the other hand, loss of bone on facial or oral tooth surfaces can seldom be detected on a radiograph.

235 Periodontal radiographic technique
Undistorted representation of the periodontal hard tissues requires the combination of long-cone and right angle techniques. Various aids (film holders etc.) are available to assist in positioning the film parallel to the tooth's long axis and positioning the central ray perpendicular to the marginal alveolar bone. The central ray should be directed at the alveolar crestal bone, not at the apices of the teeth.

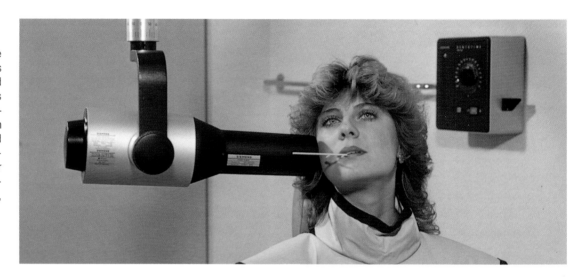

236 Periodontal radiographic survey
Fourteen periapical films are generally required in a full dentition to depict all interdental areas adequately.

This basic 14-film series should be complemented by 2–4 bitewings, especially in patients with proximal restorations and crowns, in order to detect overhangs etc.

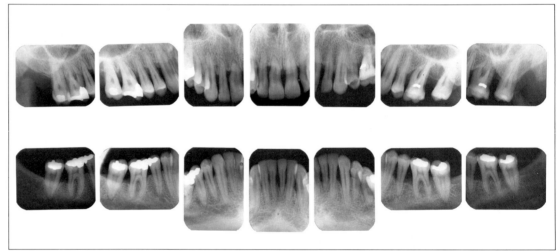

237 Right – Wrong
Left: Periapical radiograph taken with the *long-cone, right angle* technique. The compact layers of the interdental septa and the Lamina dura are clearly distinguishable.

Right: Radiograph of the same teeth using the so-called *bisected angle* technique. No sharp contours can be seen. The periodontal ligament space is not clear, and the Lamina dura is invisible.

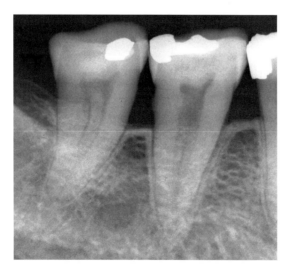
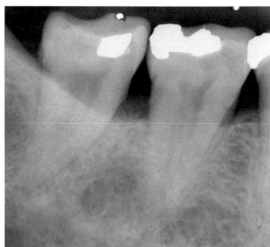

Tooth Mobility – Function

The most important causes of elevated tooth mobility are *quantitative* loss of tooth-supporting structure due to periodontitis, and *qualitative* changes in the periodontal ligament due to occlusal trauma (see Function, p. 271). It is important to differentiate between *increased tooth mobility* (stable increase; adaptation) and *progressively increasing tooth mobility* (unstable; pathologic).

A "mini" functional analysis can determine clinically the more important functional findings such as premature contacts in retruded contact position, direction and extent of shifts during intercuspation, working side interferences, balancing side interferences, parafunctions (bruxism), TMJ changes, and habits such as lip biting, tongue thrust etc.

Parafunctions related to the patient's occupation should also be recorded, e. g., holding nails between the teeth, pencil biting, or playing a musical instrument.

Degrees of Tooth Mobility (TM)

0 = normal
(physiologic mobility)

1 = detectably increased mobility

2 = visible mobility up to 0.5 mm

3 = severe mobility up to 1 mm

4 = extreme mobility, vertical, mobility; tooth no longer functional.

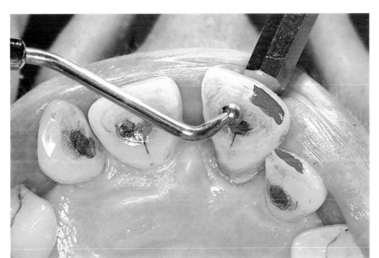

238 Tooth mobility
Increased tooth mobility is determined by applying a labiolingual force of approximately 500 g using two dental instruments. In this view, note that the central incisor can be deflected far labially.

Tooth mobility is expressed in degrees from 0–4, as shown at left.

(Physiologic tooth mobility, see p. 8)

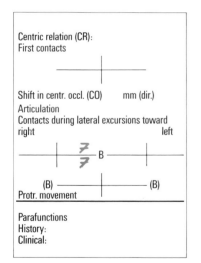

Centric relation (CR):
First contacts

Shift in centr. occl. (CO)   mm (dir.)
Articulation
Contacts during lateral excursions toward
right   left

B

(B)   (B)
Protr. movement

Parafunctions
History:
Clinical:

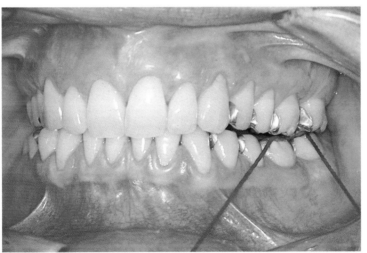

**239 Functional finding –
Balancing contact**
During lateral excursion to the right, a heavy balancing side interference is noted between teeth 27 and 37; this is recorded in red on the chart (left). A thread will not pass between 27 and 37 on the balancing side (left) during mandibular excursion to the right.

This finding is entered in Section C of the periodontal chart (see left and Fig. 244). In periodontal patients the removal of such contacts is recommended (see Function, p. 271).

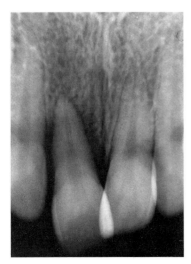

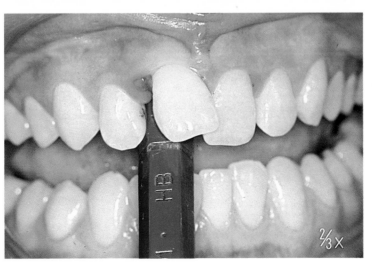

**240 Functional finding –
Parafunctions, oral habits**
In addition to occlusal dysharmonies, each patient must be examined for habits such as lip or cheek biting, pipe smoking, matchstick chewing etc.

In this 18-year-old female, the periodontal supporting structure around tooth 11 has been severely damaged as a result of gingivitis and her habit of biting pencils for hours at a time.

Diagnostic Charting

An examination of the periodontium makes sense only if the findings are permanently recorded. This can be accomplished in writing, schematically radiographically and sometimes photographically or through use of plaster models. Diagnosis and prognosis cannot be made without such records. Permanent records are also indispensable for case presentation, for treatment planning, for re-evaluation of the case during the course of therapy, as well as for later comparisons.

During the maintenance phase (recall), simplified charts may be used and only selected findings recorded. Many different charts are commercially available. The most important findings must be recorded clearly and in a standardized manner. The choice of *which* chart or *which* method is less important than making accurate and coherent entries.

241 Intraoral photography
Intraoral photographs may be indicated in periodontology, as they are in other areas of dentistry, to document the patient's condition. "Before and after" photographs can be very useful for patient motivation. A simple method is the 5-slide documentation depicted here, with anterior, R & L lateral, and occlusal views of maxilla and mandible. Use of 35 mm slides makes archiving easier.

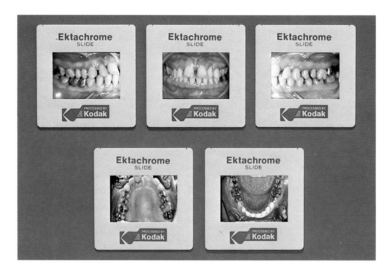

242 Chart for HYG and PBI (Hygiene and Papilla Bleeding Indices)
HYG: Plaque accumulation in every interdental area should be recorded. This will demonstrate for the patient his own level of oral hygiene proficiency, which may help correct problems in home care.

PBI: Evaluating the severity of gingival inflammation (bleeding) can provide a sensitive record of treatment successes or failures.

Both HYG and PBI are repeated regularly at every recall appointment to help motivate the patient.

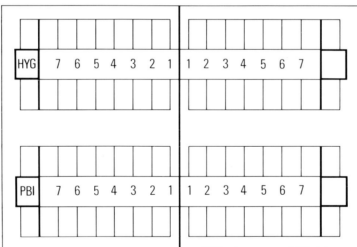

243 Radiographic survey
The radiographs from the patient shown in Figure 241 reveal the irregular distribution of attachment loss in interdental areas.
   Bite-wings provide a better view of interproximal spaces, where calculus, restoration margins and crown margins may be evaluated.

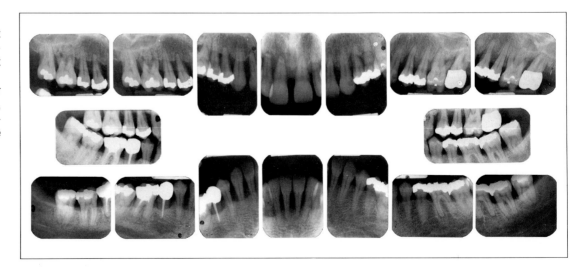

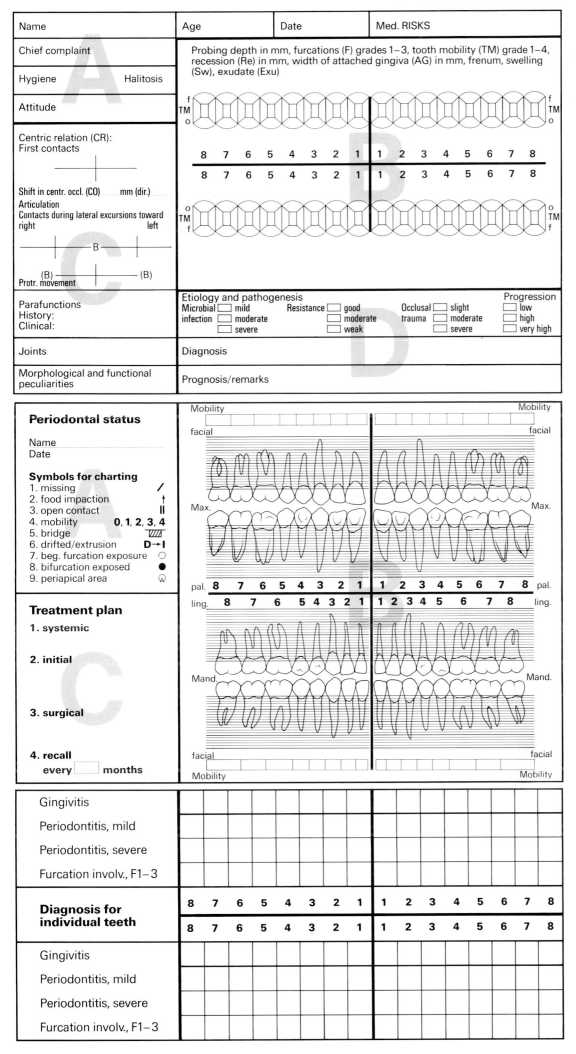

| Name | Age | Date | Med. RISKS |

Chief complaint

Hygiene   Halitosis

Attitude

Centric relation (CR):
First contacts

Shift in centr. occl. (CO)   mm (dir.)
Articulation
Contacts during lateral excursions toward
right   left

B

(B)   (B)
Protr. movement

Parafunctions
History:
Clinical:

Joints

Morphological and functional
peculiarities

Probing depth in mm, furcations (F) grades 1–3, tooth mobility (TM) grade 1–4, recession (Re) in mm, width of attached gingiva (AG) in mm, frenum, swelling (Sw), exudate (Exu)

f
TM
o

8 7 6 5 4 3 2 1 1 2 3 4 5 6 7 8
8 7 6 5 4 3 2 1 1 2 3 4 5 6 7 8

o
TM
f

Etiology and pathogenesis

					Progression
Microbial ☐ mild	Resistance ☐ good	Occlusal ☐ slight	☐ low
infection ☐ moderate	☐ moderate	trauma ☐ moderate	☐ high
☐ severe	☐ weak	☐ severe	☐ very high

Diagnosis

Prognosis/remarks

Periodontal status

Name
Date

Symbols for charting
1. missing   /
2. food impaction   ↑
3. open contact   ‖
4. mobility   0, 1, 2, 3, 4
5. bridge   ▨
6. drifted/extrusion   D→I
7. beg. furcation exposure ○
8. bifurcation exposed   ●
9. periapical area   ⊗

Treatment plan

1. systemic

2. initial

3. surgical

4. recall

every ☐ months

Mobility   Mobility
facial   facial

Max.   Max.

pal. 8 7 6 5 4 3 2 1   1 2 3 4 5 6 7 8 pal.
ling. 8 7 6 5 4 3 2 1   1 2 3 4 5 6 7 8 ling.

Mand.   Mand.

facial   facial
Mobility   Mobility

	8	7	6	5	4	3	2	1		1	2	3	4	5	6	7	8
Gingivitis																	
Periodontitis, mild																	
Periodontitis, severe																	
Furcation involv., F1–3																	
Diagnosis for individual teeth	8	7	6	5	4	3	2	1		1	2	3	4	5	6	7	8
	8	7	6	5	4	3	2	1		1	2	3	4	5	6	7	8
Gingivitis																	
Periodontitis, mild																	
Periodontitis, severe																	
Furcation involv., F1–3																	

244 Periodontal survey – I
Example of a universally applicable periodontal chart (modified from the *University of Basle* chart). It consists of 4 distinct areas (A–D):

A. History

B. Clinical findings
Probing depths, tooth mobility (TM). The blank spaces on the chart can be used for recording recession (Re), furcation involvement (F), width of attached gingiva (AG) etc.

True loss of attachment can be *calculated* easily from probing depths and recession values.

C. Functional analyses

D. Etiology, diagnosis and prognosis

245 Periodontal survey – II
This chart is a modification of the *University of Michigan* chart. It consists of 3 distinct areas (A–C):

A. Legend of symbols used in charting.

B. Clinical findings
The course of the gingival margin and the probing depths are drawn in precisely as a continuous line. This provides an excellent overview of attachment loss.

C. Treatment planning
The most important aspects of systemic and local initial therapy are entered in writing.

Planning for surgical procedures is done only after initial therapy is completed.

The recall interval is determined after completion of all therapy.

246 Chart for "Single Tooth Diagnosis"
There is no "average" diagnosis of periodontitis that applies to the entire dentition. Each tooth is an individual entity and may manifest its own degree of disease severity.

Using this chart, the dentist gleans an overview of the distribution of disease, which is helpful in assessing where emphasis must be placed in therapy (for example, on prospective abutment teeth). Single tooth diagnosis leads the practitioner to formulate a *prognosis* for each tooth (see p. 98).

Prognosis

Determining the prognosis for a new periodontitis patient is difficult, and depends on a myriad of factors. A *provisional prognosis,* made after the initial examination and diagnosis, frequently must be modified during the course of treatment. Modifying factors would include degree of patient cooperation and dexterity, and the reaction of the host to treatment in terms of wound healing and capacity for regeneration. These factors are difficult to assess at the outset of treatment.

Generally speaking, slowly progressing adult periodontitis (AP) carries a good prognosis, while the less common rapidly progressive periodontitis of young adults (RPP) has a less favorable prognosis.

The case prognosis is based on consideration of the *prognosis for each individual tooth (maintainable, doubtful, hopeless).* Great care must be exercised in the determination of prognosis for prospective abutment teeth.

A basic rule is that both general and local factors play a role in the determination of prognosis.

General prognostic factors:
– Patient's desires, demands, and ability to be motivated (don't overtreat!)
– Systemic health, host resistance, immune status
– Level of psychic stress/tension
– Age in relation to attachment loss.

Local prognostic factors:
– Speed of plaque formation, independent of quality and intensity of oral hygiene
– Amount and bacterial composition (virulence) of plaque
– Depth and localization of pockets
– Activity of pockets (bleeding, suppuration)
– Attachment loss
– Remaining attachment (root length)
– Pocket morphology, type of bone loss (horizontal bone loss = good prognosis, vertical bone loss = unfavorable prognosis)
– Tooth and root morphology (plaque-retentive areas)
– Furcation involvement or open furcation (unfavorable prognosis)
– Tooth mobility in relation to amount of bone loss
– Tooth mobility in relation to occlusal trauma
– Anomalies of tooth position.

247   Single tooth prognosis
A prognosis must be established for each individual tooth. Following initial therapy, each such prognosis should be re-evaluated and revised.

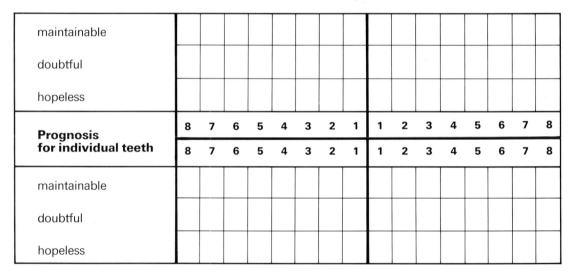

	8	7	6	5	4	3	2	1	1	2	3	4	5	6	7	8
Prognosis for individual teeth																
	8	7	6	5	4	3	2	1	1	2	3	4	5	6	7	8

maintainable / doubtful / hopeless (above and below the tooth chart)

"Tooth by tooth"

The compilation of all the various single tooth prognoses to arrive at a prognosis for the entire case will determine whether the subsequent therapy will be *radical, conservative* or only *palliative.*

If the prognosis is poor, especially in cases of rapidly progressive, advanced, active disease in a patient who cannot be motivated adequately, the practitioner must consider whether performing periodontal therapy is rational at all. In some cases it may be better to perform extractions and treat the case prosthetically.

Prevention

Maintenance of Health – Prevention of Disease...

... are the noblest goals of modern medicine. Prevention is more important, simpler and less costly than treatment.

Prevention should benefit every socioeconomic segment of society and every age group. Children and young persons in particular should be exposed to preventive measures. At the same time, they must be educated as to the importance of taking care of their own health. Over the long term, it is really the patient's own desires and persistence that must keep his preventive orientation and behaviour alive.

In *general medicine* there are many examples of pathogenic influences that are known to the layman. Preventive behaviour is encouraged worldwide: don't smoke, drink less alcohol, watch your diet, exercise more. However, too many people seldom go beyond making good resolutions.

In a similar manner, oral preventive measures including proper nutrition and good oral hygiene are acknowledged as important, but are also too often not carried out persistently over the long term. Successful *oral prevention* demands the recognition and elimination of all irritants that could damage the oral structures. Simultaneously, all possible attempts should be made to elevate the level of host resistance to the pathogenic agents or situations. The great successes in caries prevention have been known for decades. The main pillars of this success have been collective and individual use of fluorides, reduction of sugar consumption, and plaque control by means of effective oral hygiene procedures.

Within the past several years it has been demonstrated that *preventive periodontics* can also be successful if it is applied consistently and appropriately (Axelsson & Lindhe 1977, 1981a, b; Axelsson 1982). Gingivitis and periodontitis prevention is similar to caries prevention in terms of patient motivation as well as recognition and removal of plaque by means of effective oral hygiene procedures performed at least once daily. The goals of plaque control are prevention of gingival margin infection and prevention of the initiation of gingivitis and periodontitis.

From a somewhat broader perspective, prevention of periodontal disease encompasses several additional measures, which are also targeted toward elimination of plaque, but indirectly. Included under this heading are calculus removal, elimination of plaque-retentive areas by means of selective odontoplasty or orthodontic treatment, and the elimination of iatrogenic irritants. For example, an overhanging restoration or a poorly adapted crown margin make oral hygiene in the interdental area impossible. Dental floss is ineffective in such cases; it tears and becomes lodged in the defective restoration. Efficient oral hygiene leading to freedom from plaque will only be possible if crown and restoration margins are supragingival, free of overhang and free of defects. The junction between filling material and tooth substance must be smooth.

But the dentist's efforts in prevention of periodontal disease must go beyond the correction of restorative inadequacies that represent plaque-retentive areas. The dentist must fabricate and insert only restorations and reconstructions that enhance prevention, whenever possible with supragingival margins. Perfect operative and prosthetic dentistry is an important component of preventive periodontics.

An additional component of periodontal prevention is maintenance of the results achieved by periodontal therapy. Proper maintenance prevents re-infection. If total freedom from plaque is a utopian goal, reality lies in defining for each patient an individual optimum level of hygiene that can be maintained over the years. This will be dependent upon the patient's degree of motivation and above all the recall frequency. Many investigators have demonstrated that the gingival and periodontal condition post-therapy is unlikely to break down if the recall interval does not exceed 3 months (Ramfjord et al. 1975, 1982; Rosling et al. 1976a; Axelsson & Lindhe 1981a, b; Axelsson 1982).

Effective disease preventive measures are identical to the "initial therapy" regimen described in detail on pages 107–134.

Therapy of Periodontal Diseases

Gingivitis…, Periodontitis…, Recession…

… can all be successfully treated and their progression halted. The primary goals of treatment for gingivitis and periodontitis are:

- Elimination of gingival inflammation
- Elimination of symptoms of disease activity
  (exudate, pus, hemorrhage) in periodontal pockets
- Cessation of bone loss and attachment loss
- Elimination or reduction of periodontal pockets that represent
  potential sites of re-infection
- Prevention of re-infection and recurrence of inflammation
- Achieving new attachment to the root surface by means of
  regeneration of periodontal tissues
- Improvement of gingival contour
- Creation of optimal, functional occlusal relationships
- Stabilization of mobile teeth.

Towards the achievement of these treatment goals there are many clinically proven and scientifically tested concepts of therapy. All such concepts have in common the attempt to remove the supra- and subgingival microorganisms (plaque control) that elicit disease, as well as the creation of a clean, smooth, endotoxin-free and bioacceptable root surface. These are the elements of *initial therapy*.

Beyond these similarities of orientation, the various treatment concepts and treatment goals may differ according to the form and severity of disease. A variety of standard surgical procedures may be indicated. The most important aspect of surgical intervention is that it provides the opportunity for the dentist to treat the root surface with direct vision, as well as to correct morphological irregularities of gingival and periodontal structures. This is called the *corrective phase of therapy*.

Only in cases of acute, progressive forms of disease in children and young adults should administration of any systemic medications be expected to improve the results obtained with purely local (mechanical) efforts. Functional therapeutic measures such as occlusal adjustment by selective grinding or orthodontics, stabilization or splinting are only undertaken if some functional disturbance (e.g., occlusal trauma) is accelerating the progress of periodontitis and if increasing tooth mobility is noted.

Recession as a disease entity has lost much of its former status. The therapy for progressing recession is described in the chapter on mucogingival surgery (p. 228).

Treatment Planning – Sequence of Treatment

Following clinical examination and determination of prognosis, a case presentation is made. The patient is informed about the diagnosis, severity of disease, the necessity for treatment and the phases of treatment. During the case presentation, the dentist should begin to gather the subjective signs indicating the patient's desire to cooperate.

The approximate time course for the proposed therapy and the expected costs are also discussed. Emergency procedures are performed immediately.

The treatment plan depends upon the following factors:

- Clinical findings and diagnosis
- The patient's own wishes
- The patient's interest level and degree of cooperation
- Prognosis
- Financial wherewithal of the patient if there is no insurance or other coverage.

248   Basic treatment plan
Almost all periodontal therapy, regardless of the disease type, follows a similar general course. This is not to say that periodontal treatment can be done in "cook book" fashion.

1. Initial therapy
Creation of hygienic relationships in the oral cavity through the combined efforts of the dentist, his auxiliary personnel and the patient himself. Functional disturbances are eliminated. The patient's cooperation is definitively ascertained.

After *re-evaluation,* one or both of the following may ensue...

2. Surgical intervention
Correction of morphological problems that persist after initial therapy, and treatment of the root surface with direct vision.

3. Maintenance phase (recall)
The recall interval is determined for the most part by the patient's level of cooperation and motivation, by the success of the surgical phase, and by the degree of severity of the original periodontal disease process.

A. *Negative findings at re-evaluation*
If the patient's level of home care is insufficient or if the initial therapy did not achieve the expected goals, it may be repeated.

B. *Positive findings at re-evaluation*
If initial therapy alone has led to control of the periodontitis and if no morphological problems are evident, the patient moves directly into the recall phase.

C. *Recurrent periodontitis*
If signs of active periodontitis are detected during a recall appointment, the patient's oral hygiene is checked and the dentist may elect to re-institute initial therapy.

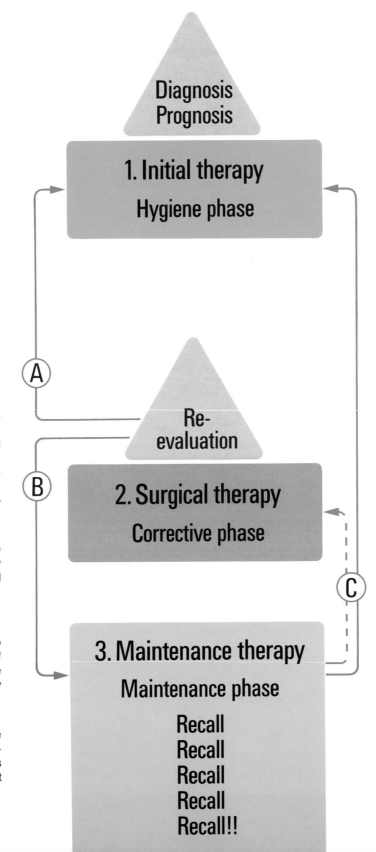

Checklist of periodontal therapy
- History and clinical exam
- Diagnosis
- Case presentation
- Information and motivation
- Provisional prognosis
- Temporary treatment plan
- Emergency treatment

Initial therapy
- Oral hygiene instruction
- Supragingival plaque and calculus removal
- Elimination of iatrogenic irritants and plaque-retentive areas
- Subgingival plaque and calculus removal
- Root planing
- Curettage
- Functional therapy
- (Systemic medication)
- Temporary restorations
- Endodontic therapy
- Orthodontic therapy
- Temporary splinting

Re-evaluation
- Definitive prognosis
- Definitive treatment plan

Surgical therapy
- Gingivectomy/gingivoplasty
- Modified Widman operation (conservative flaps)
- More radical flap operation (including osseous contouring, implants etc.)
- Combined operations
- Special surgical procedures
- Mucogingival surgery
- Temporary restoration
- Definitive restoration

Maintenance therapy (recall)
- Periodic checks:
    Bleeding Index
    Hygiene Index
    Probing depths
    Radiographs
- Re-motivation, re-instruction
- Plaque and calculus removal
- Treatment of recurrent disease

Treatment Plans for Various Forms of Periodontal Disease

The five diagrams below demonstrate how the length, intensity and frequency of treatment can vary dramatically, depending on the type of disease being treated. In every case, initial therapy consisting of local debridement, oral hygiene instruction (OHI) and motivation is performed, while surgical intervention is reserved only for more advanced cases of periodontitis. Systemic medication is employed as an adjunct to local therapy only in resistant and rapidly progressive disease (RPP), as well as in juvenile periodontitis (LJP).

Symbols for planning and treatment

△ Comprehensive evaluation and re-evaluation

△ Intermittant findings and checks

| Appointment for initial therapy

| Appointment for surgery

|R 1 First recall, maintenance therapy

 Systemic therapy as adjunct

CHX Chlorhexidine (topical chemotherapy)

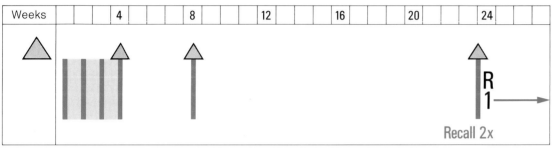

249 Time frame for therapy (5 examples)

1. Gingivitis
Successful therapy for gingivitis usually requires only a few appointments for motivation, OHI, debridement. At the first recall shortly after treatment, the definitive recall interval is determined.

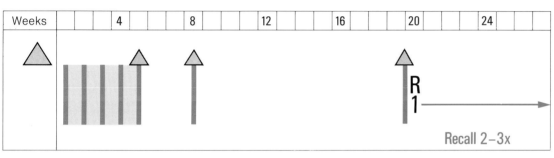

2. Mild, slowly progressive periodontitis
Periodontal disease in its initial stage does not require substantially more comprehensive treatment than does simple gingivitis. Debridement and root planing can be accomplished as therapy for the initial attachment loss. Recall 2–3 times per year.

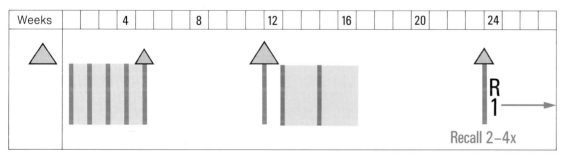

3. Moderate, slowly progressing periodontitis
In addition to a somewhat more extensive course for initial therapy, two surgical procedures in specific arch segments are planned in this case. First recall at 2–3 months postoperatively, then a regular recall interval of 2–4 times per year.

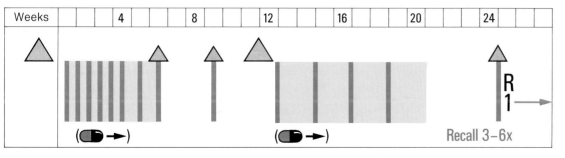

4. Severe, rapidly progressive periodontitis
Initial therapy can take 8–10 appointments. Subsequently, 4 surgical sessions with appropriate follow-up are planned. Both phases are supported by systemic administration of antibiotics. The recall interval is very short, e.g., every 3 months.

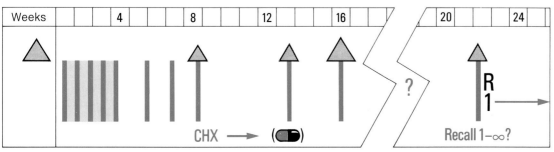

5. Most severe, "hopeless" periodontitis
Poor patient cooperation will hamper success. When the chances of success appear dim after initial therapy has already begun, treatment may have to be abandoned. Treatment in such cases simply involves frequent recall and palliative therapy only.

Emergency Treatment

Many periodontitis patients are not aware that a disease is in progress in the oral cavity. Only when an acute exacerbation occurs do these persons seek out a dentist, usually on an emergency basis. Periodontal emergencies should be handled immediately, following a brief medical history (anticoagulants? allergies? focal infections?), clinical examination and a radiographic survey.

Periodontal emergencies include:
- Immediate extraction of hopelessly mobile teeth
- Debridement of periodontal abscesses
- Treatment of pockets with acute symptoms (purulence)
- Initial treatment for acute necrotizing ulcerative gingivitis (ANUG).

**250 Hopeless tooth 11 –
Fistula and pain**
The disease process has reached the apex (see radiograph). Pus escapes via a fistulous tract and from the pocket. The tooth must be extracted immediately.

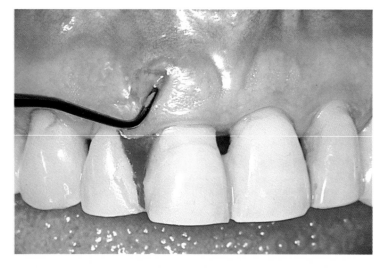 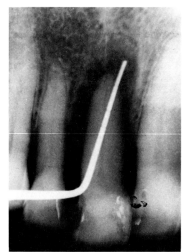

**251 Resected root
immediately after extraction**
An immediate temporary is necessary for esthetics. Following extraction, the root is severed and the crown is used as a temporary. A wire and acid-etch resin secure the crown to its adjacent teeth.

The result is esthetically acceptable. This type of temporary can generally be maintained until periodontal therapy is complete and a definitive restoration has been prepared.

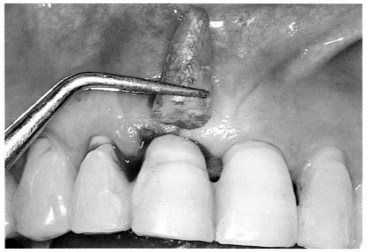 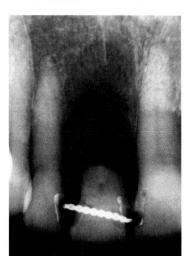

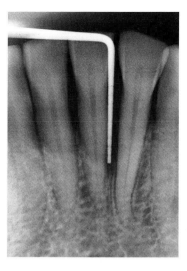

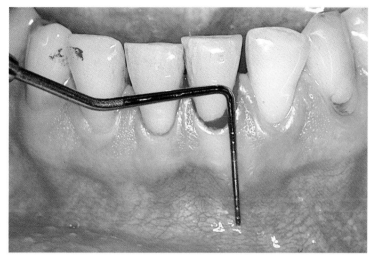

252 Acute exacerbation in a localized deep pocket
Tooth 31 is vital and should be maintained despite the 10 mm pocket.

The *radiograph* reveals that about one-fourth of the root is still anchored in alveolar bone.

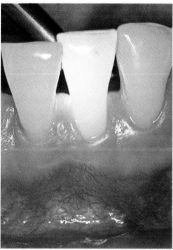

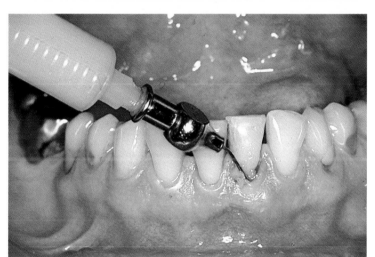

253 Emergency treatment using local medicament
As an emergency measure the pocket was first rinsed thoroughly with chlorhexidine and then filled with achromycine ointment (3%). Once the acute symptoms subside, a thorough subgingival root planing can be performed.

Left: Eight weeks after emergency therapy, the gingiva has receded somewhat. Probing depth is now only ca. 3 mm.

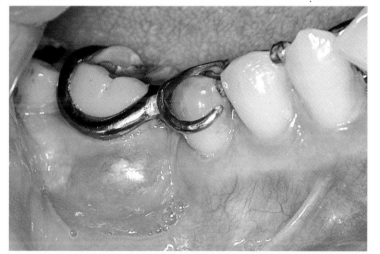

254 Pocket abscess
Originating from the deep infrabony pocket mesial to the tipped tooth 47, an abscess has developed. The buccal gingiva is distended as the abscess is about to break through the mucosa.

Tooth 47 is an abutment for a cast removable partial denture that is ill-fitting.

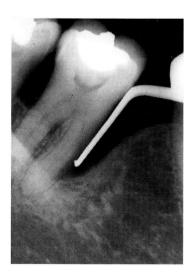

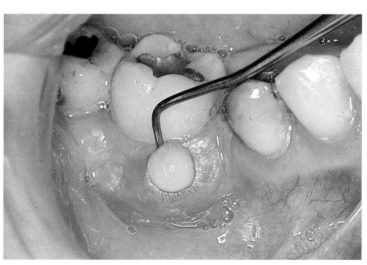

255 Opening the abscess
As soon as the mucosa was touched with a probe, the abscess opened immediately and pus exuded.

Radiographically, one observes the deep periodontal pocket on the mesial aspect. Since the furcation appears not to be involved, it is possible to think in terms of maintaining this tooth.

256 Hopeless molar (37)

Pus exudes spontaneously from the deep pocket around 37. The tooth is highly mobile and painful to percussion.

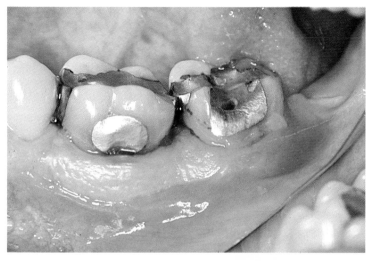

257 Radiograph of 37 before extraction

The osseous defect was localized to the facial surface (visible radiographically with probe in situ) and the distal aspect, and extended to the apex.

Right: Highly infiltrated granulation tissue remains attached to the tooth after extraction.

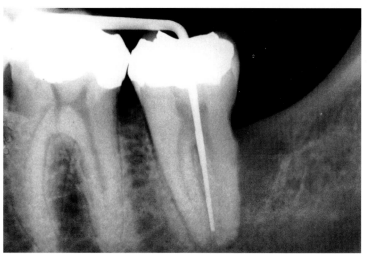
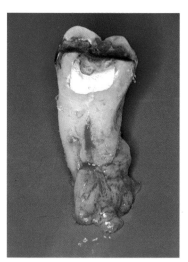

258 Acute necrotizing ulcerative gingivitis (ANUG)

The pain associated with ANUG permits only a very careful, peripheral attempt at cleansing. Following gentle debridement with 3% hydrogen peroxide, a cortisone/antibiotic ointment may be applied with cotton balls or a blunt cannula. The cortisone acts as an anti-inflammatory agent, reducing pain, while the antibiotic prevents further infection.

Some clinicians discount the need for chemotherapy, especially of cortisone at this stage of ANUG.

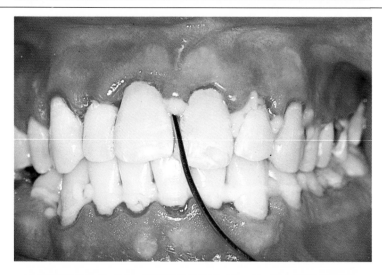

259 ANUG in a subacute stage

Several days after emergency topical application of medicaments and debridement, the signs of active ANUG have subsided.

Treatment by means of systematic subgingival scaling and root planing can now proceed. A gingivoplasty may be indicated subsequently.

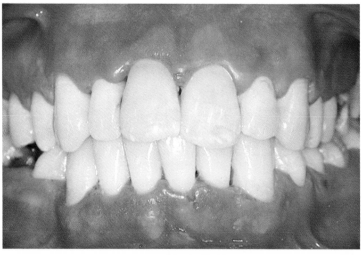

Initial Therapy

The causes of gingivitis and periodontitis are acknowledged to be microorganisms and their metabolic products. The first goal of prevention and treatment must therefore be the creation of an oral cavity that is as free of plaque and calculus as possible. The term "initial therapy" is used to describe the various procedures that are used to achieve this goal. Thus, initial therapy is truly therapy aimed at the etiology of the disease process, while the surgical treatment methods primarily serve to correct morphologic alterations and to provide access to the root surfaces.

Every patient must traverse the initial therapy phase. For gingivitis and for periodontitis, initial therapy is often the only treatment necessary. Since the clinical procedures are usually simple, but time-consuming, they are delegated as much as possible to auxiliary personnel such as the dental hygienist or dental assistant. Of course, each phase of initial therapy is performed under the dentist's direct supervision.

Each case is re-evaluated after initial therapy and a healing period. Gingival bleeding (PBI), probing depths and plaque accumulation (HYG) must be evaluated anew. Performing these evaluations provides a check not only upon the success of initial therapy but also on the patient's level of cooperation in home care. A successful result after initial therapy depends in great measure upon the intensity of the patient's cooperation.

Working together, the dentist and the auxiliary personnel must accomplish the following (see Recall, p. 269, Fig. 712):

- *Informing* the patient about his periodontal disease and its treatment (case presentation), as well as *motivating* him concerning disease control
- *Instruction* in oral hygiene, including use of the toothbrush and other aids for interdental hygiene
- *Prescription of medicaments* in special cases only, e.g., topical chlorhexidine rinses or systemic administration of tetracycline or metranidazole (see Medicaments, p. 263)
- *Supragingival calculus removal* (gross scaling and fine debridement)
- *Elimination of iatrogenic irritants,* polishing old restorations, creation of conditions that will foster interdental hygiene (access)
- *Elimination of natural plaque-retentive areas* such as grooves, depressions or irregularities on crown and root surfaces, furcations, and crowding of teeth
- *Subgingival plaque and calculus removal, root planing, and soft tissue curettage*
- *Functional treatment* (bite guard, selective occlusal grinding)
- *Arch stabilization via splinting* of excessively mobile teeth.

Motivation – Information

Maintenance or restoration of periodontal health is possible. However, this goal will only be achieved through a successful *cooperative* effort between the dentist and the patient. The patient must be interested in maintaining the health of his/her oral cavity, and must acknowledge the necessity for treatment. The patient must be motivated to work toward these goals. It is unfortunate that today we still do not possess a scientifically proven method that will ensure patient motivation and interest (Sheiham 1977). Whether or not a patient can be motivated will depend upon many factors including socioeconomic status, intelligence, personality, behaviour patterns, and the patient's own appraisal of his body and its health. The most important prerequisite for successful patient motivation is a trusting relationship between the patient and the dentist.

The recommendations presented here have their base in practical clinical experience, and not necessarily in the scientific literature. However, the following aids for patient motivation have proven to be useful:

260   Motivation during the inital examination
The patient watches in a mirror as the dentist performs the Papilla Bleeding Index, and learns to recognize gingival bleeding as a sign of "gingival disease." The PBI scores are dictated to the assistant, who makes appropriate entries in the chart (see pp. 30 & 31; Figs. 65 & 66); the patient quickly acknowledges that a "4" is bad and a "0" good!

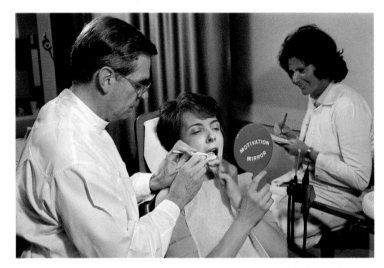

261   "Motivation Mirror"
Using a large hand mirror, the patient can see the difference between healthy papillae and diseased (bleeding) ones. The patient will remember this later when performing oral hygiene at home, and is likely to work harder in the areas that bled.

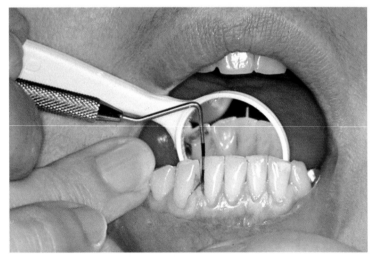

262   Descriptive brochures
A case presentation will be much easier und more meaningful for the patient when modern pictorial aids (Dental Atlas etc.) are employed. Such aids are commercially available, but the dentist may elect to prepare his own as well. Pictures and models can also be used to help the patient understand the treatment phases that will follow initial therapy.

Only an informed patient is a motivated patient!

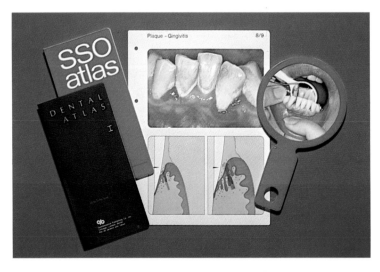

- Demonstration of bleeding gingiva as the PBI is recorded. The patient can see the hemorrhage using a hand mirror.
- Explanation of the symptoms of gingivitis and periodontitis using pictures and other visual aids.
- Presentation of the patient's own case using the records taken during examination, especially the probing depth chart and the radiographs.
- Demonstration of plaque using disclosing agents, and explanation of the microbial etiology of bleeding and inflammation ("local infectious disease").

The symptom of gingival hemorrhage has achieved heightened status as a motivating factor in recent years. Using the PBI (Saxer & Mühlemann 1975; Mühlemann 1978), the severity of gingival inflammation can be evaluated numerically. If the PBI score decreases continually during the initial therapy phase, it will serve as a motivating factor for the patient, who recognizes that the treatment and his home care have led to a lessening of his symptoms of disease.

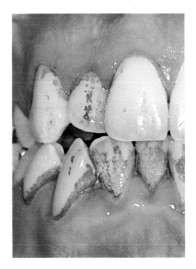
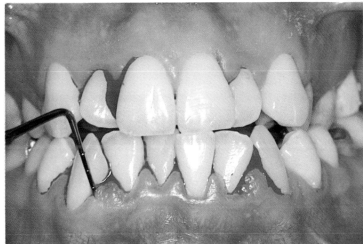

PBI as a motivating factor

263   Initial finding: Moderate gingivitis
The patient sees heavy bleeding as the PBI is recorded.

Left: Thereafter, a plaque-disclosing agent is used to demonstrate to the patient the cause of the bleeding he has just witnessed.
   The next step is oral hygiene instruction (OHI) and a professional cleaning of the teeth by the dentist or hygienist.

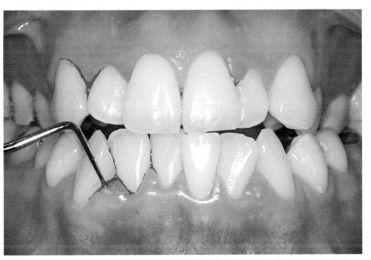

264   Clinical situation 2 weeks later
After prophylaxis and repeated OH instruction, the patient can visualize the improvement that has occurred in his gingival health, as the degree of bleeding that occurs during PBI recording is considerably diminished. This can serve as motivation toward a high level of patient cooperation.

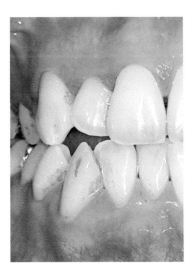
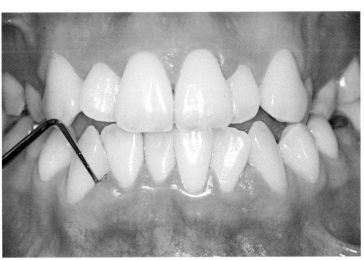

265   Clinical situation 4 weeks later
Bleeding has been reduced to almost nothing, and the disclosing agent reveals very little plaque accumulation. These two facts should convince the patient of the logic of the treatment.

Left: Additional OH instruction then is concentrated on those tooth surfaces and interdental areas that have not been perfectly cleaned by the patient.

Home Care by the Patient

Plaque control by the patient has been and remains a critical component of prevention and treatment of periodontal disease.

Without continuing home care by the patient, all the efforts of the practitioner and the auxiliary personnel in treatment of periodontitis will achieve little success and, more importantly, the success achieved will be of short duration. The critical aspect of patient home care is reduction of the amount of plaque at the gingival margin. The gingival massage that occurs during toothbrushing is of secondary importance, but may be beneficial from a physiotherapeutic standpoint. In some special cases, the patient's home care can be supported through use of anti-plaque mouth rinses (chlorhexidine) for a limited period of time.

This chapter is divided into 6 sections:

- Plaque disclosing agents
- Toothbrushes, dentifrices
- Toothbrushing techniques
- Interdental hygiene
- Special cleaning aids, irrigation devices
- Chemical plaque control (chlorhexidine, CHX).

The toothbrush is a most important tool for mechanical removal of plaque, but it can reach only the *facial, oral* and *occlusal* tooth surfaces.

This fact is important to understand because the initial lesions of gingivitis and periodontitis (as well as dental caries) usually occur in the *interproximal* areas. For this reason, the toothbrush must always be supplemented with other hygiene aids that can ensure cleaning in the interdental spaces.

There is no single method of oral hygiene that is right for every patient. The appropriate method will be determined by the type and severity of the patient's disease, the morphological situation (crowding, diastemas etc.), as well as the manual dexterity of the patient. The hygiene method may even be different for various areas within the mouth of a single patient. Furthermore, during the course of periodontal therapy, the hygiene methods may have to be modified to fit the new morphological situation (longer teeth, open interdental areas etc.).

The patient must be informed concerning the necessary frequency and duration of home care. Generally speaking, it is necessary to perform a thorough and systematic plaque removal at least one time each day (Lang et al. 1973).

In the final analysis it is not the instruments, nor the technique, nor the amount of time expended that is of prime importance; it is the result, in terms of *freedom from plaque*. Plaque control and gingival condition must be re-evaluated at regular intervals, using disclosing agents and the PBI. To accomplish this, a well-illuminated mirror is required, whether in the operatory or in the patient's bathroom.

Plaque Disclosing Agents

Many times a patient will ask questions about the causes of his periodontal condition, usually when the PBI is being recorded or during case presentation.

This is an opportune time for a demonstration of microbial plaque, the most important etiologic factor in gingivitis and periodontitis. Using vital dyes and food coloring agents, the adherent plaque on tooth surfaces and on gingiva can be selectively stained. The patient can see his own plaque in a mirror, and can watch as the dentist scrapes some off using an explorer or probe.

This demonstrates first of all that it is necessary to remove plaque and second that it is possible to do so by means of oral hygiene procedures. Thereafter, the first oral hygiene instructions fall upon receptive ears.

A disadvantage of plaque disclosing agents is that they tend to remain in the mouth for some time and can be an esthetic problem after an appointment. This disadvantage can be overcome through use of the Plak-Lite system. A solution that is invisible in room light glows bright yellow when exposed to ultraviolet light (Fig. 268).

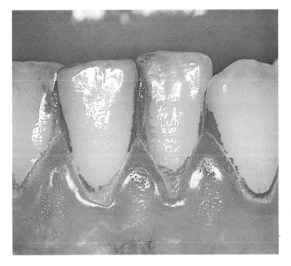
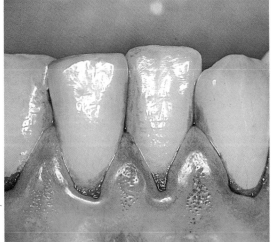

266 Red and violet disclosing agents
The classic agent for plaque disclosure is erythrosin solution (left).

Its disadvantage is that it is the same color as gingiva and the plaque is not as dramatically visible. The Dis-Plaque solution stains plaque violet, which makes it easier to discern from gingival tissues. Furthermore, Dis-Plaque stains older plaque a much deeper color than younger plaque.

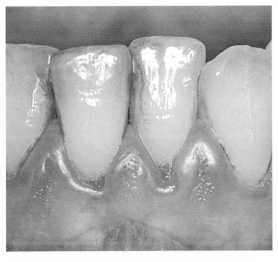
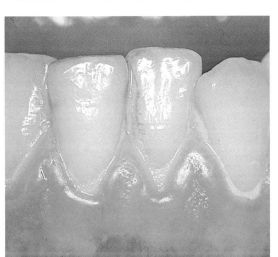

267 Blue-green disclosing agents and Plak-Lite
Vital dyes and food coloring agents such as patent blue have been used to advantage as plaque disclosing agents.

Plaque stained with the Plak-Lite solution is hardly visible in normal light (right).

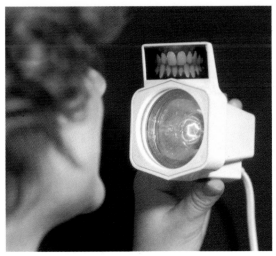
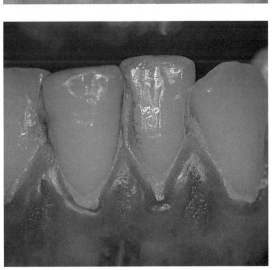

268 UV light and stained plaque
The ingredient in Plak-Lite solution glows a brilliant yellow-green when exposed to UV light. The handy mirror mounted above the UV light source permits the patient to make a close intraoral inspection of plaque accumulation sites.

Toothbrushes

For centuries the toothbrush in its variety of forms has served mankind for removal of plaque and food debris from *occlusal, facial* and *oral* tooth surfaces. Today the toothbrush is still the cornerstone of proper oral hygiene, but it cannot satisfactorily clean in the interdental areas.

There is no "ideal" toothbrush in terms of shape or size, but in the treatment of periodontal disease experience has shown that a manual toothbrush with a short head and multitufted, straight, soft bristles is effective (Riethe 1974). Hard bristles do not damage enamel or

dentin, but may well traumatize the gingivae slightly and thus enhance gingival recession. Synthetic bristles with rounded ends are recommended. The *force* with which the toothbrush bristles are applied to the tooth surface should not exceed 300–400 g.

Electric toothbrushes are no more effective in cleaning than manual toothbrushes. Use of an electric toothbrush must also be demonstrated to the patient, and proper use re-evaluated periodically.

269 Recommended toothbrushes (manual)
A short head, relatively dense bristle bundles and soft synthetic bristles with rounded ends comprise a good toothbrush.

– Bristle thickness: 0.18–0.25 mm
– Bristle length: 10–12 mm, depending on hardness (*Riethe* 1974).

Electric toothbrushes (right, below) are no more effective than hand toothbrushes.

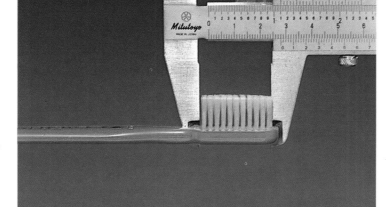 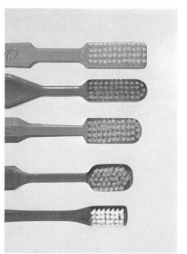

270 Proper bristle contour – Round end
Clinical view of gingiva following a single experimental brushing with a standardized, relatively heavy force (Breitenmoser et al. 1978).

Right: A scanning EM view shows that the bristle ends were *rounded* off during the manufacturing process, and thus do not cause gingival injury. White dot indicates bristle profile.

The blue acrylic block is used to standardize the photographic angulation (*Germann* 1971).

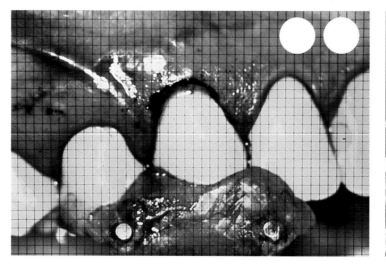 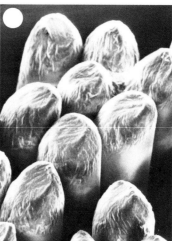

271 Improper bristle contour – Sharp end
Using the same standardized methods as above, the sharp bristles (triangle symbol) elicit easily visible gingival injury. The dark discoloration of the facial gingivae indicates erosion and epithelial damage. *Dis-Plaque* was used as disclosant (courtesy of *W. Mörmann*).

Right: Sharp-ended bristles as seen in scanning electron microscope. These bristles were not rounded during toothbrush fabrication.

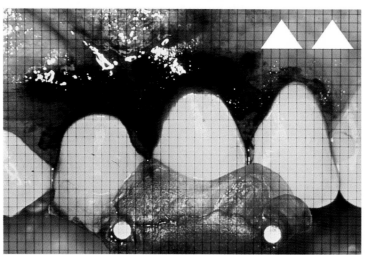 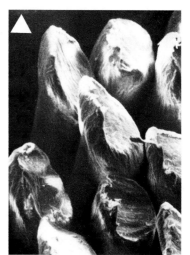

Dentifrices

Toothpastes that contain abrasive compounds improve the mechanical cleansing of the teeth by the toothbrush. Such abrasives can, however, also scratch the tooth surface. Some dentifrices containing medicaments and additives are claimed to be beneficial for the periodontium, but these claims have yet to be substantiated by clinical research.

A dentifrice contains of the following components:
– *Abrasive/polishing substance:* Calcium carbonate, calcium phosphate and sodium phosphate. Modern abrasives such as silica (SiO_2), alumina (Al_2O_3) and aluminum hydroxide ($Al[OH]_3$) are very hard substances which, depending on particle size and homogeneity, can be effective for cleaning and polishing without causing excessive abrasion.
– *Suspending substance* (e.g., carboxymethylcellulose)
– *Surfactant* (e.g., sodium N-laroyl sarcosinate)
– *Flavoring and coloring agents*
– *Fluoride compounds* (not in all products).

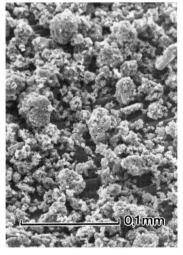
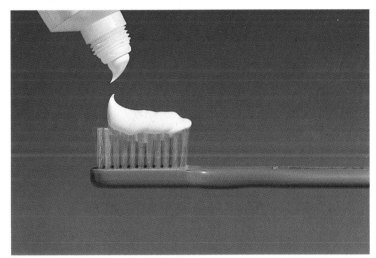

272 The dentifrice
The most important ingredient of any toothpaste is the abrasive. The abrasive effect must be a compromise between excessive abrasion and ineffective cleaning effect.

Left: Sodium metaphosphate powder. This is one of the most often employed abrasives in dentifrices. It is of moderate abrasiveness.

Courtesy of *J.-M. Meyer*

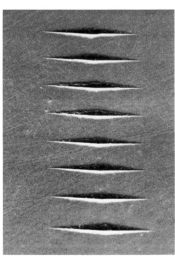
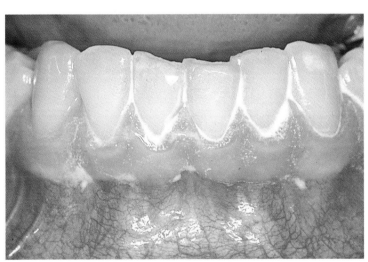

273 Good dentifrice – No enamel abrasion
The clinical picture shows the mandibular anterior area immediately after tootbrushing.
    A dentifrice must not elicit excessive tooth abrasion even after daily use for years.

Left: In experiments with various dentifrices (*Schweizer* 1978), acceptable products did not cause detectable abrasion in a test system measuring effect on artificial enamel indentations.

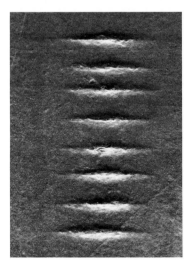
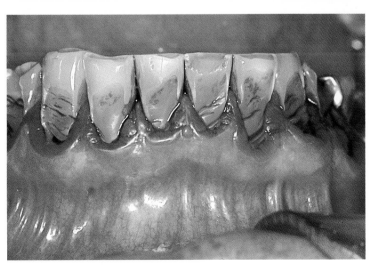

274 Poor dentifrice – Severe enamel abrasion
Highly abrasive dentifrices used with an improper brushing technique can lead to devastating consequences.

Left: The indentations in enamel in the test system (see Fig. 273) have been severely abraded after experimental brushing with a highly abrasive dentifrice.

Courtesy of *Ch. Schweizer*

Toothbrushing Techniques

The goal of toothbrushing is plaque removal. Any method and any means that achieves this goal is acceptable, as long as neither the teeth nor the gingiva are traumatized in the process.

The *"modified Bass technique"* (*Bass* 1954) has proven to be effective for patients with a healthy oral cavitiy, but it is also especially appropriate for patients with gingivitis or periodontitis. The bristles are placed onto the tooth surface at a 45° angle and small vibratory or circular motions are made, which force the bristle tips into accessible interdental areas and into the gingival sulci. Plaque removal from these particularly vulnerable areas is thus accomplished.

The *"vertical-rotatory method"* (modified *Stillman*) is appropriate for periodontally healthy patients as well as for those manifesting generalized gingival recession. The bristles are moved from the gingiva toward the tooth with a simultaneous rotatory movement around the bristle long axis.

Modified Bass technique

275 Placement of the toothbrush
Toothbrush bristles positioned perpendicular to the tooth long axis will not effectively clean the interdental spaces unless heavy force is applied. This would be accompanied by the danger of gingival injury.

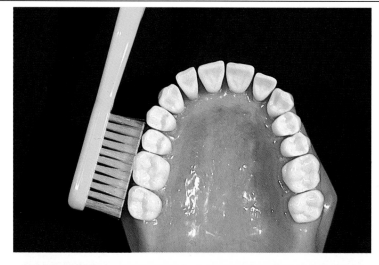

276 45° angle of the bristles
When the brush is applied at a 45° angle to the teeth, and then rotated toward occlusal plane, the bristles slip easily into the interdental areas and gingival sulci *without* excessive force. With the brush in this position, small rotary or vibratory movements can effectively remove plaque.

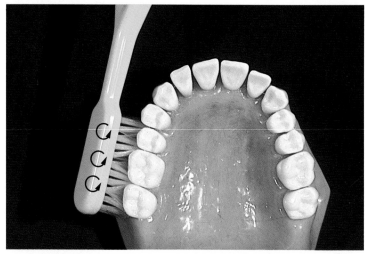

277 45° angle – Distal surface
When viewed from the distal aspect, the position of the bristles in the Bass technique becomes clear.

Contact points between teeth cannot be reached by any toothbrush nor through any toothbrushing technique. Therefore, additional oral hygiene aids for interdental cleaning are necessary.

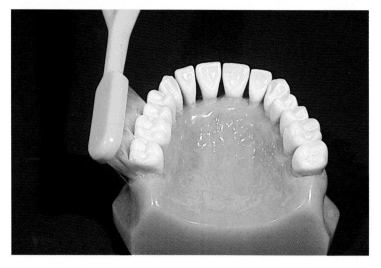

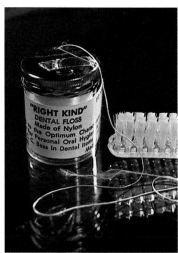

Systematic Toothbrushing

Freedom from plaque is the result of more than just the shape of the toothbrush, the dentifrice or the toothbrushing technique. It is the product of a systematic and logical tooth cleaning procedure by which each surface of each tooth is cleaned.

A systematic approach will eliminate accumulations of plaque in areas that are generally left untouched (see Plaque Indices, p. 27).

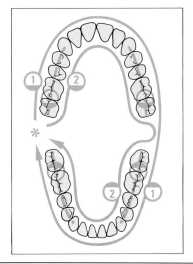

278 Systematic toothbrushing
This procedure has proven effective. The starting point is the upper right sextant (∗).

1. Facial surfaces of maxilla and mandible
2. Distal surfaces of the most distal teeth in each arch, and all oral (palatal, lingual) surfaces in both arches
3. Occlusal surfaces upper and lower

4. *Interdental areas* with special OH aids (see pp. 116–117).

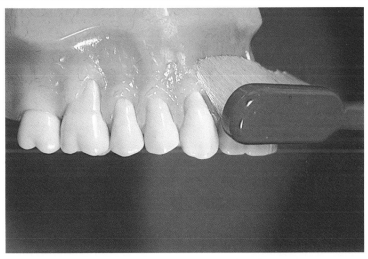

Modified Stillman Technique (vertical-rotatory brushing)

279 Initial phase of the movement – From red...
The bristles are placed onto the attached gingiva with light pressure at a 45° angle to the tooth long axis. The bristles bend and do not injure the gingival tissue.

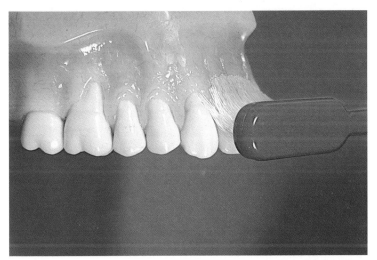

280 [Middle phase]
The toothbrush handle is now approximately parallel to the tooth surface. The bristles are still bent sharply upwards. The lateral surfaces of the bristles exert a massaging effect on the gingiva.

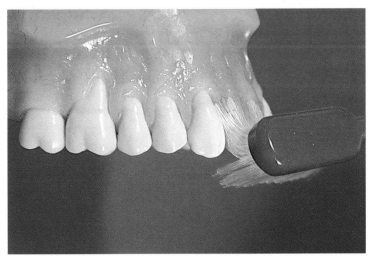

281 ...To white – Final phase of the movement
The toothbrush head is rotated under pressure away from the tooth, and the bristle tips effectively clean embrasure areas as well as the facial tooth surfaces. Plaque accumulations at the gingival margin are effectively removed.
This series of brush movements is repeated 5–10 times in the same area, then the brush head is moved either mesially or distally and the same series of movements performed on another 2–3 tooth segment of the arch.

Interdental Hygiene

Gingivitis and periodontitis are generally more severe in the interdental areas than on the facial and oral surfaces. Caries, too, is more frequent on interproximal surfaces than on facial or oral smooth surfaces. For these reasons, interdental hygiene – which cannot be achieved using a toothbrush alone – is of particular importance for the periodontitis patient.

The proper interdental hygiene aids must be selected on the basis of each patient's individual requirements. There are many different aids available commercially; the appropriate choice depends primarily upon the morphology of the interdental areas.

In a healthy periodontium, and in cases of gingivitis or crowded teeth, the use of *dental floss* should be taught and practiced.

If the interdental areas are open, for example after completion of periodontal therapy, *tooth picks* (or Stimudents) or *interdental brushes* may be appropriate for interdental plaque removal, depending upon the size of the interdental spaces.

282 Interdental space size and hygiene aids
The choice of an aid for interdental hygiene depends primarily on the size of the interdental space:

A. Dental floss: indicated for narrow interdental spaces

B. Toothpicks/Stimudents: for slightly open spaces

C. Interdental brushes: for interdental spaces that are wide open

All of these aids are associated with some advantages and some disadvantages.

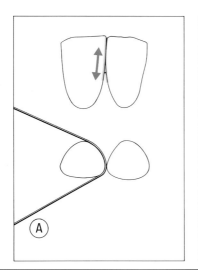
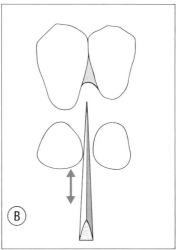
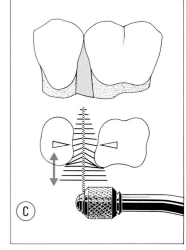

283 Dental Floss
Unwaxed or lightly waxed floss should be recommended. Dental floss is composed of numerous individual filaments.

The floss holder shown here may be useful in patients who lack manual dexterity.

For special cases such as cleansing of interdental areas beneath bridge pontics or bars, brush-like dental floss such as
"Brush and floss" (far right) and
"Superfloss" may be recommended.

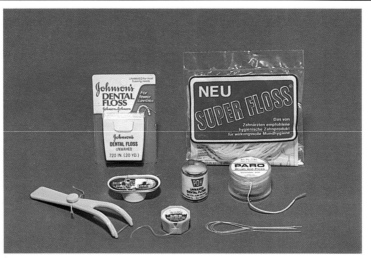
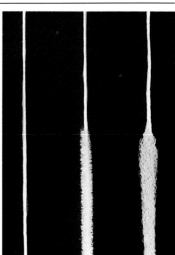

284 Use of dental floss
In order to avoid injury to the interdental papillae, the floss is guided with a sawing motion through the interdental contact point. Within the interdental area, the floss is first pulled against a tooth surface, then moved apically and occlusally (double arrow). The neighboring tooth is then cleaned identically.

Horizontal sawing motions for plaque removal are effective only with "Superfloss" or "Brush and floss."

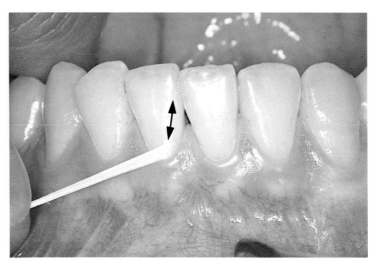

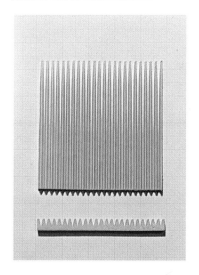

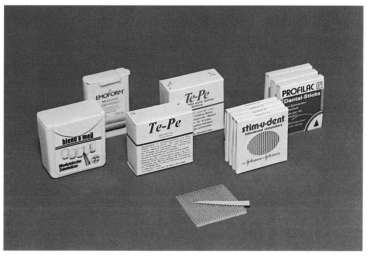

285 Wooden toothpicks

The ideal interdental toothpick has a triangular profile that approximates the shape of the interdental area. Different manufacturers use woods of varying hardness (balsa, birch, linden). Most commercially available wooden stimulators are effective as interdental hygiene aids if used properly.

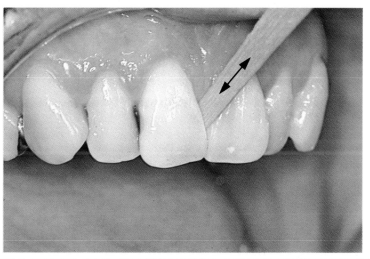

286 Use of wooden toothpicks

The tip is inserted into the interdental space from a slightly oblique angle, as shown.

Plaque removal is accomplished by horizontal back-and-forth movement (double arrow). If the interdental space is wide, the surface of one tooth is first cleaned by applying slight pressure to one side, then the adjacent tooth is similarly cleaned.

Remember: The contact point itself cannot be cleaned using these wooden aids (caries!).

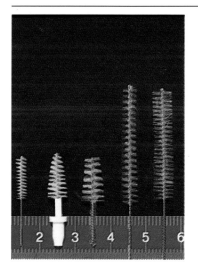

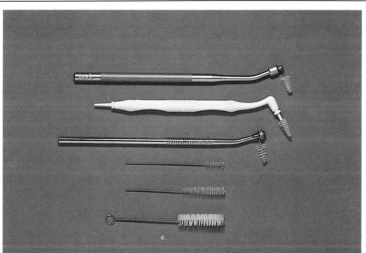

287 Interdental brushes

If interdental spaces are wide open, the interdental (spiral) brush is the ideal hygiene aid.

Many different varieties of interdental brushes are available, some with interchangeable heads and others with extended metal handles. If the cervical areas of the teeth are sensitive, an interdental brush with a plastic coating over the wire is advisable.

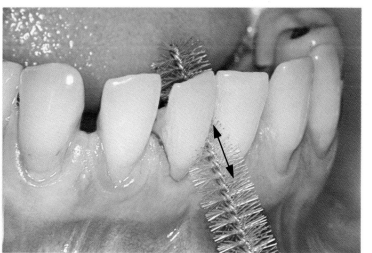

288 Use of interdental brushes

The brush is inserted obliquely from an apical direction, as with wooden toothpicks, accommodating the morphology of the interdental papilla.

Cleaning is accomplished by back-and-forth movements. Usually no toothpaste is used, to preclude abrasion of exposed dentin. However, if staining is a problem, a dentifrice with a mild abrasive may be used once daily or weekly.

Special Cleaning Aids – Irrigation Devices

In general, two hygiene instruments are necessary for plaque control: *One* toothbrush and *one* instrument for interdental hygiene.

It is often counterproductive to recommend half a dozen "special instruments" for the patient, because these will be neither regularly nor systematically employed. Nevertheless, for patients with fixed bridgework and partial dentures there are additional hygiene aids for removal of plaque and food debris.

The *oral irrigator* is only an adjunct in oral hygiene. The stream of water cannot remove adherent microbial plaque, and therefore cannot replace the toothbrush or the interdental hygiene aid. An irrigator can, however, effectively remove some non-adherent plaque and food debris from the oral cavity.

For patients with extensive reconstructions, the oral irrigator may be indicated. It is generally used with water, but this can be replaced with a dilute chlorhexidine solution for prevention of plaque accumulation (Lang & Ramseier-Grossmann 1981).

289 Special cleaning aids
These may be beneficial as adjuncts to the toothbrush and interdental aids for cleaning difficult-to-reach areas, plaque-retentive areas and peculiar morphological situations.

– **Interdental/marginal brushes**
– **Rubber and plastic stimulators**
– **Round toothpicks in a holder** (Perio-Aid)
– **Superfloss** with a stiff end for insertion
– **Threaders** for dental floss.

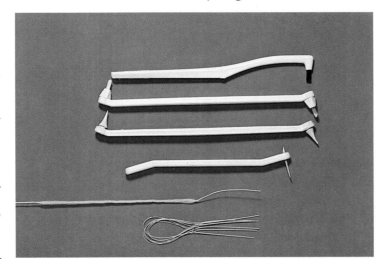

290 Use of special cleaning aids
– *Interdental/marginal brush:* Beneath bridge pontics, bars etc., the use of special hygiene aids is frequently mandatory.

– *Threading devices for floss:* In areas with soldered contact points and beneath bars, normal dental floss is inserted using a threading device. In this way, even soldered interdental areas can be maintained plaque- and inflammation-free.

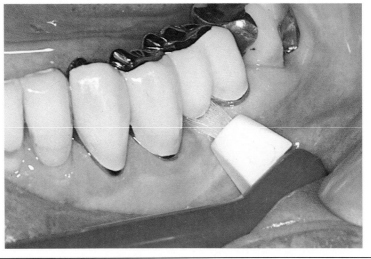
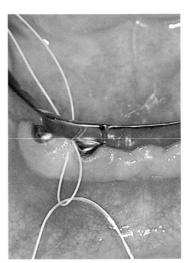

291 Irrigators
Single-stream (e.g., Aquapik) or multi-stream (e.g., Broxojet) irrigators cannot remove adherent microbial plaque. However, following mechanical plaque removal with toothbrush and other instruments, an irrigator can effectively rinse the oral cavity free of particulate matter, including removed plaque accumulations loosened by the toothbrush or floss.

A dilute chlorhexidine solution (CHX = 0.05%) may be used in an irrigator to effect a significant reduction in plaque accumulation.

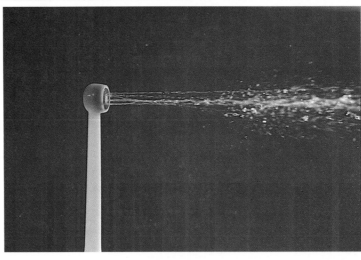

Chemical Plaque Control – Chlorhexidine (CHX)

Removal of plaque by the patient or by the dentist using mechanical means is never 100% effective.

For decades, therefore, a goal of dental research has been to discover a rinsing solution that would inhibit plaque formation. With the introduction of chlorhexidine by Davies et al. in 1956, a topical chemotherapeutic agent became available that to a great degree achieved the goal of chemical plaque control.

Because of its side effects, CHX should be used only for short periods of time.

1. Chlorhexidine digluconate (water soluble)
Because of its cationic characteristics, chlorhexidine has a high affinity for the cell wall of microorganisms, and depending upon its concentration it may be either bacteriostatic or bactericidal. It has an extended effectiveness because of its anionic bonding to pellicle and salivary glycoproteins which coat the entire oral cavity. Rinsing twice daily with 0.2% chlorhexidine solution will lead to almost total inhibition of plaque formation in the long term (Löe & Schiött 1970).

Chlorhexidine
digluconate

Chemical formula

$$C_{22}H_{30}Cl_2N_{10}, 2C_6H_{12}O_7$$

Gluconic acid

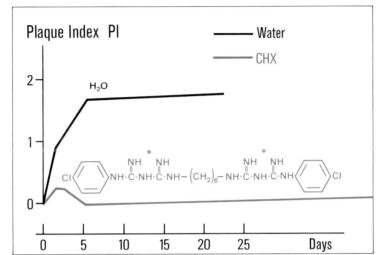

292 Chlorhexidine (CHX)
The basic substance of chlorhexidine is a water-insoluble powder with highly basic properties.

Chlorhexidine digluconate
The water-soluble, neutral digluconate of CHX is frequently used as a mucosal and skin disinfectant (formulae see left side).

If routine oral hygiene measures are replaced by water rinsing alone, microbial plaque accumulates within a few days. If CHX (0.1–0.2%) is used twice a day (30 sec.) for rinsing instead of water, no such accumulation occurs.

293 Staining by CHX
If CHX rinsing is performed for weeks, the teeth (pellicle) and tongue take on a brownish discoloration that is reversible if CHX rinsing is halted.

The unesthetic staining may become so heavy in enamel fissures and on dentin that it can be removed only through use of highly abrasive substances, or with the Prophy-Jet (p. 124).

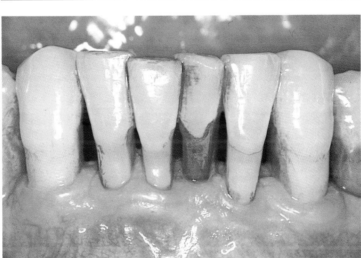

**294 High concentration –
Mucosal desquamation**
Use of excessively high CHX concentrations may elicit severe, painful desquamation. The lesions heal spontaneously and rapidly if CHX rinsing is halted. Desquamation almost never is observed with use of commercially available CHX oral rinses containing normal, low (0.1–0.2%) chlorhexidine concentrations.

Indications for CHX digluconate:
- Disinfection of the oral cavity before each dental treatment
- ANUG (Gingivitis ulcerosa)
- As an adjunct during initial therapy, especially in cases of RPP and LJP
- Following periodontal surgery
- In handicapped patients.

Side effects of CHX digluconate:
- Staining of teeth and tongue
- Taste disturbances
- Mucosal desquamation.

2. Chlorhexidine dihydrochloride
As its hydrochloride (–HCl), chlorhexidine is a practically *water-insoluble* white powder of neutral pH, which is quite easy to incorporate into most periodontal packs and dressings. Tooth and root surfaces beneath such periodontal dressings are significantly cleaner after 5 days than when dressings without CHX-dihydrochloride are used (Plüss et al. 1975).

Chlorhexidine rinses should not be routinely prescribed for extended periods of time, since they contain residues of *chloraniline* from the manufacturing process.

295   Plaque inhibition beneath periodontal dressing
Clinical picture immediately after removal of a periodontal dressing, 7 days after a gingivoplasty.
The CHX-HCl incorporated into the dressing almost completely inhibited plaque accumulation. The coronal portions of the teeth were not covered by the dressing, and a disclosing agent reveals gross plaque accumulation.

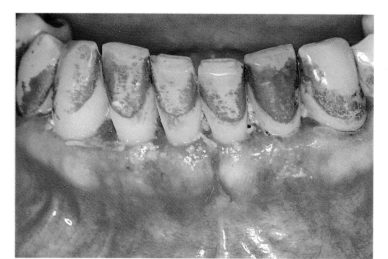

Chlorhexidine – Dihydrochloride

Chemical formula

$$C_{22}H_{30}Cl_2N_{10}, 2HCl$$

296   Normal wound healing in a standardized mucosal wound after rinsing with Ringer's solution
A standardized 2 mm wide punch biopsy on the rat palate (dashed lines indicate wound) was rinsed twice daily with Ringer's solution for one week. Healing was without complications when evaluated clinically and histologically (Goldner, × 40).

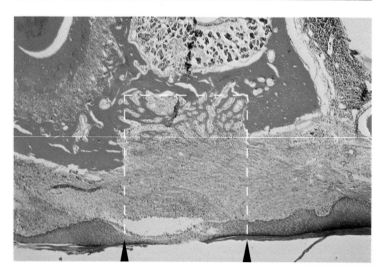

297   Disturbed wound healing in a standardized mucosal wound after rinsing with 0.5% CHX solution
The standardized wound in the rat palate was rinsed twice daily with a high concentration CHX digluconate solution (0.5%). Wound healing was severely impaired. Note that the wound is filled with granulation tissue and fibrin, and exhibits no re-epithelialization even after 7 days (Goldner, × 40; *Bassetti & Kallenberger* 1980).

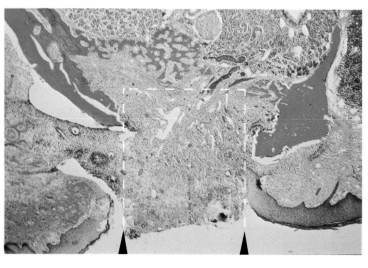

Professional Care – Creating Conditions that Enhance Hygiene

This phase of therapy coupled with good patient home care is often all that is required for treatment of gingivitis and initial periodontitis. For treatment of advanced periodontitis, creation of hygienic relationships is the most important phase.

Active professional treatment should begin even as oral hygiene instruction, patient motivation and evaluation of home care are ongoing. The patient cannot be expected to improve his oral hygiene if the preconditions for good hygiene are not simultaneously created. Professional prophylaxis is particularly important in this regard, as well as elimination of plaque-retentive areas and harbors for bacterial accumulation. The following pages contain details concerning:

- Gross debridement – Supragingival calculus removal
- Fine debridement – Definitive and complete removal of supragingival plaque, calculus and stain
- Removal of iatrogenic irritants – Creation of conditions conducive to oral hygiene
- Removal of natural plaque-retentive areas
- Extraction of "hopeless" teeth
- Odontoplasty – The "opening" of grooves, irregularities and furcations
- Morphologic selective grinding in cases of crowding.

- Subgingival plaque and calculus removal
- Root planing
- (Soft tissue curettage; the transition to surgery).

The various treatments performed during initial therapy cannot be strictly separated from one another, either in the presentations that follow in this book, or in the practice of dentistry. At a single appointment, calculus removal, elimination of amalgam overhangs, minor odontoplasty and occlusal equilibration may be accomplished together.

Subgingival treatment may include simultaneous calculus removal, root planing and perhaps even soft tissue curettage.

Soft tissue curettage is really an initial phase of surgical therapy, but it cannot always be separated entirely from root planing, and is therefore considered in this book as part of initial therapy.

Gross Scaling – Supragingival Calculus Removal Instruments and Materials...

The removal of calculus, deposits and stains is a pains-taking, routine endeavor. For decades it has been accomplished by means of hand instruments as well as polishing pastes applied with rotating brushes and rubber cups.

The dental marketplace offers an innumerable variety of scalers and curettes, which, if properly used, will accomplish the task of removing deposits. Many manufacturers produce high quality steel instruments with excellent form, balance and sharpness. But success of treatment depends more on the operator's skill and manual dexterity than on the instrument.

For supragingival gross debridement, the most useful instruments are straight and angled *scalers, chisels* and perhaps a *lingual scaler. Curettes* may also have to be used during gross scaling procedures, especially in bicuspid and molar areas, in grooves and in irregularities on the crown and on exposed roots.

298   Scalers
Sharp, pointed scalers in various shapes are indicated for supragingival calculus removal and for accretions that lie only a few millimeters below the gingival margin. From left to right (color coded):

- **Chisel** (white)
- **Scalers,** straight and paired L and R (blue)
- **Lingual scaler** (black)

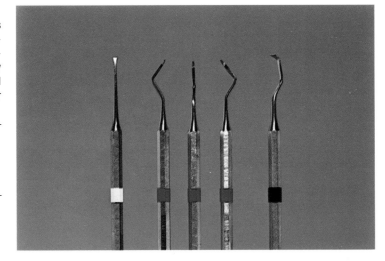

299   Curettes
For subgingival accretions that can be removed without anesthesia, the scaler armamentarium may be enhanced by curettes (see also p. 138, Figs. 342 & 343). From left to right (color coded):

- **Universal curettes** (yellow), 1.2 mm wide
- **Anterior curettes** (orange)
- **Posterior curettes** (red) Anterior and posterior curettes are 0.95 mm wide

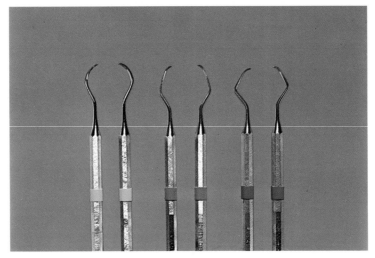

300   Abrasive prophy pastes
During gross debridement, the dental prophylaxis begun by the use of scalers and curettes is completed using polishing pastes of moderate to heavy abrasiveness.
   The figure depicts a scanning EM view of the abrasive in a typical highly abrasive prophy paste (Nupro Red).
   In principle, only the least abrasive paste that is effective in cleaning should be used, due to the possibility of scratching and abrading the tooth surface.
SEM courtesy of *J.-M. Meyer*

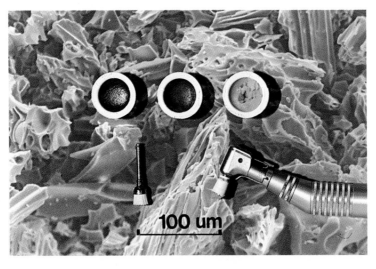

100 um

...and Their Uses

Curettes may also be used if subgingival deposits are to be removed during the initial gross scaling. In many patients this is possible without local anesthesia.

If calculus is covered by thick soft deposits, these should be removed with brushes and coarse cleaning paste before gross scaling begins, to lessen the severity of the bacteremia that inevitably follows scaling and root planing. A pre-scaling rinse with disinfectant (e.g., chlorhexidine) is also advisable.

Following calculus removal, the teeth are always polished using a rubber cup and prophy paste. Polishing of the crowns and exposed root surfaces may also be performed using a dentifrice. The rubber cup can be used with care to polish tooth surfaces *below* the gingival margin; the sulcus should be thoroughly irrigated afterwords.

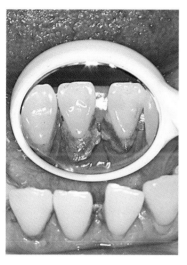
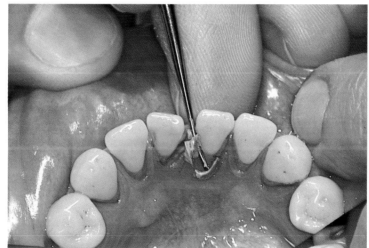

301 Supragingival calculus removal
The chisel is the only instrument that is used with a pushing motion. It is effective for removal of gross lingual supragingival calculus in the mandibular anterior, cuspid and premolar areas by pushing from the facial aspects through the interdental spaces.
    After the collar of calculus is removed with the chisel, straight and curved scalers are used to remove remaining deposits.

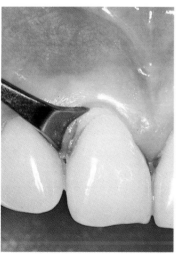
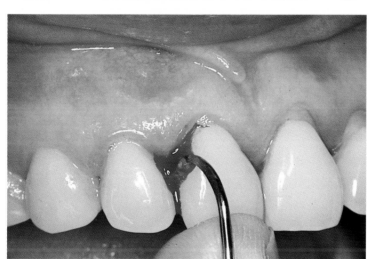

302 Removal of subgingival accretions
Using scalers, calculus adherent to the tooth just below the gingival margin (left) can often be removed without local anesthesia during the initial gross scaling appointment. Curved curettes can accomplish this more effectively.
    Even a careful operator will injure the ulcerated pocket epithelium when removing subgingival deposits, resulting in gingival hemorrhage.

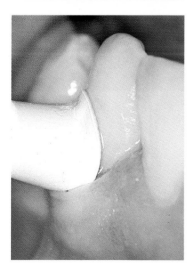
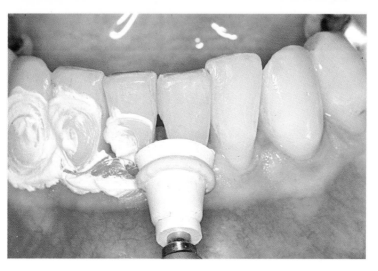

303 Polishing with rubber cup and prophy paste
Each time scaling is performed, the teeth must be polished, otherwise remaining rough surfaces will enhance re-accumulation of plaque bacteria. The rubber cup with prophy paste is the best polishing method, since rotating brushes are not as "kind" to the gingival tissues. When applied carefully, a rubber cup can also clean the clinical sulcus 1–2 mm below the gingival margin.

Fine Scaling and Polishing Instruments and Materials...

Removal of all deposits and stains via scaling, root planing and polishing is a modality utilized in initial therapy of gingivitis and periodontitis, as a preventive measure in periodontally healthy individuals, and as maintenance therapy following periodontal treatment.

This preventive therapy "without end" necessitates effective utilization of auxiliary personnel such as the dental hygienist. It also demands practice rationalization, standardization, work simplification and innovation in the use of instruments.

Soft deposits that are difficult to remove, e. g., stains from tobacco, chlorhexidine, tea, wine and foodstuffs, as well as microbial plaque, may be quickly removed from tooth surfaces with an abrasive spray (Prophy Jet). The sodium bicarbonate ($NaHCO_3$) that is added to the water is rather abrasive to dentin (Atkinson et al. 1984). For this reason, the Prophy Jet should not be directed at a single spot on a tooth for too long. Superficial injuries of the gingiva are also possible. The cleaning efficiency is not as high in the interproximal areas.

304 Prophy Jet
The abrasive powder is composed primarily of sodium bicarbonate, which is mixed with water and sprayed onto the stains destined for removal.

Use of a high capacity evacuation system is advisable because of the Prophy Jet's high efflux volume.

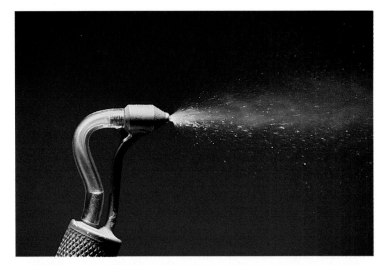

305 Ultrasonic scaler
Various ultrasonic instruments for dental prophylaxis are available. The necessary water coolant is directed onto the working tip either through a separate tube or through the working tip itself.

Ultrasonic instruments have an output of 25,000–50,000 oscillations per second (Hz) at very small and regulable amplitude (resonance frequency).

Ultrasonic instruments can also be used to advantage for gross scaling.

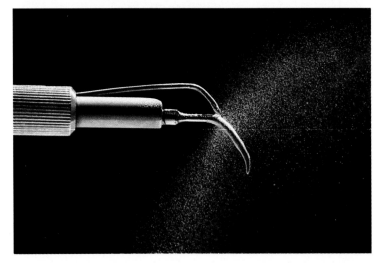
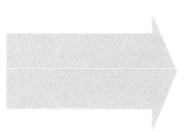

306 Standardized prophylaxis pastes
These pastes are available in various degrees of abrasiveness, and all contain fluoride (Svedia Dental).

The standardization is based on their relative dentin abrasion (RDA):

RDA 40: Mild abrasion
RDA 120: Normal abrasion
RDA 170: Moderate abrasion
RDA 250: High abrasion

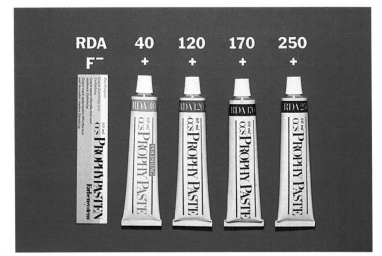

...and Their Uses

Calculus that becomes visible after a Prophy Jet cleaning can be removed either with an ultrasonic instrument (e.g., Cavitron) or with fine hand instruments. Subsequently, the teeth must be polished using a rubber cup and an abrasive paste, which is now available in various forms (Fig. 306), based on *relative dentin abrasion (RDA)*. Interdental areas are finished using very fine polishing strips (Fig. 309).

Gross and fine debridement overlap to some degree in practice and may often be accomplished at a single appointment.

The *effect* of professional tooth cleaning in gingivitis cases is a massive reduction of supragingival plaque flora and, as a result of this, healing of the marginal gingiva with disappearance of inflammatory symptoms.

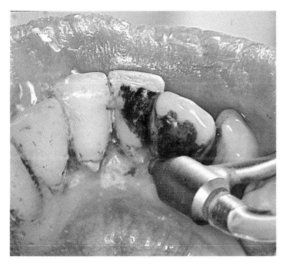
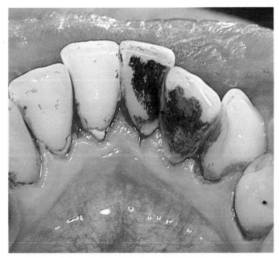

307   Removal of soft deposits and stains with the Prophy Jet
Tough deposits, microbial plaque and stains from tobacco, tea, wine, CHX etc. can be easily removed from accessible tooth surfaces using the Prophy Jet. Cleaning in interdental areas is not adequate; the Prophy Jet is not the instrument of choice for this area.

The spray stream should be directed at a 45° angle to the tooth surface. The chairside assistant removes detritus and water with a high capacity evacuation system.

The spray should never be directed into the sulcus or pocket.

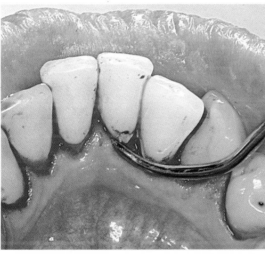
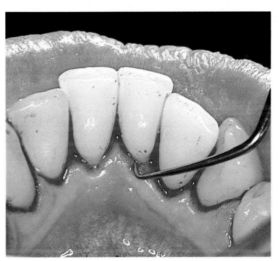

308   Removal of hard supragingival deposits on the crown using an ultrasonic instrument
Left: After stains and soft deposits are removed, the ultrasonic instrument is used to completely remove any remaining calculus. In narrow, difficult-to-reach areas, fine hand instruments must also be employed after the Cavitron.

Right: Using a fine explorer, the operator checks to be sure that all accretions have been eliminated, especially at the cementoenamel junction.

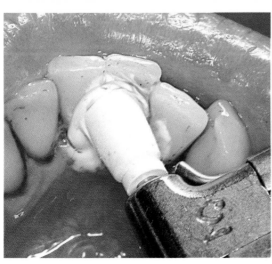
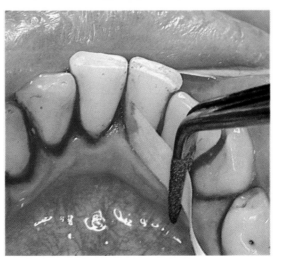

309   Polishing
Left: Polishing of the teeth is performed using progressively milder abrasive pastes (RDA 170 – 120 – 40).

Rubber cups and paste are used on occlusal, facial and oral tooth surfaces.

Right: Interproximal surfaces and contact points are cleaned and polished using polishing strips and paste.

Removal of Iatrogenic Irritants – Amalgam Overhangs – Creation of Conditions that Enhance Good Oral Hygiene

Concurrent with gross scaling, all imperfect dental restorations are corrected with the goal of creating smooth supra- and subgingival tooth surfaces as well as impeccable transition areas between natural tooth structure and the margins of restorations and crowns. Only when this is achieved will it be possible for the patient to practice effective interdental hygiene. It is not the overhanging margin *per se* that causes periodontal injury, it is the fact that the area is not accessible for plaque removal.

Amalgam overhangs can be removed using flame-shaped diamonds and periodontal files, but Proxoshape files (EVA System) accomplish the task with greater ease (Mörmann et al. 1983). Contact points are smoothed using special abrasive strips.

Deep caries is a reservoir for bacteria and should be excavated immediately and restored temporarily.

Massive irritants such as depressable partial denture clasps and saddles may traumatize the periodontium directly.

310 Amalgam overhang – Prime symptom of careless dentistry
Inadequate restorations, especially pronounced on tooth 24, create plaque-retentive areas and thus foster gingivitis, periodontitis and caries. Such restorations render interdental hygiene impossible. Dental floss catches and shreads despite proper technique.

The radiograph clearly reveals the exceptionally poor amalgam margins.

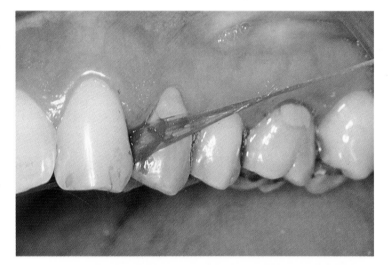 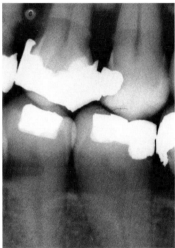

311 Initial occlusal view
The old, rough, corroded amalgam surface must be smoothed and polished. Note the improper contact with adjacent tooth, overcontoured margin, secondary caries, supra- and subgingival calculus, and gingivitis.
    Very poor or broken down restorations should be removed immediately and replaced with either a temporary or a definitive restoration.

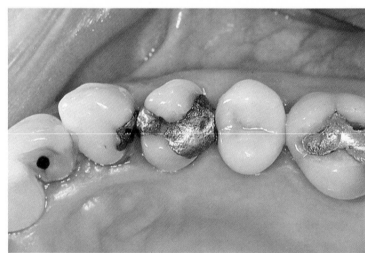

312 Initial removal of overhang
Following recontouring and polishing of the restoration surface, the gross overhang is removed by means of a flame-shaped coarse diamond. Then a fine diamond is used to achieve a final smoothing of the margin.

Right: Enlarged view of diamond burs, one with 75 μm particle size, the other with 15 μm.

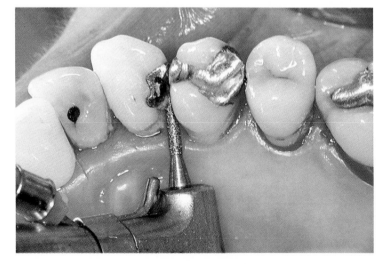 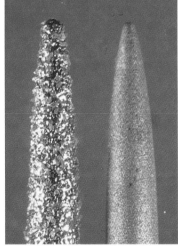

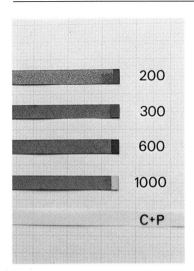

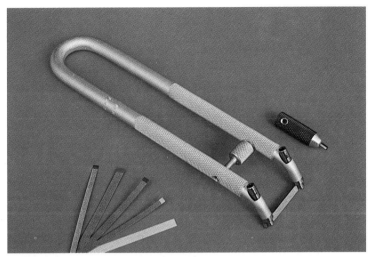

313 Strip holder – Strips with standardized abrasiveness

The task of removing amalgam overhangs can be greatly simplified through use of a strip holder, with which diamond-coated strips can be held either loosely (for filling margins) or tightly (for smooth surfaces).

Left:

- **Diamond-coated steel strips**
  Standardized thin strips with graded coarseness (GC/Fuji)
- **Fine polishing strip** (3M)

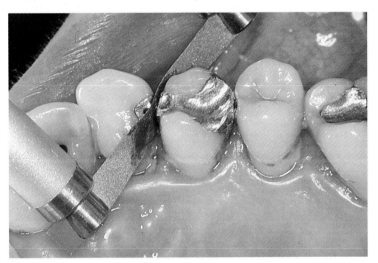

314 Contouring the proximal surface of an amalgam restoration

Using diamond strips, the rough mesial surface of the amalgam restoration is contoured and smoothed.

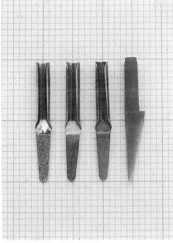

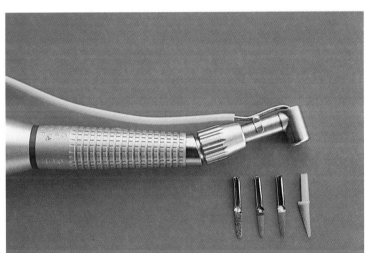

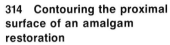

315 EVA System and Proxoshape files

Since the introduction of the EVA handpiece, mechanical filing for recontouring of restorations has been possible. The water-cooled, flexible Proxoshape files easily remove overhangs and polish narrow interdental areas (*Mörmann* et al. 1983).

Left:

- **Proxoshape files**
  (Intensiv Co.)
  Diamond coatings of 75 µm, 40 µm (yellow) and 15 µm (red)
- **EVA polishing file** (plastic)

316 Polishing the proximal surface of a restoration

Using the finest file (15 µm, red), the junction of amalgam with tooth surface is polished.

The radiograph of tooth 24 depicts the absence of any overhang (compare Fig. 10). The secondary caries on 25 was excavated and a temporary restoration placed.

Proper contouring of proximal restorations and crown margins makes it possible for the patient to practice optimum interdental hygiene.

Removal of Iatrogenic Irritants – Overhanging Crown Margins

The open margins of full cast crowns that extend below the gingival margin represent particularly massive iatrogenic irritants that can lead to destruction of periodontal tissues. Every subgingival margin is a potential plaque-retentive area that can foster caries and periodontal disorder (Hammer & Hotz 1979). Compromises should only be tolerated for esthetic reasons in the anterior area.

The removal of a subgingival and/or open crown margin during initial therapy is generally only a temporary measure. Thereafter the old crowns or bridges serve as fixed temporary restorations. Following completion of periodontal therapy, these restorations are usually replaced.

Removal of overhanging crown margins is accomplished using diamond burs. An attendant problem is the incorporation of gold fillings into the gingival tissues. Severely open or overhanging crown margins may be removed through use of a finishing bur or a round bur supragingivally (Fig. 317).

317 Subgingival overhanging crown margins
Iatrogenic irritants are easy to recognize both clinically and radiographically (arrows). Plaque accumulates beneath the open margin, and gingivitis may persist for years.

The overhang may be removed with a diamond *supragingivally,* or a round bur may be used to remove the entire crown margin, as depicted here.

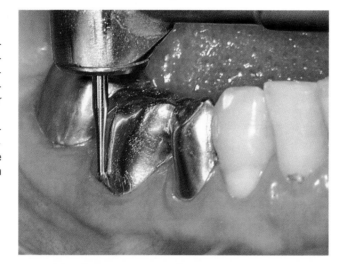
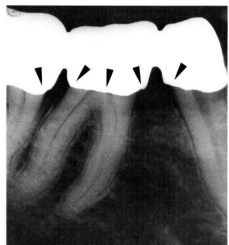

318 Overhanging crown margin removed
Caries is often encountered following radical removal of an overhanging subgingival crown margin. Before initial therapy, this carious process could not be diagnosed either radiographically or clinically.

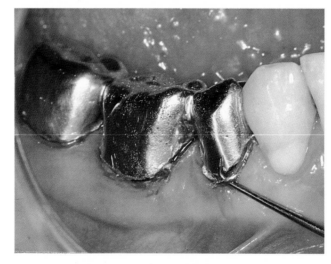
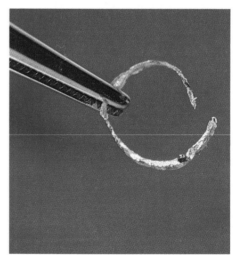

319 Crown margins now supragingival
The old crowns serve nicely as "temporaries" following treatment of the cervical caries. Interdental hygiene can be accomplished using Stimudents.

These crowns will be replaced following completion of periodontal therapy. There is no reason to splint these well-supported teeth using soldered crowns.

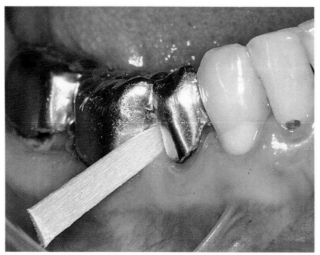
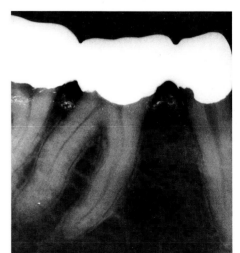

Correction of Iatrogenic Irritants – Bridge Pontics

Pontics in the *anterior area* should lightly contact the attached gingiva but not the mucosa. There must be no pressure exerted upon the marginal gingiva of the adjacent abutment teeth. In *posterior areas,* where esthetics is not a consideration, it is often beneficial to leave ca. 2 mm of space beneath pontics to facilitate use of hygiene aids in the removal of plaque *under* the pontic.

A facetted pontic makes it easier to use interdental brushes, Stimudents or Superfloss to clean abutment teeth, because of the guidance that is absent when the pontic is far removed from the gingiva or when a bar-like pontic is used.

Improperly constructed bridge pontics may be corrected on an emergency basis using flame-shaped diamonds. The undersurface of pontics treated in this manner can be polished almost to laboratory smoothness using Proxoshape files (15 μm abrasiveness).

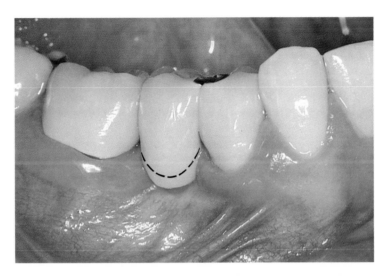

320 Improper bridge pontic form
This pontic is too long and its saddle shape contacts both attached gingiva and mobile oral mucosa on the facial aspect. It is also too wide, contacts the mesial abutment over a broad expanse, encroaches on the mesial gingival papilla, and precludes any interdental hygiene.
The planned shortening and contouring is indicated by the dashed line.

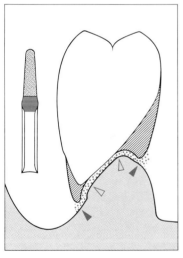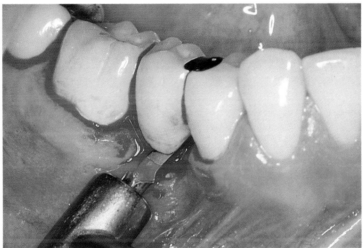

321 Correction of the pontic
The fixed bridge is otherwise clinically acceptable. Thus the indicated procedure is to use flame-shaped diamonds to shorten and recontour the improper pontic especially at its mesial and distal aspects. Proxoshape files are used after recontouring to smooth the undersurface of the pontic where the diamonds were used.

Diagram: The massive plaque retention area beneath the pontic (solid arrows) is reduced considerably (open arrows) by the recontouring process (hatched areas).

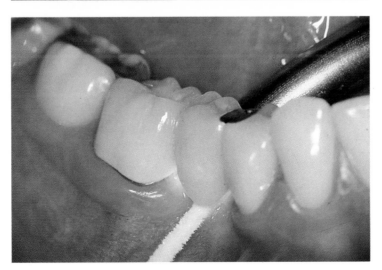

322 Pontic area accessible for hygiene
After the soft tissues heal, optimal hygiene is possible in the interdental areas and under the pontic using Superfloss or Brush and Floss.

The fiber optic light used from the lingual aspect reveals healthy keratinized gingiva.

The cervical extent of fixed restorations, from a simple amalgam to extensive bridgework should be located supragingivally whenever possible, and should exhibit optimum closure at the margins. Correction of inadequate fixed restorations can be difficult, and does not always lead to the desired success.

In addition, attempting to correct subgingival inadequacies in fixed restorations is almost always accompanied by gingival trauma. Metal dust or fine particles of metal may become sequestered within the soft tissue, usually without any clinical sequelae.

Silver amalgam lodged in soft tissue often presents as a clinical "tatoo" that is esthetically undesirable. Histologically a foreign body reaction can be observed. Amalgam particles may be phagocytosed by connective tissue cells, decomposed and transported within the tissue, leading to an expansion of the clinical tatoo.

Amalgam **Gold**

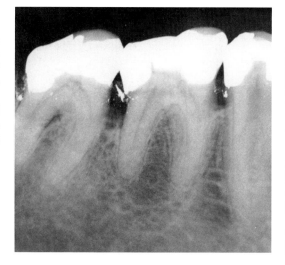
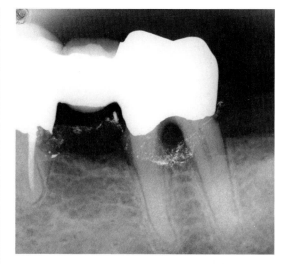

323 Metal pigmentation viewed radiographically
Large particles of amalgam (left) and gold dust (right) are visible in the radiographs after removal of overhangs. Some particles are expelled from the tissue.

It is impossible to remove all metal fragments, even by means of curettage of the sulcus/pocket wall.

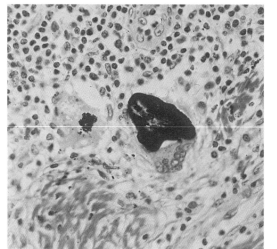
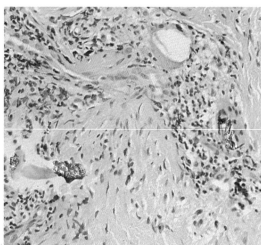

324 Reaction of gingival tissue
Left: Two amalgam particles surrounded by an infiltrate of multinucleated foreign body giant cells (Masson, ×250).

Right: Gold particle in the gingiva without any visible reaction of the tissue (H&E, ×250).

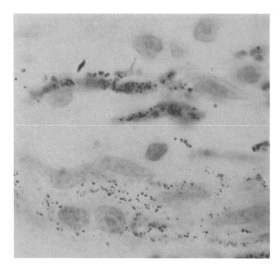
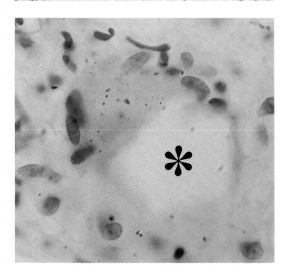

325 Phagocytosis – Foreign body reaction
Left: Amalgam can be degraded within connective tissue, whereupon fibroblasts phagocytose the amalgam dust (Masson, ×1000)

Right: A large gold particle (✳) was lost from the tissue during sectioning for histological examination. Multinucleated foreign body giant cells surround the area (H&E, ×1000).

Removal of Natural Plaque-Retentive Areas – Extraction

If hopeless teeth are not extracted on an emergency basis, then the extraction should be performed at the latest during the hygiene phase of therapy. The deep and usually active periodontal pockets surrounding such teeth represent enormous bacterial reservoirs. These endanger the interdental septa of adjacent teeth and therefore the periodontal support of these mesial and distal teeth may continue to be compromised. Before extraction of the hopeless tooth, any restorations in the adjacent teeth should be polished. Immediately after extraction, the interproximal crown and root surfaces of the adjacent teeth can be cleaned and polished.

Excess gingival tissue in the interproximal area can be removed by means of a wedge excision during the extraction appointment, and sutures placed (see Figs. 326–328 below, and Extraction and Revision, p. 204). Temporary replacement of an extracted tooth in the posterior segment is not necessary immediately.

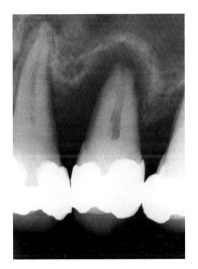
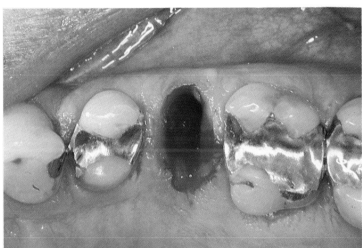

326 Elimination of a plaque-retentive area through extraction
The radiograph depicts a hopelessly involved tooth with all support lost to the apex.
The osseous support of the adjacent teeth is endangered. After recontouring of the amalgam restorations on the adjacent teeth, 25 was extracted.

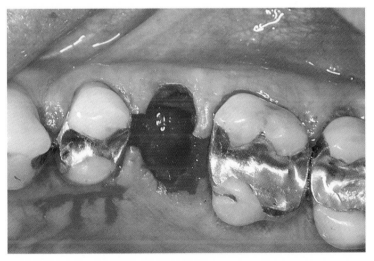

327 Gingival excision and scaling of adjacent teeth
Inflamed gingival and pocket tissue around adjacent teeth is excised as a wedge. The interproximal surfaces of these teeth can now be cleaned and smoothed under direct vision.

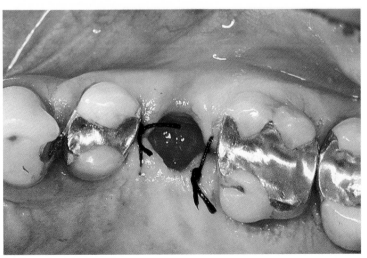

328 Suture placement
Individual sutures partially close the extraction wound mesially and distally, and also serve to adapt the tissues to the adjacent teeth.

Removal of Natural Plaque-Retentive Areas
Odontoplasty of Grooves, Ridges, Irregularities...

The natural morphology of a tooth manifests grooves, irregularities, depressions etc. on both the crown and the root. In a healthy dentition, these can usually be cleaned adequately with the toothbrush and interdental hygiene aids. However, morphological anomalies that represent plaque-retentive areas are to be found at the cervical area of some teeth. Frequently encountered are *narrow grooves* that extend apically from the lingual pit of an incisor far down the root surface (Fig. 330).

Fused roots of multirooted teeth may exhibit an irregular profile, with *large grooves* that may extend deeply into the subjacent dentin. Following initial periodontal pocket formation, such grooves are exposed and become plaque-retentive areas that are difficult to ascertain clinically. They may assume an etiologic role in localized, progressive destruction of periodontal supporting structures.

329 Diamonds for odontoplasty
Fine flame-shaped diamonds with long shafts are ideal for subgingival debridement, contouring (odontoplasty) and final polishing. Such special diamonds are available in various shapes and degrees of abrasiveness.

— **Perio-Set**
(Intensiv Co.)
75 µm, 40 µm (yellow), 15 µm (red)

The size of these instruments is shown here against the profiles of natural teeth.

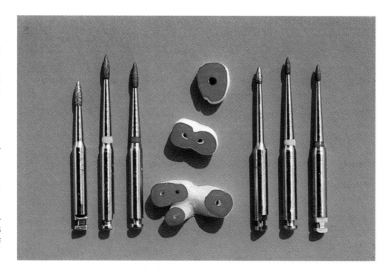

330 Recontouring a depression on tooth 22
Apical to the lingual pit amalgam on this lateral incisor, a fine groove that could be detected clinically with an explorer extended 5 mm into the periodontal pocket.

The groove was so narrow that its depth could not be probed with either a scaler or a curette. An odontoplastic modification was indicated, which included widening, rounding and polishing with a 15 µm diamond.

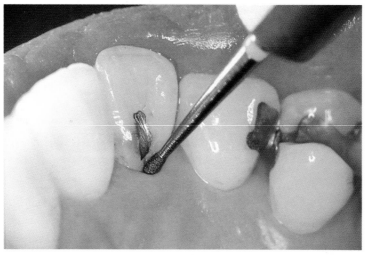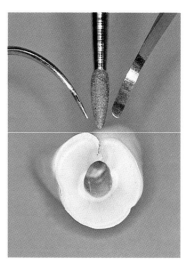

331 Tooth 22 after odontoplasty
The narrow groove was opened up using diamond burs. The depth of the groove can now be reached with fine hand instruments (e.g., an 0.8 mm wide curette), making adequate hygiene possible.

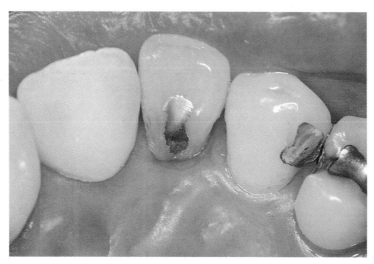

... and Furcations

Furcations can pose a clinical problem after even minor loss of periodontal supporting structure, because the entrance to a furcation may be located immediately apical to the crestal bone margin, e.g., in mandibular molars. When such an entrance is exposed, it becomes a plaque-retentive area that is impossible to reach with any hygiene aid. The enamel pearls and enamel projections frequently located at the furcation entrance just apical to the CEJ represent potential weak links in the attachment apparatus.

During the combined clinical and radiographic examination of each individual tooth, such anomalies must be diagnosed. In most cases, they can be corrected easily by means of minor odontoplasty, making the plaque-retentive areas accessible for hygiene. Teeth that have undergone odontoplasty must be carefully polished and treated with topical fluoride. It is not uncommon for a patient to experience sensitivity of the cervical area for some time following odontoplasty.

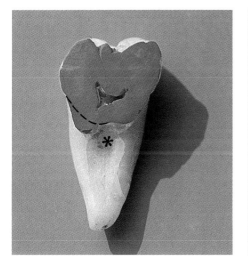
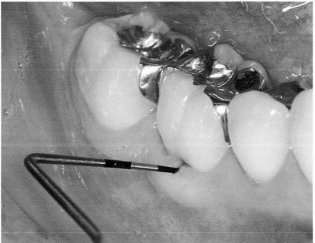

332 Furcation (class F 1) as a plaque-retentive area
This mandibular molar furcation can be probed 3 mm horizontally from the buccal aspect. A cavernous hollow is located behind the slightly overhanging enamel (dashed line). Without odontoplasty this kind of plaque-retentive area is impossible to clean.

Left: For demonstration of this situation, a similar mandibular molar was sectioned through the furcation area. The interradicular "cave" (✱) and the planned odontoplastic procedure are shown.

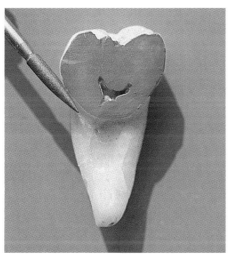
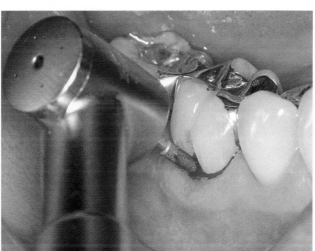

333 Odontoplasty of the furcation entrance
Using coarse diamond burs, the overhanging buccal enamel is removed and the entrance to the furcation area opened.
  Subsequently the area is smoothed and polished using 15 μm diamonds. The furcation is now accessible for professional plaque control (scaling, polishing, root planing).

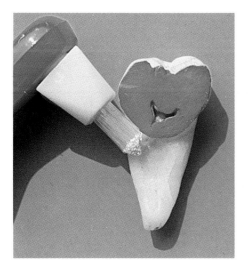
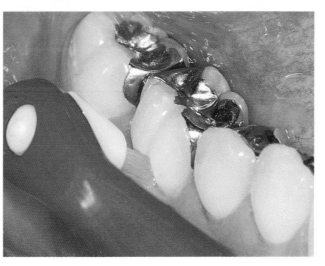

334 Hygiene with the marginal/interdental brush
The furcation entrance can now be cleaned easily by the patient using, for example, the Lactona no. 27 brush.
  At each recall appointment, this area must be carefully re-evaluated.

Reduction of Natural Plaque-Retentive Areas Caused by Crowding – Odontoplasty

Crowding of teeth is one of the few tooth positional anomalies that can be of significance indirectly in the etiology of gingivitis and periodontitis. This has less to do with functional occlusal factors than with the accumulation of plaque that occurs around crowded teeth, coupled with the fact that the patient has difficulty keeping the area clean.

Extensive orthodontic treatment including selective extractions is often refused by adults due to the cost in time, effort and money.

Careful *odontoplasty* of crowded teeth is an alternative to orthodontic treatment, albeit a limited alternative. Such grinding also may enhance the esthetic situation. The corrections are performed *only in enamel* using fine diamonds. Tooth surfaces must subsequently be smoothed, polished and treated with topical fluoride.

335 Crowding – Plaque retention
In this severe case of mandibular anterior crowding, a disclosing agent reveals heavy plaque accumulation on tooth surfaces that cannot be reached by the normal self-cleansing mechanisms, i.e., the labial surfaces that are precluded from lip contact and the lingual surfaces that are not touched by the tongue. This clinical situation can be improved by careful morphologic grinding.

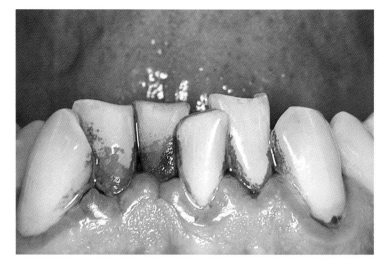 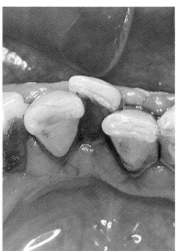

336 Odontoplasty
The incisal edges were first evened somewhat for esthetic reasons, but incisal contacts were left intact (red). The labial tooth surfaces were then selectively recontoured, as indicated by the black markings, to eliminate the plaque-retentive area as much as possible.

The interdental spaces were filed using abrasive strips to permit the use of dental floss.

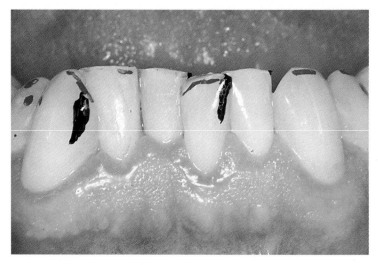

337 After grinding and initial therapy
The plaque-retentive areas are less dramatic, as indicated by the disclosing agent, which reveals only minor plaque accumulation. Interdental hygiene by means of dental floss is now possible for the patient.

Initial therapy and optimum home care have eliminated inflammation for the most part. The gingiva has shrunk, but the contour remains imperfect.

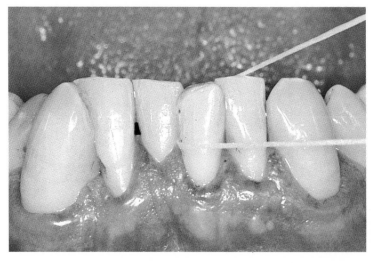 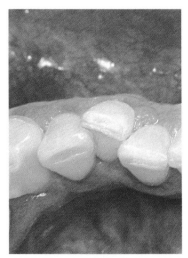

Scaling
Root Planing
Curettage

After removal of supragingival deposits and iatrogenic irritants, treatment of the periodontal pocket may begin. The goals of this treatment include 1) elimination of the microorganisms that elicit inflammation, 2) the creation of a clean, smooth root surface that will accept a new soft tissue attachment and 3) removal of diseased or infiltrated tissues (Frank 1980; Saglie et al. 1982; Allenspach-Petrzilka & Guggenheim 1983). Several interrelated procedures are used to achieve the desired results:

- Scaling
- Root planing
- Endotoxin removal
- Soft tissue curettage.

Subgingival scaling and root planing are the two procedures most often employed in initial periodontal therapy. The dividing line between root planing and supragingival plaque and calculus removal is often not distinct, since even during supragingival procedures the scalers, ultrasonic instruments and curettes often enter the subgingival area, thereby removing calculus and cementum from the root surface.

Successful performance of subgingival procedures can lead to the elimination of inflammation and to true healing of the periodontal lesion, with tissue shrinkage and regeneration of lost attachment.

Definitions
The nomenclature for the methods described is not internationally uniform. The following definitions are presented for clarity in this book:

- *Scaling:* The process by which plaque and calculus are removed from both supra- and subgingival tooth surfaces.
- *Root planing:* The process by which residual embedded calculus and portions of the cementum are removed from the roots to produce a clean, hard, smooth surface that is free of endotoxin.
- *Gingival curettage (soft tissue curettage, closed curettage):* The process by which the pocket epithelium and infiltrated subepithelial connectives are removed without reflecting flaps, i.e., without direct vision of the surfaces being treated. Gingival curettage is classified as a surgical procedure.
- *Open curettage:* The process by which thorough scaling, root planing, and removal of diseased pocket epithelium and connective tissue are accomplished with direct vision, after an inverse bevel incision and conservative reflection of marginal gingiva (see Modified Widman procedure, p. 179).

Indication

Closed curettage without subsequent surgical intervention is indicated in cases of mild to moderate periodontitis with pockets of 6 mm or less. During a re-evaluation of the case several weeks or months later, the dentist can decide whether local surgical intervention may be required. In severe, advanced periodontitis, curettage in the form of subgingival debridement may be considered as pretreatment for the subsequent surgery, as wound healing is enhanced.

Contraindication

There are really no contraindications, although certain patients with severe systemic diseases deserve special attention; for example, patients taking anticoagulants should have a bleeding time performed, and a consultation with the physician is advisable. If there is a danger of focus of infection, the patient should be covered antibiotically because curettage always elicits a transient bacteremia (see Medicaments, p. 263).

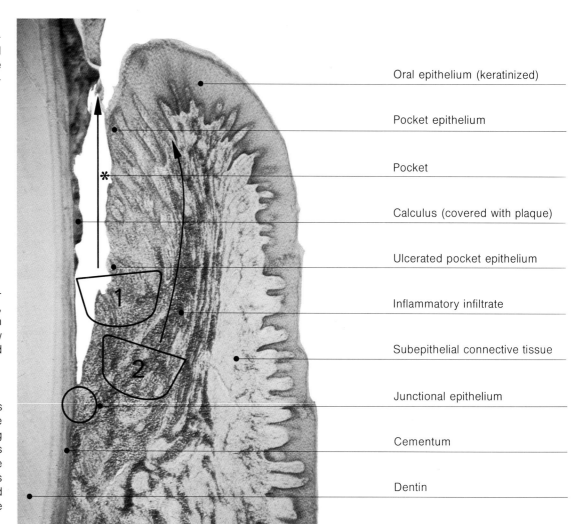

337 Principle of "curettage"
This stained (H & E, × 20) histologic section through a periodontal pocket will be used to illustrate root planing and soft tissue curettage.

Oral epithelium (keratinized)

Pocket epithelium

Pocket

Calculus (covered with plaque)

Ulcerated pocket epithelium

Inflammatory infiltrate

Subepithelial connective tissue

Junctional epithelium

Cementum

Dentin

1. Root planing
The unilaterally sharp Gracey curette (1) removes plaque, calculus, cementum and sometimes dentin from the tooth surface. The arrow indicates the direction toward which the curette tip is pulled.

2. Gingival curettage
A Gracey curette sharpened on its other edge (2) is used to remove pocket epithelium and remaining (apical) junctional epithelium, as well as the infiltrated connective tissue (destroyed collagenous matrix) that is sharply demarcated from the intact, healthy connective tissue.

Advantages

Closed curettage causes less trauma and hemorrhage than a radical surgical intervention. Thus, gingival shrinkage during the healing phase is less than after invasive surgery, and this may be important for esthetics.

In terms of maintenance of attachment, the results achieved with closed curettage are good if comprehensive maintenance therapy (recall) is followed (see p. 151, also Knowles et al. 1979; Lindhe et al. 1984).

Disadvantages

Several studies have shown that, when therapy is performed without direct vision, some root surfaces are totally missed and others are not completely freed of plaque and calculus (Waerhaug 1978; Thornton & Garnick 1982; Eaton et al. 1985). In *deep and narrow pockets, in furcations* and when *root irregularities* are present, closed curettage or root planing cannot ensure 100 % success. There is always the danger of recurrence. The manual dexterity of the operator is also of significance in closed curettage.

Treatment Goals

Absolute cleanliness of the root surface is the most critical goal. All substances must be removed from the root surface including plaque, calculus and endotoxin. Endotoxin (lipopolysaccharide from gram-negative bacteria) is found in the superficial layers of cementum, and can inhibit reattachment of epithelium and regenerated connective tissue to the root surface. For this reason, the root surface must be planed and smoothed until only healthy (hard) cementum or dentin remains.

Once the root surface is treated, the "peeling out" of the pocket epithelium and infiltrated connective tissue

is accomplished. If the curettes used for root planing are sharp on both edges, some soft tissue curettage will be accomplished inadvertently even as the hard tooth structure is planed.

The goals of these procedures are the elimination of pocket infection and the healing of the periodontal lesion (see pp. 260–261).

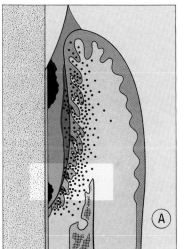
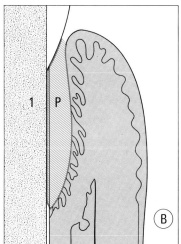
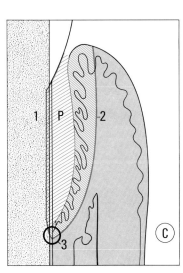

339 Root planing versus curettage – Principles

A. Pocket
Calculus (black), adherent (blue) and nonadherent plaque (red).

B. Scaling and root planing
Only the tooth surface is treated (1). Plaque (P) is removed from the pocket (essential procedure).

C. Curettage
The pocket epithelium / infiltrate (2) and junctional epithelium (3) are removed (never as sole procedure).

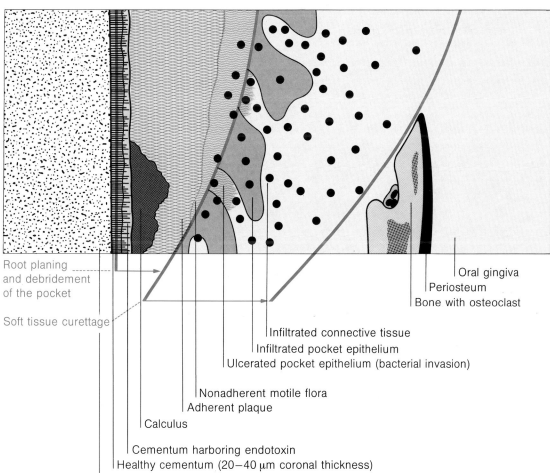

340 Root planing versus curettage – Details
Enlargement from Figure 339 A: The various structures that would be removed or treated during subgingival treatment for plaque and calculus elimination, root planing and soft tissue curettage are depicted.

Root planing
and debridement
of the pocket

Soft tissue curettage

Oral gingiva
Periosteum
Bone with osteoclast

Infiltrated connective tissue
Infiltrated pocket epithelium
Ulcerated pocket epithelium (bacterial invasion)

Nonadherent motile flora
Adherent plaque

Calculus

Cementum harboring endotoxin
Healthy cementum (20–40 µm coronal thickness)
Dentin

Instruments for Root Planing and Curettage...

For the removal of large accumulations of subgingival calculus, *hoes* and *curettes* are the instruments of choice. For plaque removal, root planing and soft tissue curettage, curettes exclusively are indicated.

The dental marketplace offers innumerable instruments of various designs and varying quality. Every dental school and every dental practitioner have favorites. This *Atlas* makes no recommendations as to brand names, but it is important that the assortment of curettes selected must be able to reach all root surfaces. In practice, the instrument should be used with its working tip at an angle of 80° to the root surface. All instruments must be sharpened before each use.

Note that the common universal curettes are sharp on both sides of the working tip, while the special Gracey curettes are sharp on only one side of the tip. Graceys are used more often for root planing than for soft tissue curettage.

341 Hoes

– Ash TC 210–213

These hoes have carbide steel tips and are useful for removal of hard subgingival accretions even in deep pockets. These instruments can cause deep scratches, however, and are therefore not indicated for root planing.

Right: The carbide tip cannot be sharpened by the dentist! If it becomes dull after long use, it must be returned to the manufacturer for sharpening or replacement.

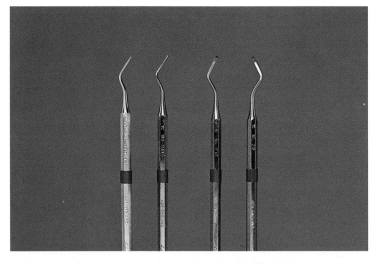
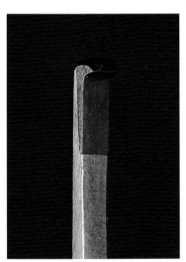

342 Curettes
Three paired (L & R) instruments will usually suffice for almost all areas of curettage. Those depicted are from Deppeler.

– Universal curette ZI 15
   (yellow)
– Anterior curette M 24 (orange)
– Posterior curette M 23 (red)

Sharpening (right)
These instruments are sharpened on both edges (red arrowheads). With universal curettes, the face of the working tip is at 90° to the shaft of the instrument.

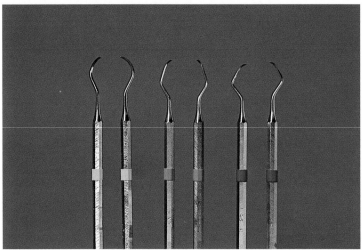
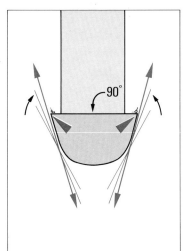

343 Gracey curettes
A complete set consists of 14 instruments (GRA 1–14, e.g., from Hu-Friedy), each indicated for a different area of the oral cavitiy. Practically, the following selection is sufficent:

– 7/8 (white) anterior area
– 11/12 (blue) mesial surfaces
– 13/14 (black) distal surfaces

Sharpening (right)
Only one side of the working tip is sharpened (blue arrows).

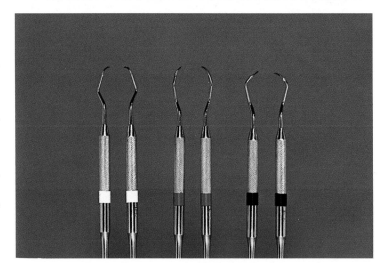
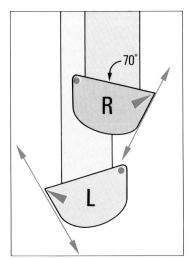

...and Their Use

Closed curettage can only be a successfull procedure if it is performed systematically, generally by quadrants or sextants and using local anesthesia. The operator must be aware of the probing depths and attachment loss on all root surfaces of each tooth to be treated.

The procedure can be performed *"tooth by tooth"* or *"instrument by instrument."* Here, the degree of precision demanded by the procedure is pitted against a rational approach. It is more rational, more time-effective and easier to treat all tooth surfaces in a dental segment with one instrument, and then switch to the next instrument.

However, when probing depths vary greatly from one tooth to another, and when teeth exhibit root fusions, furcation involvement or other anatomical peculiarities, it often makes more sense to treat all surfaces of one tooth, even though it requires several instrument changes. This is the only way to ensure that every root surface is appropriately treated.

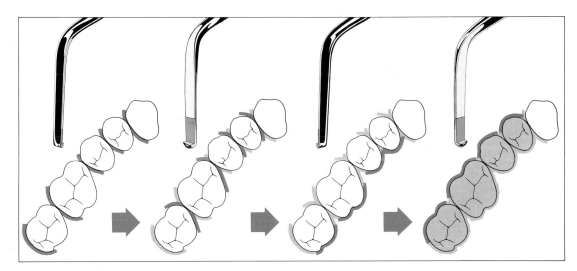

Systematic procedure

344 Tooth surface by tooth surface – Hoe instruments
The operator holds a double-ended hoe scaler (Ash TC 210–211) in his hand and treats first all distal surfaces of teeth in the maxillary right sextant. He then turns the instrument over and treats all mesial surfaces of the same teeth.

The same procedure is performed on buccal and palatal surfaces using the TC 212–213 hoe.

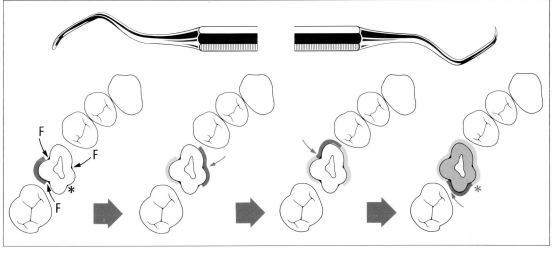

345 Tooth by tooth – Posterior curette
In the example depicted, a molar (16) with a palatal depression and initial furcation involvement is completely curetted.

Using one side of a double-ended curette (M 23, Deppeler), the distobuccal aspect of the tooth is treated first, then the mesiopalatal. With the other end of the instrument, the mesiobuccal and finally the distopalatal root segment are treated. Note the depression (✳) and the furcation entrances (F).

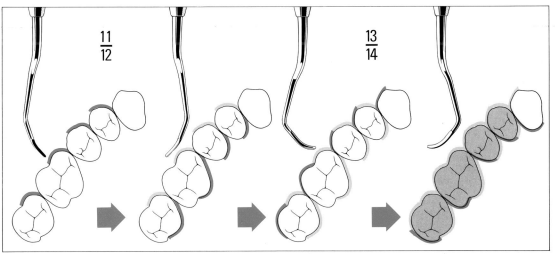

346 Tooth surface by tooth surface – Gracey curettes
The approach when using Gracey curettes is different as they are sharp on only one side, as compared to universal curettes, which have two sharp edges.

The double-ended (paired) instruments are used as depicted here to treat the mesiobuccal (GRA 11) and the mesiopalatal (GRA 12) surfaces, then GRA 13/14 is used to treat distobuccal and distopalatal surfaces in this sextant.

Rest Position – Position of the Operator

The dentist in a modern practice today usually works according to the principles of ergonomics, and generally with a chairside assistant (4-handed dentistry). The assistant doesn't merely hand the dentist the proper instrument, she (he) also maintains a clean operating field by means of continuous rinsing and evacuation of blood, especially from the entrance to periodontal pockets.

Closed curettage is performed *without direct vision* into the pocket; the root surface being curetted is never seen. The entire procedure depends upon the tactile sensitivity of the operator. Clearly then, closed curettage is one of the most difficult procedures in periodontal therapy to accomplish perfectly. Use of appropriate finger rests for stabilization during the procedure, and excellent illumination of the field will enhance the results. The operator's position in relation to the patient's head and to the quadrant being treated is also important.

Presented here are three examples of instrument use, rest position and operator location.

Root Planing and Curettage

347 Maxillary right, buccal
The left hand is used to reflect the lip and cheek, to provide a clear view of the field of operation. The right hand is stabilized by placement of the ring finger on the occlusal surfaces of teeth in the upper right quadrant.

"9 o'clock" position for curettage in this segment, with direct vision, is appropriate.

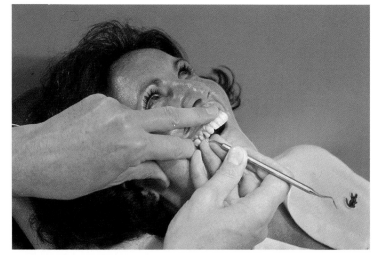
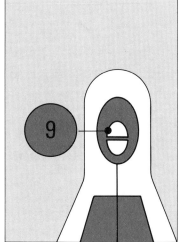

348 Maxillary left, palatal
For curettage on upper molars, it is often not possible to have a triangular rest of the operating hand on the occlusal surfaces of teeth in the quadrant. Support is gained indirectly on the mandible and with the left hand.

"8 o'clock" position is ideal for the dentist working in this quadrant with direct vision.

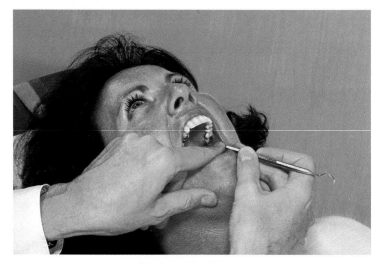
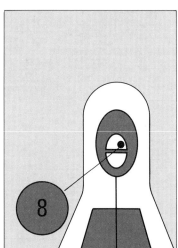

349 Mandibular anterior, lingual
The left hand is used to reflect the lip and cheek. The working hand is supported via a finger rest with the ring finger. Lingual surfaces of the anterior teeth are illuminated by reflected light from the mirror, which also serves to deflect the tongue away from the field.

"11 o'clock" position for curettage with direct vision in the mandibular anterior segment.

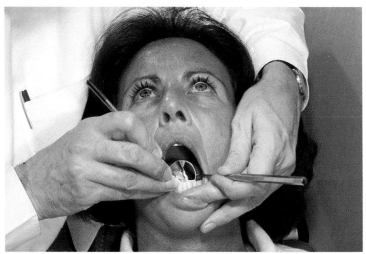
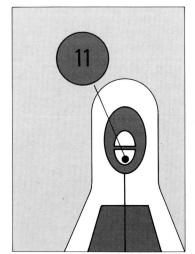

Root Planing and Curettage

Operative procedure

A curettage procedure in the maxillary right sextant will be presented in detail. The procedures to be performed will include subgingival plaque and calculus removal, root planing and gingival curettage. The photographic sequence depicts complete treatment of tooth 14.

Re-evaluation: After the first phase of initial therapy (motivation, hygiene, debridement) the following values were recorded:

HYG 65%   PBI 1.7   TM 1–2

Figures 350 and 351 depict the clinical situation, probing depths, gingival contour and radiographs of the quadrant to be treated.

The patient is a 39-year-old female with generalized, moderate periodontitis. Her motivation and cooperation in home care are average.

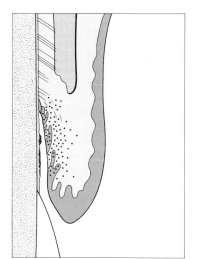 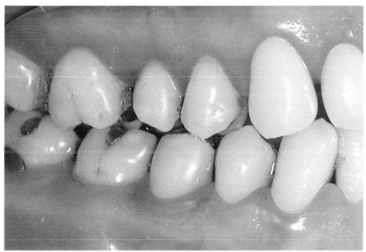

350 Clinical situation following supragingival plaque and calculus removal (debridement)
Following this portion of initial therapy, active pockets up to 6 mm in depth remained (see Fig. 351).

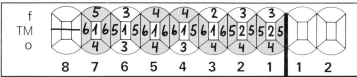

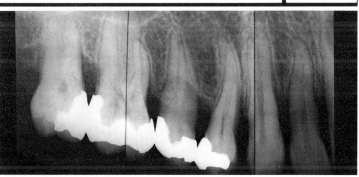

351 Pockets and radiographic findings
Attachment loss is particularly pronounced in the interproximal areas. A crater-like defect appears to exist around tooth 15.

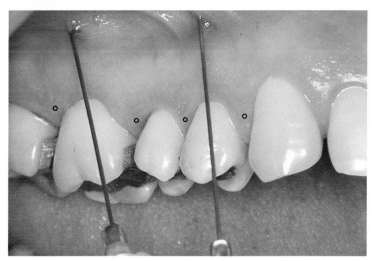

352 Anesthesia
Scaling, root planing and curettage are performed under local anesthesia.

Injections of anesthetic solution are made in the buccal vestibule and on the palate.

In order to prevent excessive hemorrhage, anesthetic is infiltrated directly into individual papillae (circles).

353 Debriding the root surface – Insertion of the hoe scaler

Using light pressure, the instrument is inserted into the pocket until resistance is encountered. When the shaft of the instrument is parallel to the long axis of the tooth, the working end is positioned at an angle of 90° to the root surface. The hoe is used with a pulling motion from apical to coronal, while applying lateral pressure to the tooth.

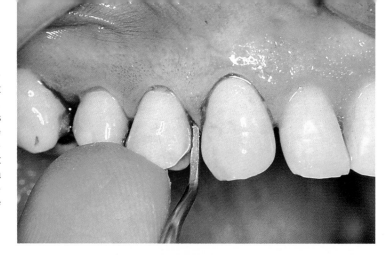

354 Hoe within the pocket

In the radiograph and in the schematic the size of the instrument in relation to the gingiva and the interdental space is clearly depicted. Where crowding exists, for example the mandibular anterior area, carbide-tipped hoes are not always useful, as they are relatively gross instruments. Grooves in roots cannot be effectively reached with hoe scalers.

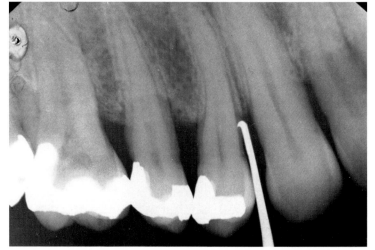
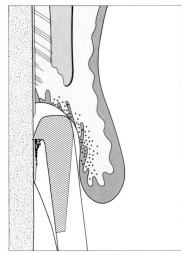

355 Use of the hoe in buccal segment

A finger rest is established with the ring finger on the tooth (bicuspid) being treated. The working movement is the same as above.

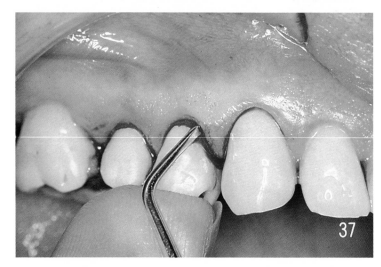

356 Use of the hoe scaler on palatal surfaces

The shank of the instrument is placed parallel to the long axis of the tooth. In this case the bend in the shank curves back over the occlusal surface. An angle of about 90° between root surface and cutting edge is maintained during the working stroke.

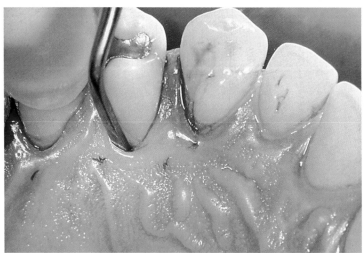

Curettes

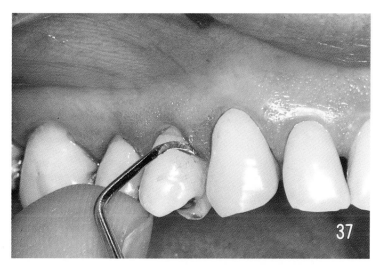

357 Root planing, mesial of tooth 14
The curette is inserted into the depth of the pocket until resistance is encountered. The working stroke is performed with pressure exerted against the root surface. The curette will remove additional plaque and calculus, and will serve to smooth out any scratches made by the hoe scaler.

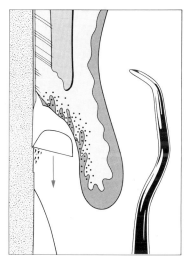

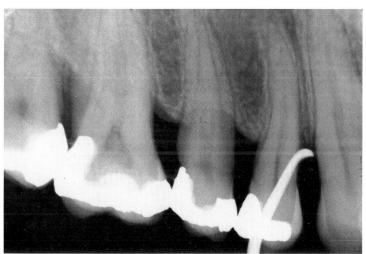

358 Working angle of the curette blade
For the removal of subgingival accretions and for planing away endotoxin-containing cementum (red arrow in diagram), the cutting edge of the curette is placed at an angle of about 80° to the root surface. For definitive root planing (smoothing) after all accretions have been removed, a blade angle of 50–60° is used.

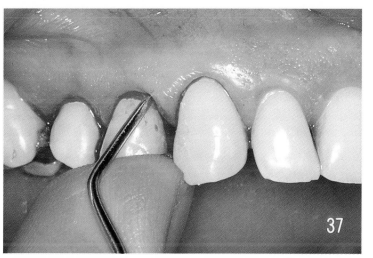

359 Planing a depression on the mesial of tooth 14
Although shallow depressions and grooves on root surfaces can be easily reached using fine curettes (0.8 mm width), it is questionable whether or not curettes can completely clean and smooth narrow depressions and grooves. In such cases, it is often necessary to open up the grooves with fine diamond burs (see Fig. 329).

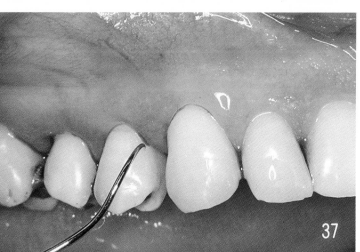

360 Checking the planed surface using an explorer
After each treatment, the planed root surface should be scrutinized using a fine explorer point, to evaluate absence of deposits and root surface smoothness.

361 Soft tissue curettage, supporting the tissue

When attempting to remove the pocket epithelium and diseased subepithelial tissues, it is often necessary to exert light finger pressure on the gingival surface against the curette in the pocket, as depicted here clinically and in the schematic. Excessive force should be avoided so that tissue is not torn during the procedure.

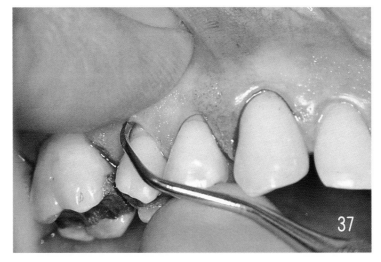 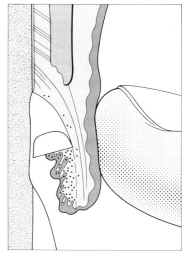

362 Removal of the soft tissue of the pocket wall

During gingival curettage the working stroke of the curette is directed against the pocket wall (arrow).

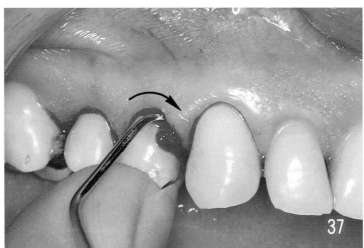

363 Granulation tissue

Pocket epithelium and granulation tissue are removed, but there is no way to determine clinically whether all of the diseased soft tissue has in fact been eliminated. Because of this, the significance of this treatment procedure (closed gingival curettage) for healing of the periodontal pocket is disputed.

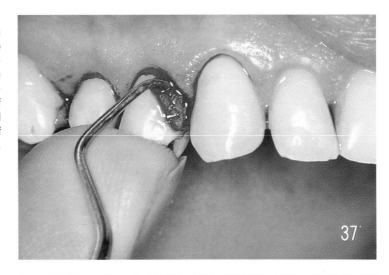

364 Rinsing the pocket – Adaption of soft tissue

During the soft tissue curettage procedure, the area should be rinsed repeatedly with Ringer's solution, hydrogen peroxide or CHX solution. When curettage is completed, the pocket should be thoroughly rinsed.

Right: Frequently following curettage the gingival tissues must be readapted (arrow) using sutures or a periodontal dressing. This helps to keep the blood clot (red) minimal between the tooth surface and the soft tissue.

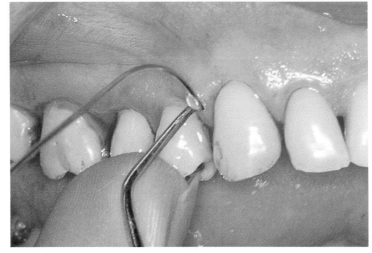 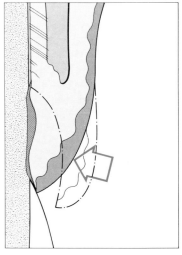

Root Planing and Curettage

Summary

A 39-year-old female demonstrated only average motivation and manual dexterity during initial therapy (debridement, repeated OH instruction and re-evaluation). Nevertheless, the clinically pronounced gingival inflammation she manifested initially (PBI 3) was reduced significantly by the initial therapy (PBI 1.7). Subsequent treatment consisting of subgingival calculus removal, root planing and gingival curettage led to further improvement (PBI 0.9).

At a re-evaluation appointment 2 months later, probing depths were reduced and there were no symptoms of active periodontal disease. The reduced probing depth measurements were due, in part, to gingival shrinkage. The quality of the periodontal regeneration could not be evaluated clinically (see Periodontal Healing, Reattachment – New Attachment, pp. 260–261). The clinical result in terms of gingival contour remained unsatisfactory, and her OH remained suboptimal.

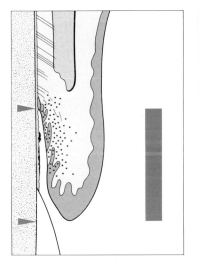
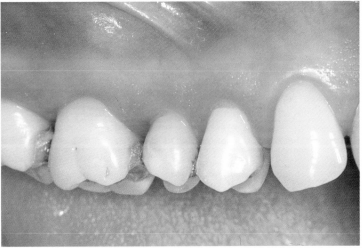

365 Clinical situation before curettage
The level of inflammation and edema has already been remarkably reduced as a result of supra- and subgingival plaque and calculus removal. Probing depths have been reduced somewhat due to the reduction in gingival edema (see red arrows). Residual plaque and calculus are still present.

Before

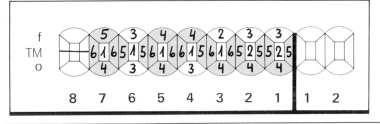

366 Probing depths and TM before curettage
In the upper right quadrant the probing depths are 6 mm in interproximal areas and up to 4 mm facially and orally (see also the radiographic findings, Fig. 351).

After

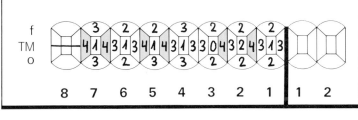

Probing depths and TM 2 months after curettage
After treatment the probing depths were 3–4 mm interproximally and 2 mm facially and orally.

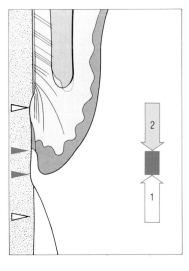
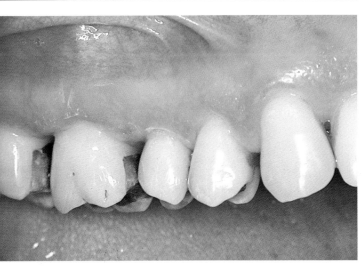

367 2 months after treatment
Considerable shrinkage of the tissue is observed (note clinically between teeth 15 and 16; arrow 1 in diagram).

New attachment (2) composed of epithelium and also possibly of connective tissue lead to a marked reduction in probing depth (red zone).

Gingival contour and stippling, however, remain unsatisfactory.

Treatment of Mild Furcation Involvement (Class F 1)

Class F 1 furcation involvements (see Diseases of the Periodontium, p. 60) are usually treated conservatively by means of root planing and curettage (Ramfjord & Ash 1979). In order to ensure that optimum hygiene will be possible for the patient after postsurgical healing in the area, root planing of the furcation must often be enhanced by odontoplasty. The depression at the entrance to the furcation must not remain as a plaque-retentive area. Full coverage crowns, as depicted by the case below, must be contoured so that natural crown and root form is duplicated. The furcation entrance is an "endangered area"; crown margins in this area should not be located subgingivally.

Following the surgical procedure (curettage), the gingiva must be well adapted onto the root surface in order to provide optimum conditions for regeneration, especially if odontoplasty has been performed in the furcation area. Tissue adaptation can be accomplished with a periodontal dressing or with tissue adhesive (cyanoacrylates, e.g., Histoacryl).

368   Curettage and root planing in a case of mild furcation involvement (F 1)
During supragingival debridement the open crown margin is corrected as much as possible. During curettage the crown margin is definitively smoothed and polished and the buccal furcation is widened slightly coronally (odontoplasty).

This *radiograph* was taken before revision of the overhanging crown margins.

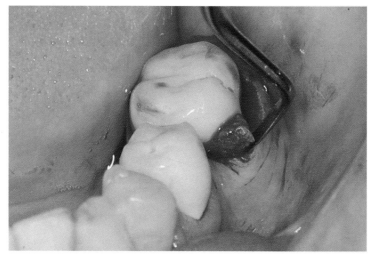
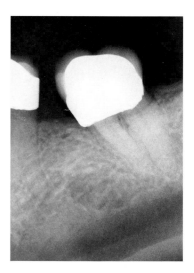

369   Adaptation of the gingiva using tissue adhesive
Following curettage the gingiva must be adapted closely into the furcation area that has been altered via odontoplasty. The tissues are first formed and pressed against the tooth using finger pressure, then sealed to place using the tissue adhesive Histoacryl. The adhesive must *not* be permitted to flow into the furcation entrance; this would render new attachment impossible and could elicit a severe foreign body reaction.

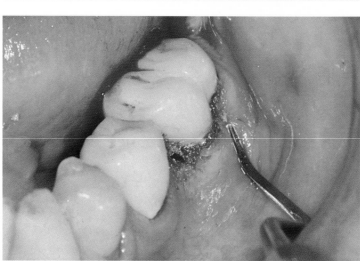

370   6 weeks after curettage
The pocket is almost completely healed via shrinkage and regeneration. The crown margin is supragingival and follows the contour of the root surface depression in the furcation area.

Special hygiene aids (e.g., the Lactona no. 27 interdental brush) must be used in this area to enhance the toothbrush (Bass technique).

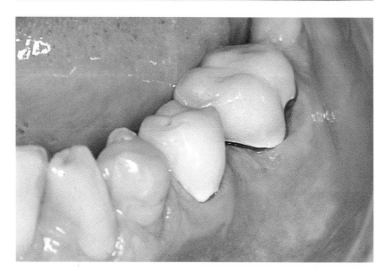

Treatment of Moderate Furcation Involvement (Class F 2) – Odontoplasty

It is common for the roots of a multirooted tooth to converge at the furcation area with the creation of very narrow interradicular space (Fig. 371). Even the finest curette cannot gain entrance to such an area, rendering debridement and root planing impossible.

Teeth with furcation involvement that are not essential in terms of the treatment plan for the entire case may be considered for extraction. On the other hand, if a particular tooth is critical to the success of a total treatment plan, odontoplasty may be the treatment of choice. With a fine diamond bur, the furcation area is opened to such an extent that the finest curette can gain entrance for debridement. In the case of a Class F 2 furcation involvement, such odontoplasty can only be performed with direct vision, i.e., after reflection of the gingiva (see Open Curettage, Modified Widman Procedure, p. 179).

Any time odontoplasty is performed, there is the danger of increased caries susceptibility and dentin hypersensitivity. For this reason, the furcation that has undergone odontoplasty must be accessible for routine hygiene and home fluoride treatment.

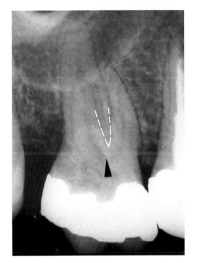

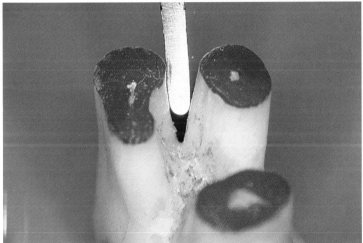

371 Narrow buccal furcation entrance
Even the finest curette, only 0.8 mm wide, cannot effectively reach the involved furcation.

Left: The radiograph reveals the closely spaced buccal roots (arrow). The severity of the furcation involvement (periodontal pocket, plaque, calculus), however, cannot be ascertained radiographically, especially in 3-rooted maxillary molars.

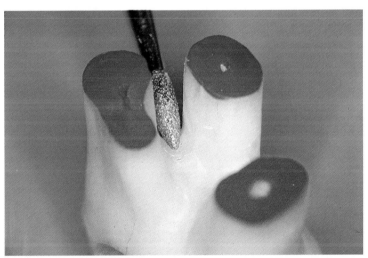

372 "Furcation-Plasty"
Using flame-shaped diamonds (coarse 75 μm and medium 40 μm particles), the involved furcation can be opened just enough so that a fine curette can enter for debridement and root planing.

It is important to remember that furcations that have been treated via odontoplasty are especially susceptible to caries! Once opened, they must be polished with the finest diamond bur (15 μm, see Fig. 329) and treated with topical fluoride.

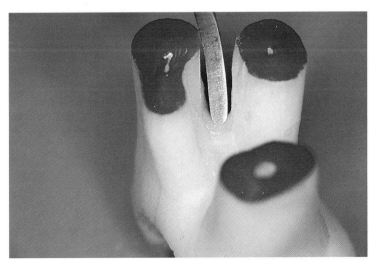

373 Furcation now accessible for cleaning
Debridement and root planing with fine curettes can now be performed during the course of periodontal therapy as well as at each recall appointment after therapy is completed.

In such cases, cervical sensitivity may be particularly troublesome and persistent. The patient should be warned of this possibility before performing the odontoplasty. The area must be treated with topical fluoride to enhance remineralization, prevent plaque accumulation, and reduce sensitivity.

Open Curettage and Root Planing

Complete planing of a root surface is extremely difficult during *closed curettage (without direct vision)* because root surfaces exhibit such a variety of irregularities, depressions and grooves. Good results can only be achieved with a systematic procedure, a fine tactile sense, a talented operator and the expenditure of considerable time.

Open curettage (with direct vision), on the other hand, simplifies considerably the task of perfect root planing and debridement. Marginal incisions are made facially and orally, and the gingivae reflected only to the crest of the alveolar bone. This procedure exposes the root surfaces, which can be planed with direct vision.

After the operation the wound margins are repositioned and adapted around the teeth by means of interdental sutures. Following open curettage, gingival shrinkage and postoperative bone resorption will be more pronounced than after closed curettage.

If the releasing incision for open curettage takes the form of an internal gingivectomy (inverse bevel), open curettage is very similar to the Ramfjord technique (see Modified Widman Procedure, p. 179).

374   Open curettage
A marginal incision is made and the gingiva is reflected. Pocket epithelium and granulation tissue are removed and the flaps are thinned internally using fine scissors. Thinning the flap enhances its subsequent adaptation. The root surfaces are cleaned and planed with direct vision.

Right: Using an extracted tooth it is possible to demonstrate that in an area with 9 mm of attachment loss, only the coronal 5 mm of the root surface can be effectively treated by means of closed curettage.

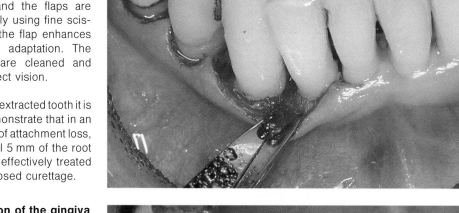
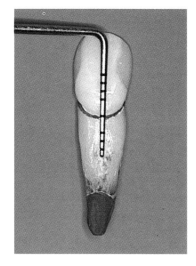

375   Adaptation of the gingiva
Following open curettage the gingival flaps must be readapted and repositioned, then sutured to place. Sutures should be placed using atraumatic straight or curved needles and thin suture material (3−0 or 4−0).

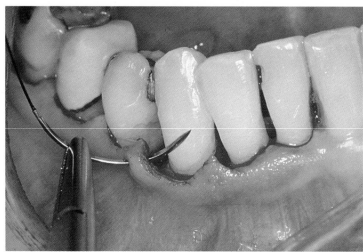

376   Wound closure after open curettage
It is not always possible to completely close the interdental space, and small interdental soft tissue craters may persist after healing. With intensive interdental hygiene (e.g., Butler no. 614 interdental brush) and frequent recall such craters will close with time. It may be necessary to perform a minor papilloplasty to improve gingival contour. Electrosurgery is often used for such minor revisions.

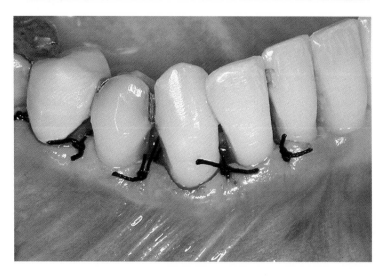

Open Curettage, Root Planing – Correction of Undercontured Crown Margin

Plaque-retentive areas that exist around overhangs and overbulked margins of crowns are usually corrected during the first appointment for initial therapy.

In the esthetically important anterior region, correction of a crown margin without injuring the gingival margin can often be accomplished only by means of open curettage. In order to avoid replacing a restoration that has clinically unacceptable marginal relationships, the dentist may attempt, as shown in the clinical example below, to recontour the restoration or the tooth itself by grinding with direct vision. Once the adaptation of the margins is complete, the ground surfaces of both tooth structure and restoration must be smoothed with fine diamonds, polished with mild abrasive paste and treated topically with fluoride.

If there is a gap between the restoration margin and the margin of the prepared tooth ("open margin"), no amount of grinding will adequately correct the situation. In such cases, the crown will have to be replaced.

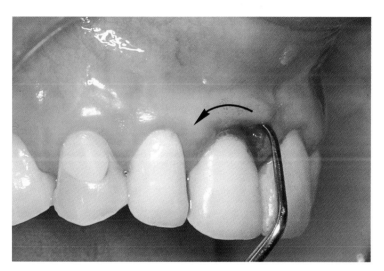

377 Curettage in the area of a jacket crown
On the labial surface of the two incisor jacket crowns, the gingivae are inflamed and swollen. Closed curettage was attempted, but it was quickly evident that the margin of the jacket crown on tooth 11 was short of the preparation margin, creating a plaque-retentive area.

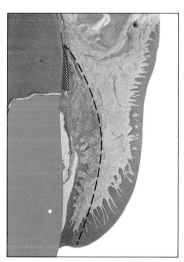
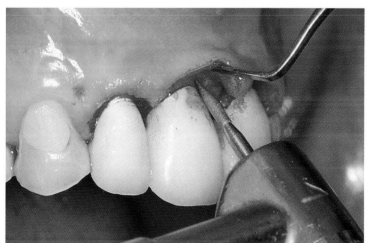

378 Open curettage, correction of the marginal inadequacy
Reflecting the gingiva revealed a discrepancy between the crown margin and tooth structure. Coarse (75 μm, then 40 μm) diamonds were used with direct vision to reduce the tooth structure until it met the crown margin.

In the histological section (left), the odontoplasty on the tooth root (hatched area) and the soft tissue curettage are indicated. A tiny cement line remains between the jacket crown (blue) and the preparation.

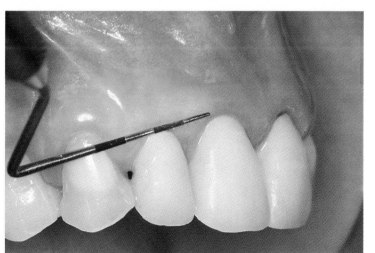

379 Two years later
Despite the crown margin that is still located somewhat subgingivally (an esthetic compromise), the gingiva is well adapted and inflammation-free two years after treatment. The probing depth is 2 mm.

What does "Root Planing" Really Mean?

Root planing, i.e., the definitive treatment of the root surface, is the most important component of periodontal therapy. Following subgingival plaque and calculus removal and elimination of cementum layers that are saturated with endotoxin, the root surface must be planed and smoothed. The rationale for this procedure is the assumption that a smooth root surface will be less plaque-retentive and that therefore the danger of re-infection and recurrence of disease should be less. Some have also espoused the theory that reattachment of either epithelial or (ideally) connective tissue would be more likely on a smooth root surface than on a rough one. Other factors, such as root treatment with citric acid, could also enhance regeneration of a new attachment, and many clinical studies are currently underway to evaluate this possibility.

The photographs below demonstrate clearly that the term "planing and smoothing" is, indeed, relative, regardless of whether it is performed with curettes or with the finest rotating diamonds (Schwarz et al. 1984).

380   Dentin planing with curettes
Using a standardized method (250 gm pressure, 10 strokes downward) for evaluating conventional mechanical root planing, parallel grooves with an average depth of 2 µm were created.

Right: A factory-new curette (CUR) is shown at high magnification (above). Note the irregularities and spurs of metal, which can never be completely eliminated.

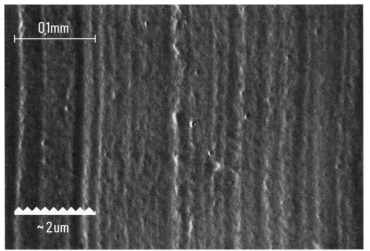
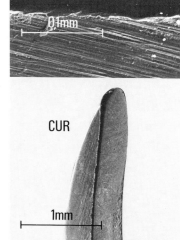

381   Dentin planing with a 15 µm diamond
Compared to the curettes, the diamond leaves scratches that are a bit deeper and less regular. This standardized test employed 60 gm pressure and 10 passes with the flame-shaped diamond rotating at 6000 rpm.

Right: Diamond for root planing (D 15). The magnification reveals the fine surface structure of the 15 µm diamond.

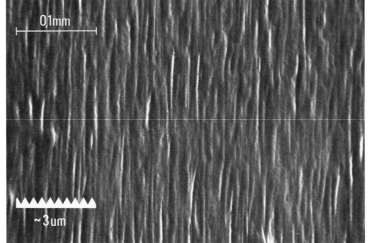
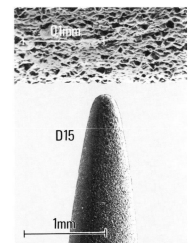

382   Dentin roughening by a 75 µm diamond
The coarse 75 µm diamond, commonly used for tooth preparation, leaves deep grooves and irregularities in the dentin. Scratches are as deep as 15 µm. The test conditions were the same as for the 15 µm diamond (Fig. 381).

Right: The 75 µm diamond (D 75), normal for tooth preparation, is unacceptable for root planing.

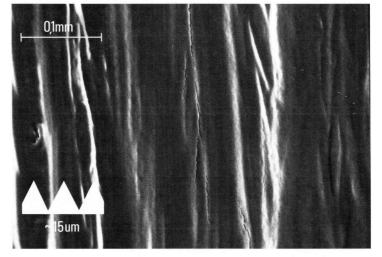
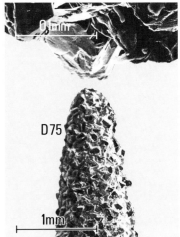

Initial Therapy – Possibilities and Limitations

Initial therapy (plaque control, debridement, root planing, curettage) is considered to be the most important phase of complete periodontal treatment. In the truest sense it is "causal therapy," since it is etiologic factors that are eliminated. Periodontal surgery, on the other hand, is targeted mainly toward correction or elimination of the *consequences* of the disease process.

In cases of *gingivitis*, initial therapy is usually the only treatment necessary. An exception is fibrous gingival overgrowth, which may persist even after inflammation is eliminated. Overgrowth may occur in cases of severe gingivitis, in patients who are mouth breathers, and with certain systemic medications such as phenytoin or cyclosporine-A (p. 50). In these situations, initial therapy must be complemented by gingivectomy/gingivoplasty.

Initial therapy alone may also bring satisfactory results in cases of *mild periodontitis*.

There are certain limitations to the success that can be achieved by initial therapy alone in cases of *moderate and severe periodontitis*. It has already been stated that non-surgical removal of subgingival plaque and calculus (closed curettage) becomes more and more difficult with increasing pocket depth. It is impossible to completely plane root irregularities, grooves, furcations and fusions; removal of diseased cementum and smoothing of the root surface can at best be accomplished imperfectly without direct vision. The result of this is a lack of new attachment (regeneration) postoperatively. Remaining pockets can become re-infected despite the patient's best efforts in home care.

For all these reasons it is imperative to re-evaluate the case 6–8 weeks after initial therapy to determine whether surgical intervention is required or whether the patient should be re-treated during a recall visit, for example, by repeated subgingival scaling, root planing and curettage.

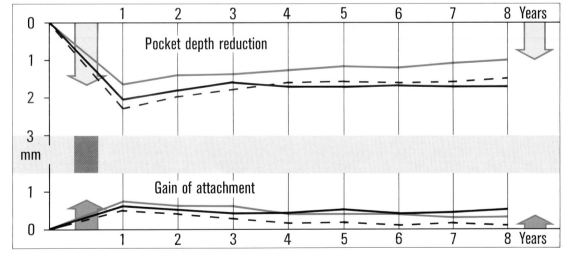

383   Pocket depth reduction and gain of attachment after various treatment methods in 4–6 mm pockets (Knowles et al. 1979)

——— Root planing and curettage
——— Modified Widman procedure
– – – Surgical pocket elimination

The Michigan long-term study

Ramfjord and his coworkers performed an 8-year longitudinal study to evaluate the long-term effects of three treatment modalities (Knowles et al. 1979, 1981):

1. Root planing and curettage
2. Modified Widman procedure
3. Surgical pocket elimination
   (flaps, ostectomy, apical repositioning).

The results of this landmark study revealed that with pocket depths of 4–6 mm all three treatment methods

gave similar results (see Fig. 383), although *closed curettage* led to slightly less reduction in pocket depth than the two surgical techniques. On the other hand, *attachment gain* after closed curettage was similar to the result obtained with modified Widman surgery, and somewhat more when compared to radical pocket elimination (ostectomy).

In cases of advanced periodontitis with probing depths of 7–12 mm, the modified Widman technique was superior to closed curettage in terms of both pocket elimination and attachment gain (p. 157).

384 Severe, plaque-elicited gingivitis

Before initial therapy, the clinical picture was one of severe inflammation, especially in the maxillary anterior region, with pronounced edematous enlargement of interdental papillae. The PBI score was 3.8.

The mandibular inflammation was less severe (PBI 3.0).

No attachment loss was detected in either area.

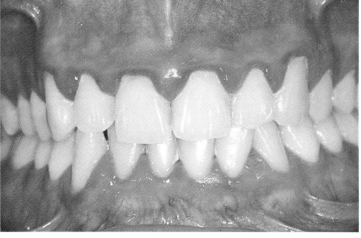

Before

Gingivitis

385 Findings 2 months after initial therapy

Severe gingivitis has been completely eliminated. The patient's level of motivation and dexterity using the Bass technique and dental floss rendered any further treatment unnecessary.

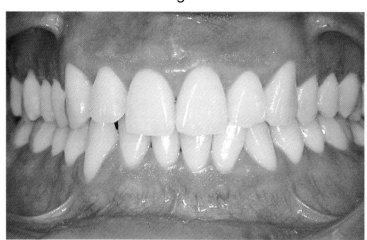

After

386 Generalized moderate periodontitis with pronounced gingivitis

In addition to the severe manifestations of gingivitis in papillary and marginal areas (PBI 3–4), pockets to 6 mm were detected (attachment loss).

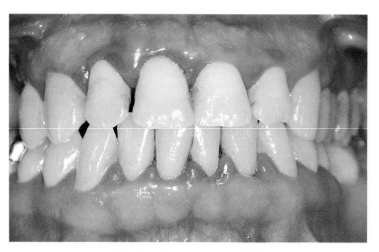

Before

Moderate periodontitis

387 Findings 2 months after initial therapy

The inflammation has been reduced (PBI 1.8). Probing depths were generally half of the original values. The gingivae have shrunk, and exhibit irregular fibrous thickening.

A subsequent surgical procedure was indicated to improve gingival contour.

Replacement of defective anterior restorations would considerably simplify interdental hygiene.

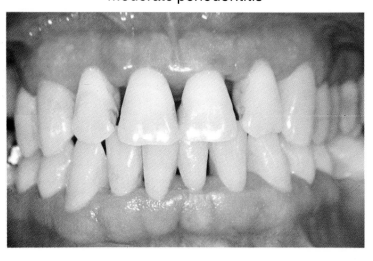

After

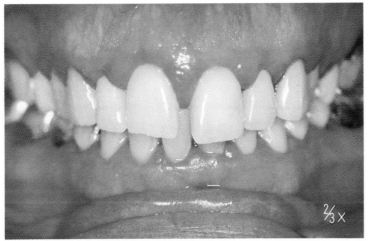

388 Moderate periodontitis – Diastema caused by the drifting of teeth
The patient reported that the 3 mm space between his front teeth had developed over the course of the previous 2 years.

Drifting of the maxillary anterior teeth could be due to the severe gingival inflammation and the localized deep periodontal pockets, as well as functional forces from premature contacts, overbite and a shift during intercuspation.

Tooth migration during periodontitis

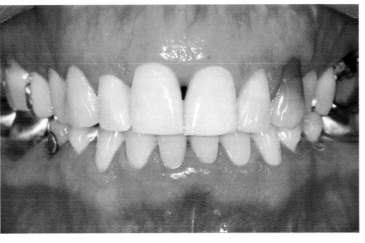

389 Findings 9 years after initial therapy
The only treatment provided for this patient was initial therapy, occlusal equilibration and slight shortening of tooth 21. The gingival inflammation remained under control despite the patient's less than optimum motivation and cooperation with home care. The diastema closed *spontaneously* six month after initial therapy, without any orthodontic measures.

Tooth 23 became dark after endodontic treatment for pulpitis.

390 Advanced periodontitis (RPP)
Pronounced marginal inflammation, hemorrhage at the lightest touch (PBI 4), 10 mm pockets with suppuration. The margins of posterior full crowns are at least 2 mm apical to the gingival margin.

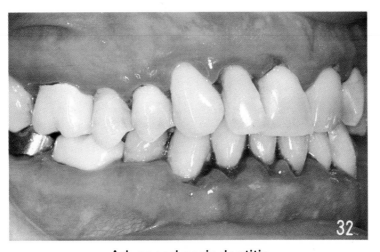

Advanced periodontitis

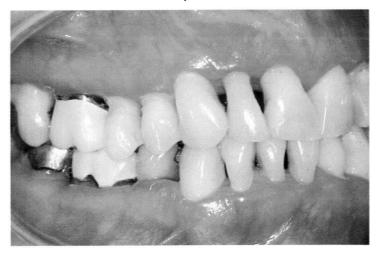

391 Findings 3 months after initial therapy
Inflammation is absent for the most part. Gingival tone has returned after tissue shrinkage that resulted in irregular contour. Crown margins are now supragingival. Some deep pockets (cratering) persist, some with signs of active disease.

Re-evaluation of this case clearly demonstrates that without surgical intervention the deep active pockets cannot be expected to disappear.

392 Acute stage of Gingivo-periodontitis ulcerosa
The gingivae are severely inflamed (PBI 3–4) and exhibit pronounced ulcerations in the interdental areas. Gingival contour is "inverted" (reverse architecture) as a result of attachment loss associated with osseous interdental cratering. Probing depths are relatively shallow (4–5 mm) due to loss of interdental papillae.

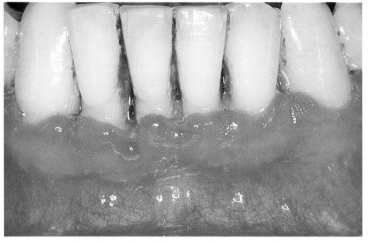

Before

Gingivoperiodontitis ulcerosa (ANUG)

393 Findings 6 months after initial therapy
The acute phase was completely eliminated by initial therapy. A surgical procedure is nonetheless required in the mandibular anterior region in order to create a morphological situation that the patient can keep clean. Frequent recall will be necessary thereafter if the results achieved are to be maintained.

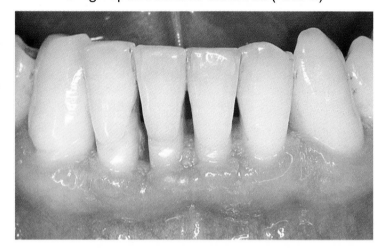

After

394 Stillman's cleft with secondary inflammation
Calculus is visible in the gingival cleft on tooth 21. Use of erythrosin disclosing solution also revealed a small accumulation of microbial plaque. This patient practiced oral hygiene vigorously but incorrectly, using a horizontal scrubbing technique with a hard-bristled toothbrush. Thus, the etiology of the Stillman's cleft could involve both plaque-elicited inflammation and trauma from toothbrushing.

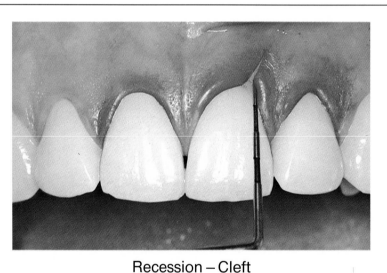

Before

Recession – Cleft

395 Findings 3 months after initial therapy
The Stillman's cleft closed spontaneously solely as a result of repeated careful scaling of the root surface in the area of the cleft, and "freshening up" of the edges of the soft tissue. The patient's brushing technique was changed to modified Stillman (vertical rotatory). Sulcus depth at the location of the former cleft is completely normal!

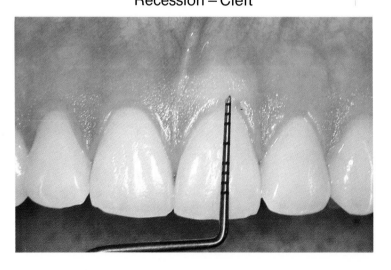

After

Periodontal Surgery

Periodontal surgical therapy is only a *part* of complete periodontal treatment. If surgery is necessary at all, it is usually performed as part of a second phase of therapy. The patient must have first demonstrated appropriate motivation and home care.

When all periodontal treatment is completed, a regular recall interval must be established (maintenance phase). If this is not done, every periodontal surgical procedure will eventually fail (Rosling et al. 1976 b; Nyman et al. 1977; Westfeld et al. 1983).

The art and science of periodontal surgery will be presented as follows:

- Purpose and goals of periodontal surgery
- Indications for and methods of periodontal surgery
- Re-evaluation and surgical planning after initial therapy
- Preparation for a periodontal surgical procedure
- Various surgical techniques.

Purpose and goals of periodontal surgery

Periodontal surgery, its goals and its purposes, can only be considered in conjunction with complete periodontal treatment. For example, initial therapy and surgery are two entities with identical goals, but which use different methods to achieve those goals. Similarly, initial therapy may represent complete therapy for one case, while for a more complicated case initial therapy is really only a preparatory pre-surgical phase.

The purpose and goal of periodontal surgery may be summarized as follows:

1. Thorough cleaning and smoothing of the root surface, with direct vision
2. Reduction or elimination of plaque-retentive areas, especially periodontal pockets, that enhance disease progression
3. Elimination of inflammation and pocket activity
4. Enhancing the regeneration of periodontal tissues
5. Creation of physiologic morphology of the marginal periodontium and the mucogingival border.

1. Cleaning and smoothing the root surface (root planing)
The root surface is exposed to clinical view either by laying mucoperiosteal flaps or by simple gingivectomy. The root surface, including its depressions, irregularities and the furcation area, is then debrided of plaque and calculus, insofar as this was not accomplished completely during initial therapy. Endotoxin-containing cementum is planed away and the root surface is smoothed. These measures make possible the healing and regeneration of periodontal structures.

2. Reduction or elimination of plaque-retentive areas (pockets)
The most important retentive areas for microbial flora are periodontal pockets. Additional areas include open furcations, root depressions, anomalies of tooth position and iatrogenic irritants such as poor margins on restorations and crowns.

Pockets with persistent signs of activity may be treated by means of a flap procedure (conservative or radical) or with gingivectomy.

Furcations can be treated by odontoplasty and rendered accessible for oral hygiene, or a root resection may be performed to eliminate the furcation problem entirely.

3. Elimination of inflammation and pocket activity

The main goal of periodontal surgery is not always to totally eliminate the pocket itself, but to eliminate any signs of pocket activity (infection), such as exudate, hemorrhage or suppuration. The goal is to halt the progression of the disease process.

4. Enhancing regeneration of periodontal tissues

The results of a periodontal surgical intervention should be "healing" and regeneration of periodontal tissues. A new soft tissue attachment should form; this is usually in the form of a long junctional epithelium with an epithelial attachment. In the depth of the operated pocket, connective tissue fibers should attach anew to the root surface. Formation of new alveolar bone is possible (see Periodontal Healing, p. 260).

5. Creation of physiologic morphology of the marginal periodontium and the mucogingival border

A physiologic contour of the marginal periodontium can be achieved by means of gingivectomy/gingivoplasty, flap surgery with internal gingivectomy and possibly minor osteoplasty.

Mucogingival surgery may be employed to enhance the width of attached gingiva or to correct unphysiologic frenum attachments that extend into the marginal gingiva. Gingival recession can be prevented by mucogingival procedures.

Indications for and methods of periodontal surgery

The choice of a periodontal surgical technique depends on the type and severity of the periodontal disease, as well as on the pathomorphologic situation at the site to be operated.

Periodontal surgery may be categorized as:

- Gingivectomy/gingivoplasty (GV/GP)
- Flap procedures with conservative flap reflection (Modified Widman flaps/Ramfjord technique)
- Flap procedure with flaps reflected completely, permitting various possibilities for flap repositioning
- Combinations of methods and special operations
- Mucogingival surgery.

The indication for gingivectomy/gingivoplasty is limited. GV/GP is used in cases of pronounced gingival enlarge-ment/overgrowth, shallow suprabony pockets, localized "minor operations," and in combination with flap surgery.

The GV/GP is *contraindicated* for treatment of infrabony pockets and osseous thickening, and when attached gingiva is narrow or absent.

The *modified Widman procedure* (Ramfjord technique, partially reflected flap) *is the most universally applicable periodontal surgical modality*. It is particularly indicated for treatment of mild to moderate periodontitis.

The fully reflected mucoperiosteal flap (with or without vertical incisions) is indicated in severe periodontitis with irregular bone loss within an arch segment and for advanced furcation involvement. In such cases, osteoplasty may also be performed, as well as intraosseous implants.

Special periodontal surgery includes wedge excisions, implants of various types into bony pockets, treatment of isolated furcation involvement, and extraction of hopeless teeth with simultaneous revision of periodontal supporting tissues of the adjacent teeth. These procedures are usually performed in conjunction with flap operations.

Mucogingival surgery is indicated only in cases exhibiting advanced gingival recession where attached gingiva is lacking or where frenum attachments radiate into the marginal gingiva.

Re-evaluation and surgical planning after initial therapy

Eight to ten weeks after initial therapy has been completed, maximum periodontal regeneration will have occurred. This is the *time to re-evaluate* the entire case: Probing depths, attachment loss, gingival inflammation (PBI) and plaque accumulation (HYG) are evaluated anew and recorded. The necessity for surgical intervention is determined by considering these new clinical findings. The patient's own cooperation and motivation are also important considerations. Surgery should only be considered if the HYG index is at least 80% and gingival bleeding on probing is essentially absent. Exceptions to this rule are patients lacking manual dexterity, retarded individuals, the handicapped, and elderly persons who, despite their best efforts and consciensciousness cannot achieve the otherwise mandatory hygiene levels. In these special patients, more frequent postsurgical recall must compensate for the deficiencies.

Following re-evaluation, the *definitive planning* of the surgical phase of therapy can be done, with consideration for the chances of success (pocket elimination, attachment gain) associated with the various operative methods (see Michigan study, Figs. 383 & 396). A decision is made concerning which areas of the dentition must be operated, what techniques are to be used, and which teeth are to be extracted. In doubtful situations it may be necessary to make a decision *during* the operation as to whether or not a tooth can be saved by periodontal therapy. Temporary replacements may have to be fabricated.

The type of prosthetic treatment planned for the patient may also influence the surgical planning when specific teeth are to be used as abutments.

Another critical factor is the *general systemic health* of the patient. This may also influence decisions concerning the extent or complexity of periodontal surgery. Of particular concern in this regard are patients with diabetes, hematologic disorders, hypertension, hemorrhagic diathesis, focal infection or elderly persons with a history of poor healing. Patients undergoing radiation therapy and those on anticoagulant medication should not be treated surgically.

Preparations for a periodontal surgical operation

Surgery is usually performed per sextant, less seldom per quadrant. The patient should always have one side functional for chewing after surgery.

The preparations for periodontal surgery are similar to those for routine small oral surgical procedures, and include the usual hand disinfection, mouth mask, operatory disinfection and instrument sterilization. It is prudent for the dentist and his auxiliary personnel to be immunized against Hepatitis-B, since the danger of infection is quite high in dental practice. Finally, the entire dental practice team should be well schooled in how to handle emergency situations (Schijatschky 1979).

Premedication is usually not necessary in patients with good oral hygiene. It is advisable, however, to have the patient rinse thoroughly (30 sec) with chlorhexidine solution (0.1–0.2%) immediately before the surgery begins. This elicits a reduction in the quantity of microorganisms in the oral cavity for several hours. Prophylactic administration of systemic medications is generally reserved as supportive therapy in distinct types of periodontal disease (RPP, LJP; see p. 283).

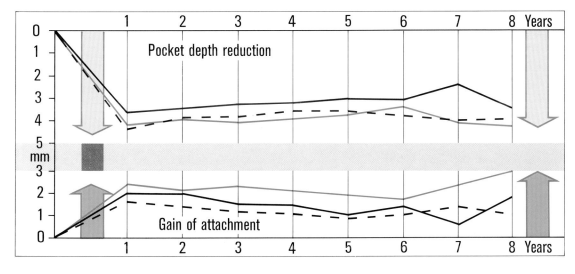

396 Pocket depth reduction and attachment gain following various treatment methods for 7–12 mm pockets (Knowles et al. 1979)

——————— Modified Widman procedure
——————— Root planing and curettage
– – – Surgical pocket elimination

Surgical techniques described in this Atlas

The most important periodontal surgical methods are described in the following pages both "in principle" and "step-by-step."

Indications and contraindications, as well as advantages and disadvantages of each surgical procedure are discussed.

Anesthesia

Nerve block anesthesia

Only in the mandibular posterior segments is true nerve block anesthesia used for periodontal surgery (inferior alveolar nerve block).

Terminal anesthesia

An advantage of terminal anesthesia is that it provides a degree of vasoconstriction for the field of operation and provides the surgeon better vision because of reduced hemorrhage.

Direct infiltration

Injection of anesthetic solution directly into interdental papillae, for example prior to a gingivectomy, can enhance the anesthetic effect and provide tissue ischemia.

Vasoconstriction

Most anesthetic solutions contain 0.5–1 mg% epinephrine. If there is a contraindication for epinephrine in a particular patient, it may be substituted by an alternate vasoconstrictor (e.g., vasopressin).

397 Surface anesthesia
A topical anesthetic is used at the site of injection to reduce the discomfort of needle penetration.

Reducing the pain of an injection can contribute greatly to the patient's psychic well-being during the entire operation.

Procaine-free topical agents reduce the chance of an allergic reaction.

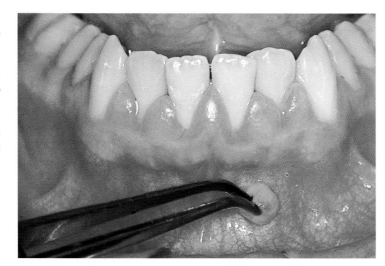

398 Terminal anesthesia in the vestibular fold
On the facial surface, anesthetic solution is injected near the periosteum in the loose submucosal connective tissue.

The diagram indicates where the anesthetic should be administered on the *lingual* aspect of the mandible.

On the *palate*, anesthetic solution should be infiltrated 5–10 mm from the gingival margin.

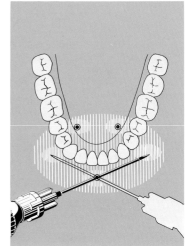

399 Infiltration into interdental papillae
Immediately before surgery the dentist may choose to inject directly into the papillae. In addition to increasing the anesthetic effect, this procedure will also greatly reduce hemorrhage.

Precaution: Direct infiltration should *never* be attempted into severely inflamed tissue.

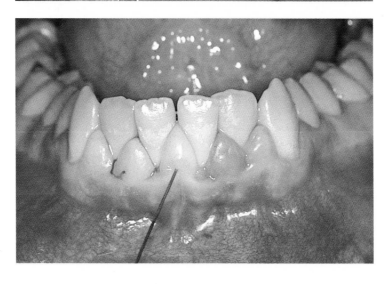

Gingivectomy (GV) and Gingivoplasty (GP)

Gingivectomy (GV) refers to a surgical procedure in which gingival pockets are eliminated by removal of gingival tissue. Gingivoplasty (GP) refers to surgical recontouring or remodeling of the gingival surface. The GV is practically always enhanced by subsequent GP. During a single operation, gingival pocket depths are reduced and the remaining attached gingiva is given a physiologic contour. Often GV/GP is combined with other surgical procedures, particularly flap operations.

The GV/GP has several disadvantages and contraindications that limit its application as sole surgical technique in certain types of cases. Nevertheless, GV/GP retains its usefulness for localized procedures to correct gingival contour (p. 172).

Indications

- Gingival enlargement or overgrowth
  (e.g., that elicited by phenytoin)
- Idiopathic gingival fibromatosis
- Pseudopockets
- Shallow suprabony pockets
- Areas with difficult access
- Minor corrective procedures.

The GV/GP *can* be employed in all these situations. However, the modified Widman procedure is a superior technique for suprabony pockets.

Contraindications

- Narrow or absent attached gingiva
- Infrabony pockets
- Thickening of marginal alveolar bone.

Advantages

- Technically simple; good visual access
- Complete pocket elimination
- Predictable morphological result.

Disadvantages

- Very limited indications
- Gross wound; postoperative pain
- Healing is by secondary intention
  (ca. 0.5 mm per day)
- Danger of exposing bone
- Loss of attached gingiva
- Exposes cervical area of tooth
  (sensitivity, esthetics, caries)
- Phonetic and esthetic problems in anterior area.

Principles of the operation

- Continuous incision at 45° angle at the base of the pocket
- Sharp dissection of tissues in the interdental area
- Smoothing of the incision edge
- Contouring the gingival surface (GP)
- Scaling and root planing
- Wound coverage (periodontal dressing).

Instruments for Gingivectomy/Gingivoplasty...

Practically every manufacturer of dental instruments offers many varieties that fulfill the requirements of a gingivectomy procedure. The original GV/GP instruments are decades old (e.g., Kirkland knives), but continue to be modified and improved. The main function of the instrument is to provide the operator with the ability to perform an uncomplicated, rapid and clean procedure. This will be determined primarily by the size, shape and angulation of the working tip, and also by the handle, which should be comfortable.

Generally speaking, a GV/GP procedure requires a gingivectomy knife and a papilla knife, each of which may be singly or doubly angled.

400 Pocket marking forceps
The paired pocket marking forceps (Deppeler; L & R) is used exclusively in the GV/GP procedure for indicating the location of the base of the pocket. Pocket depths can also be similarly marked using a fine periodontal probe.

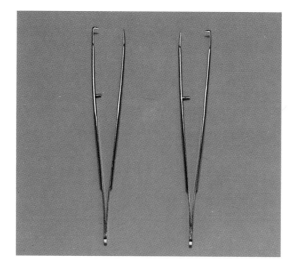
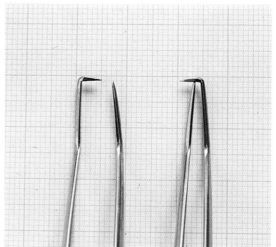

401 Gingivectomy knives

GV knife (Kirkland; L & R), single bend
Papilla knife (Orban, L & R), single bend
Universal knife, single bend

These knives are also available with two bends, and as double-ended instruments.

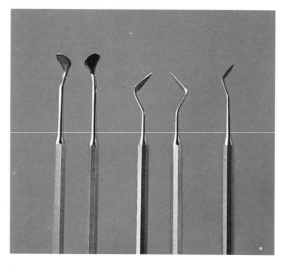
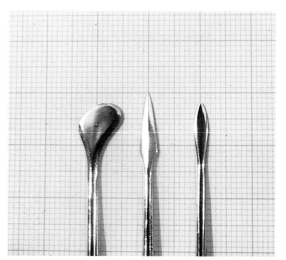

402 Electrosurgery apparatus and tips (Martin, Ellman)
Electrosurgery finds its primary function in the gingivoplasty procedure, where it is useful for contouring soft tissues, for papillectomy, for smoothing out abrupt edges, and for exposing the margins of restorations. Electrosurgery is not recommended for the primary gingivectomy incision because of the possibility of injury to the tooth root, periosteum or bone.

The high frequency current for electrosurgery should be either fully rectified or fully filtered.

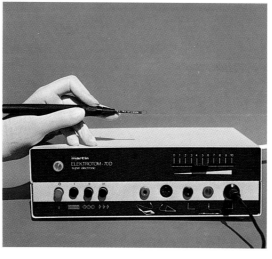
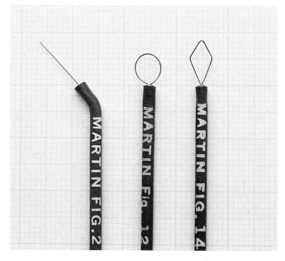

...and Their Use

More important than design and manufacturer is the sharpness of the instruments. Gingivectomy knives must be sharpened using an Arkansas stone with oil before each operation. This requirement can only be avoided through use of instruments with disposable blades.

For contouring the gingival surface (GP), fine electrosurgical tips are indicated. Electrosurgery is also indicated for minor procedures such as exposing the margin of a tooth preparation before taking the impression, or before seating a restoration. Because electrosurgery exerts a certain hemostatic effect, it may be used to advantage for excision of highly vascular soft tissues.

The typical use of some gingivectomy instruments is depicted below. A complete clinical procedure (pp. 163–169) presents their detailed use.

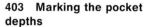
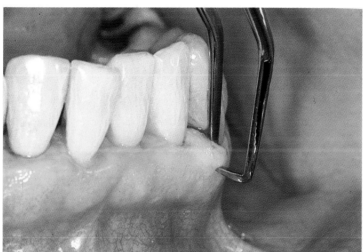

403 Marking the pocket depths
The straight arm of the forceps is guided into the buccal pocket on tooth 33, much as a periodontal probe would be. When the base of the pocket is encountered, the forceps is pinched together, causing the horizontal forceps tip to mark the depth of this 4 mm pocket.

By repeating this procedure at each tooth surface, a series of "bleeding points" is created, which are used subsequently as a guide for the incision.

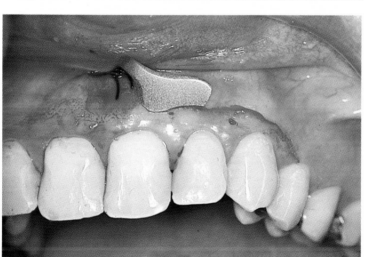

404 Gingivectomy
The blade is positioned at a 45° angle to the tooth long axis and a continuous incision is made. Here, the single-bend Kirkland knife is used in the anterior area.

For a gingivectomy on the less accessible palatal or lingual areas, a double-angled instrument is often useful.

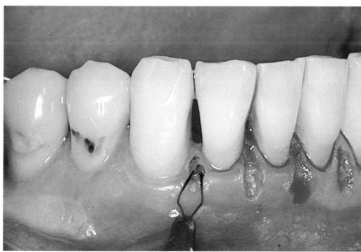

405 Gingivoplasty with the electrosurgical wire loop
The small rhomboid electrode is used here to reduce the bulbous marginal gingival contour while creating a more physiologic morphology.

Periodontal Dressings and Tissue Adhesives

In almost every case, a gingivectomy wound must be covered with a dressing, more for patient comfort than for acceleration of wound healing. A dressing can significantly reduce postoperative pain during the first few days.

Only eugenol-free dressings are recommended. Coe-pak, for example, is a 2-component dressing composed of zinc oxide and fatty acids, while Peripac comes ready-to-use from the container and has a gypsum base.

A periodontal dressing can prevent colonization of the wound surface by plaque microorganisms, if it is mixed with a disinfectant, e.g., chlorhexidine powder (Plüss et al. 1975).

Minor injuries such as those created by an electrosurgical procedure to expose the margin of a crown or restoration can be coated with a cyanoacrylate tissue adhesive (Fig. 408).

The periodontal dressing is generally left in situ for 7–10 days. A second dressing may be indicated if healing is inadequate.

406 Eugenol-free dressings

Peripac (left)
A ready-to-use dressing composed of gypsum and acrylic. It sets quickly upon contact with saliva. There is a danger of pressure aphthous ulcer formation due to its hard edges.

Coe-pak (right)
A two-component dressing composed of zinc oxide and fatty acids. Coe-pak remains pliable even after the setting reaction is complete; no irritating edges are created.

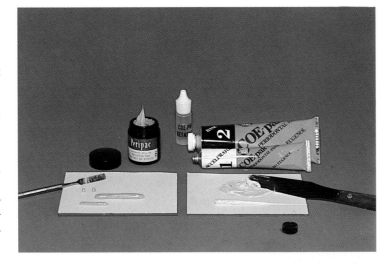

407 Chlorhexidine powder (CHX)
Periodontal dressings can be rolled in the water-insoluble CHX-HCl powder immediately before placement over a wound. This will serve to reduce plaque formation beneath the dressing. Wound healing progresses without inhibition (see pp. 120 & 264).

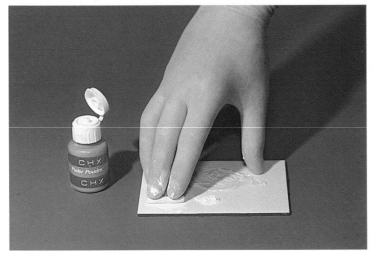

408 Tissue adhesives
(Cyanoacrylate)

– **Histoacryl** (Braun, above)
– **Bucrylate** (Ethicon, below)

For minor GV/GP wounds, tissue adhesive may be used instead of a periodontal dressing. Adhesives may also be used instead of sutures for stabilization of repositioned flaps or free gingival grafts, and for covering the palatal donor site (see p. 237).

Adhesives are applied by means of plastic tubes, brushes or cannulae.

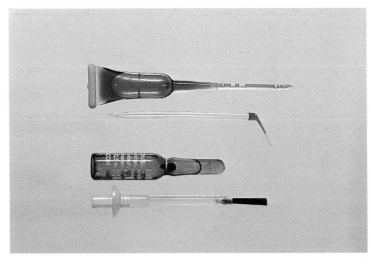

Gingivectomy/Gingivoplasty

Operative procedure

The systematic procedure for a GV/GP operation is depicted below in the case of an 18-year-old male who exhibited severe hyperplastic gingivitis without any history of phenytoin medication. Abundant plaque accumulation, maxillary anterior crowding, malocclusion and mouth breathing were all factors in the etiology of this condition.

Orthodontic therapy was recommended, but not accepted at that time by the parents or the patient; initial therapy therefore included minimal occlusal equilibration by means of selective grinding.

Initial findings:
HYG 0%   PBI 3.5   TM 0–1
Findings after initial therapy:
HYG 75%   PBI 1.5

The clinical picture, gingival contour, probing depths and radiographs are presented in the Figures below.

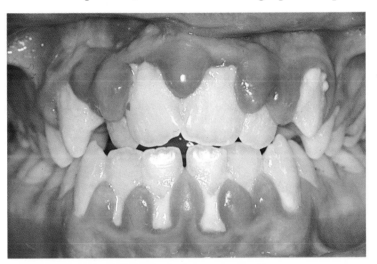

409   Clinical picture before initial therapy
Extreme gingival hyperplasia with pseudopockets to 6 mm. Heavy plaque accumulation, especially in anterior area; mouth breathing, malocclusion.

The situation prevented the patient from performing effective home care.

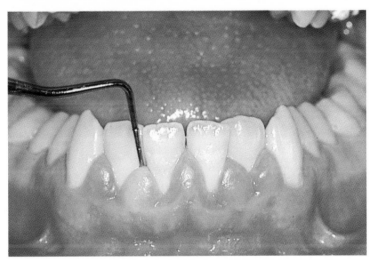

410   Mandible after initial therapy
Elimination of inflammation reduced the pseudopocket depths to 3–5 mm. The gingivae remain fibrotically enlarged and home care is still difficult.

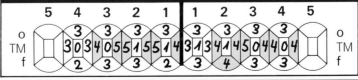

	5	4	3	2	1	1	2	3	4	5	
o	3	3	3	3		3	3	3	3		o
TM	3 0 3 4 0 5	5 1 5 5 1 4				3 1 3 4 1 4	5 0 4 4 0 4				TM
f	2	3	3	2		3	4	3	3		f

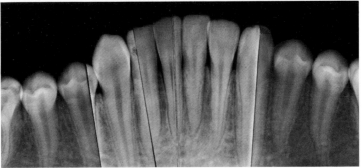

411   Probing depths, tooth mobility, radiographic findings
The remaining pseudopockets are the result solely of redundant tissue; there is no true attachment loss or osseous defect. Tooth mobility (TM) values are normal.

In the radiograph, no bone loss is detectable.

412 Gingival hyperplasia and pseudopockets

A blast of air from the syringe reflects an enlarged papilla away from the tooth surface.

Right: Histology of the area indicated by the black line in the clinical view demonstrates that the apical extent of the junctional epithelium is at its normal position at the CEJ. A mild inflammatory infiltrate is still apparent after initial therapy (H & E, × 10)

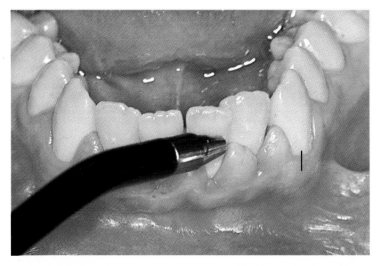
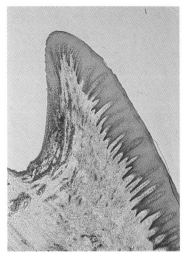

413 Anesthesia

Profound anesthesia is accomplished by injections in the mucobuccal fold. To reduce hemorrhage during the procedure, each interdental papilla destined for resection is injected directly.

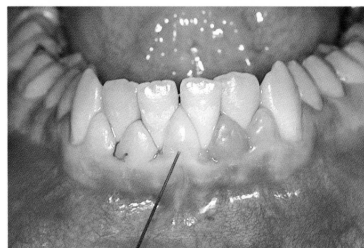

414 Marking the base of pockets

The pocket marking forceps is used on papillae and on the midfacial marginal gingivae to indicate the course of the sulcus base between teeth 43 and 33.

An incision at this level would yield a blunt ledge of tissue; therefore, the incision must be made slightly apical to the bleeding points.

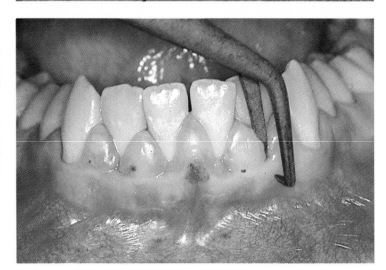

415 Marking the incision line

A periodontal probe (e.g., Michigan-0) is used to mark the incision line. The probe is inserted through the gingiva at a 45° angle to the tooth long axis (see schematic), apical to the bleeding points created by the marking forceps. The incision line must be in attached gingiva.

The skilled operator may elect not to mark the incision line in this way, but simply to use the bleeding points as a guide, in which case the incision is made 1–3 mm apical to the bleeding points.

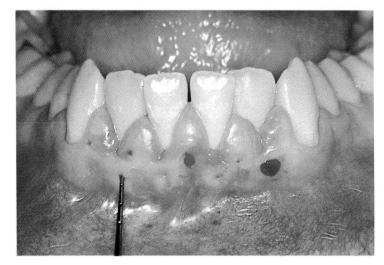
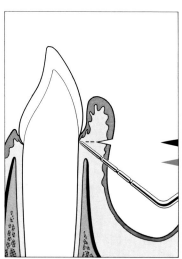

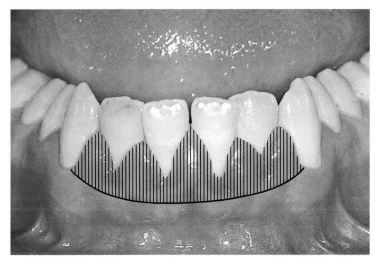

416 Planned excision
On the *labial surface,* the incision will be continuous at a 45° angle to the vertical, from 43 to 33.

No surgery is planned for the *lingual aspect* because no pseudopockets persisted after initial therapy.

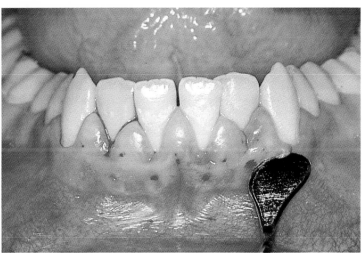

417 Proper position of the Kirkland gingivectomy knife
The GV knife is placed at a 45° angle to the tooth long axis, at the first marking point near tooth 33. From here a...

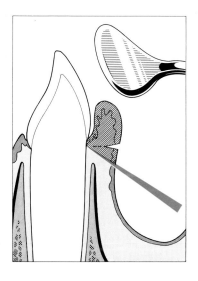

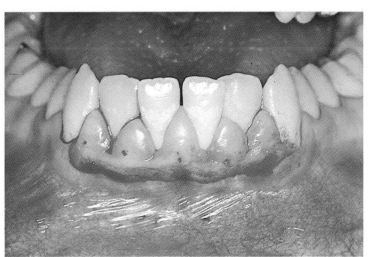

418 ... continuous incision is performed
The incision line is totally within the attached gingiva, and the mucogingival line is not approached.

The knife is generally carried through the incision one or two times to insure that the tissue is freed at the bottom of the sulcus.

419 Incision completed
The tissue to be excised is still firmly attached in the interdental areas, where the gingivectomy knife cannot reach.

420 Use of the Orban papilla knife
The pointed, rigid papilla knife is used at the same 45° angle as the GV knife to release the excised tissue by cutting through the papilla to the col region. The tissue should *not* be torn away!

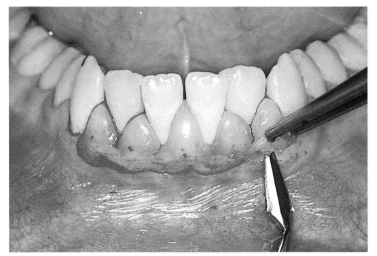 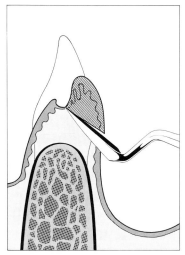

421 Removal of the tissue
The gingival segment is lifted gently with a forceps, and the papilla knife is used to severe any remaining tissue.

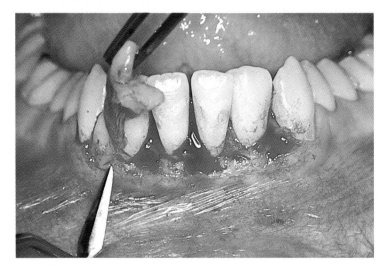

422 Excised tissue
In this case it was possible to remove the redundant tissue as a single piece. If the etiology of the lesion is known, there is no need for a histopathological assessment of the specimen.

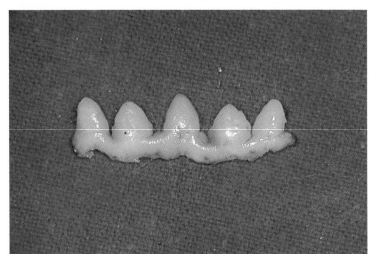

423 Scaling and root planing with direct vision
Any plaque and calculus remaining in the pseudopocket after initial therapy becomes visible once the redundant tissue is removed, and can be eliminated completely during root planing.

Thus, the most important component of the gingivectomy procedure is the thorough cleansing and smoothing of the tooth. This will insure a bioacceptable surface as the new epithelial attachment and junctional epithelium form during the healing process.

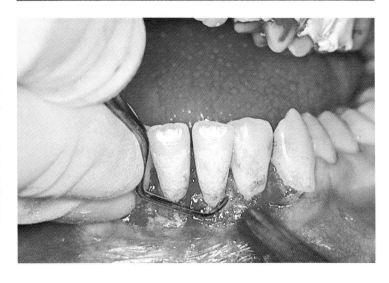

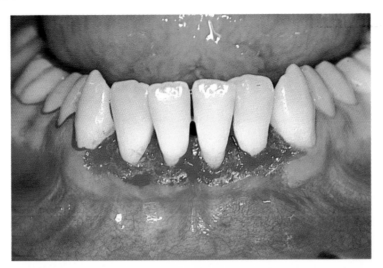

424 Gingivectomy wound after scaling
Despite the 45° angulation employed during surgery, the wound margin is still at a relatively sharp angle. This edge must be rounded in order to provide ideal gingival contour after healing.

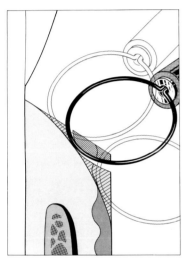

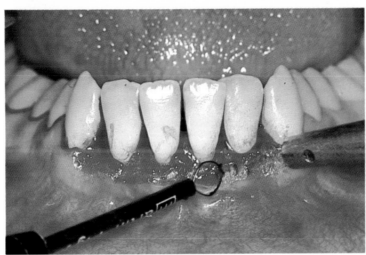

425 Smoothing the "sharp edge"
An electrosurgical loop is indicated for this fine contouring procedure.

Schematic: The motion should be "sweeping" in nature, and actual tissue contact of short duration, in order to avoid overheating and thus damaging the osseous tissues or the tooth itself.

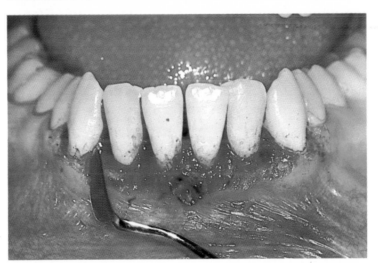

426 Cleansing the wound
The Kirkland knife is used to scrape away residual tissue tags or debris. This procedure also provides the final gingival contour.

In this case, recontouring extended bilaterally to the first bicuspids.

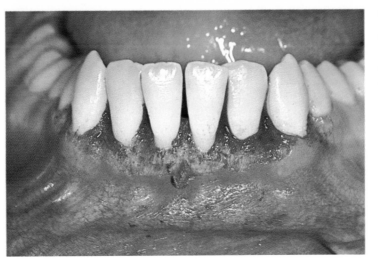

427 Clinical view immediately following GV/GP
The surgical procedure has resulted in a relatively expansive open wound surface which must be covered and protected with a periodontal dressing.

428 Wound treatment before dressing placement

An antibiotic ointment may be applied to the wound surface before the dressing is placed.

Right: Achromycin ophthalmic ointment (1%) in a disposable syringe. Such ointments do not enhance wound healing, but reduce microbial plaque colonization of the wound surface.

An alternative is incorporation of chlorhexidine-HCl powder into the periodontal dressing (Fig. 407).

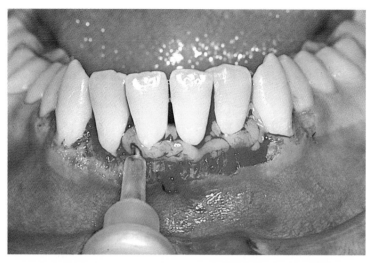
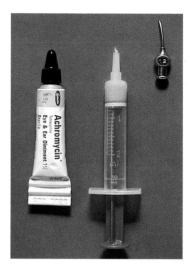

429 Dressing in place

In this case, Peripac was used. This is a rigid dressing which must not encroach upon the mobile mucosa, to prevent formation of pressure areas and ulceration. The dressing should be left in situ for 7–10 days without changing it.

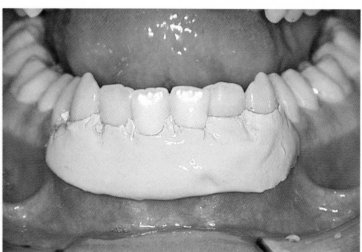

430 Dressing removal and dental prophylaxis after 7 days

The dressing is carefully removed and the teeth gently cleaned using a rubber cup and a minimally abrasive prophy paste (or dentifrice). The wound surface is cleansed using hydrogen peroxide solution (3%) on cotton pellets, then sprayed with the water syringe. The patient can be dismissed with the recommendation that oral hygiene be practiced regularly, but carefully at first.

A second dressing application is indicated only if epithelialization appears to be retarded.

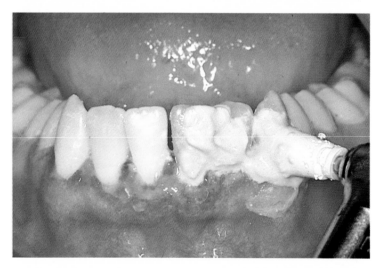

431 6 months after GV/GP

The gingivae are inflammation-free and exhibit a generally physiologic morphology. A very slight recurrence of gingival hyperplasia can be detected between 43, 42 and 41 (papillae).

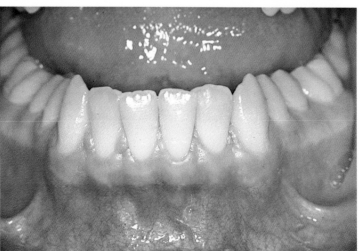

Gingivectomy/Gingivoplasty

Summary

This 18-year-old patient presented with a very severe hyperplastic gingivitis. Oral hygiene, especially in maxillary interdental areas, ranged from hopeless to non-existant. The anterior crowding contributed to the poor situation. During initial therapy, it became clear that the young man was very difficult to motivate. Both the patient and his parents initially refused orthodontic treatment, and for this reason selective occlusal grinding was employed to improve the malocclusion as much as possible. Despite these unfavorable circumstances, the surgical procedure led to an acceptable result in terms of gingival contour and freedom from gingival pockets. A short recall interval was mandatory to maintain the results of treatment.

Two years later, and motivated by the success of the treatment, the patient sought orthodontic therapy to correct the malocclusion!

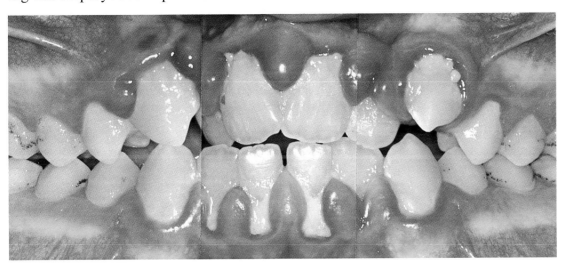

432 Initial clinical view
Extreme hyperplastic gingivitis, plaque, calculus, absence of home care.

The symptoms of disease are limited primarily to the labial surfaces of maxillary and mandibular anterior segments.

Factors contributing to the gingival condition included malocclusion, crowding in the maxilla, and mouth breathing.

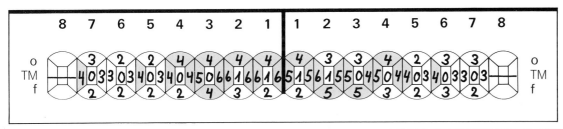

433 Probing depths and tooth mobility (TM) in the mandible before treatment
Pseudopockets, but no attachment loss.

Before

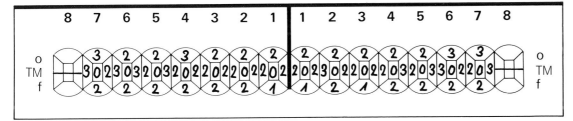

After

Probing depths and tooth mobility (TM) 2 years later
Normal probing depths after periodontal therapy and orthodontic treatment.

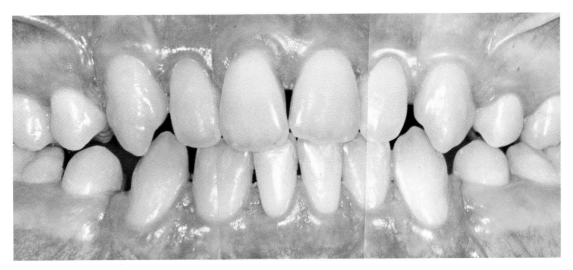

434 Clinical findings 2 years postoperatively
Thanks to a frequent recall schedule, there was no recurrence of the hyperplastic gingivitis despite only moderate home care by the patient. The patient has been able to maintain the area with only minor inflammation. The orthodontic result, while less than optimum, is satisfactory.

The upper arch was also treated by means of GV/GP (see next page).

GV/GP in the Maxilla – Buccal and Palatal

The patient documented on the previous pages also underwent a gingivectomy procedure for treatment of the extreme hyperplastic gingivitis on labial as well as palatal aspects in the maxillary arch. The surgery was carried to the distal aspect of the second bicuspids on both sides. The occlusal photographs (Figs. 435–437) depict the problems associated with this case, not the least of which was severe anterior crowding.

A GV/GP operation can be performed routinely if the palatal vault is high; however, if the palate is flat a GV with a 45° angulation results in an expansive open wound surface that heals slowly (epithelialization occurs at ca. 0.5 mm per day).

Hemorrhage from the incisive foramen can be readily controlled by means of electrocoagulation or injection directly into the canal of a vasoconstrictor-containing anesthetic solution, under pressure.

435 Before initial therapy
The hyperplastic gingivitis is enhanced on the palatal aspect by the anterior crowding, which also renders oral hygiene very difficult and leads to plaque accumulation and retention.

The *schematic* depicts the anticipated GV incisions labially and palatally. The incision on the labial aspect must not encroach upon the mucogingival line.

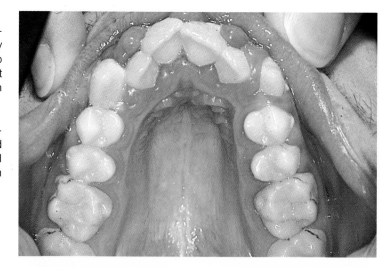 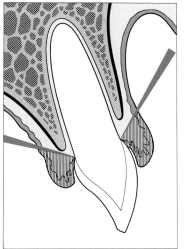

436 After gingivectomy
The ideal 45° angle incision is also applied in the palatal area if the anatomical situation permits. This can result in expansive open wound surfaces, which are painful and take longer to heal completely.

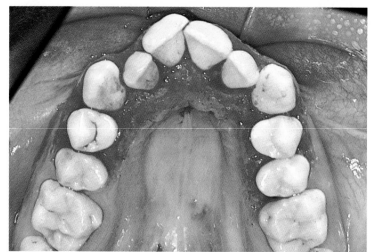

437 3 months after gingivectomy
The patient's home care has been inadequate, particularly in difficult-to-reach areas occasioned by tooth positional anomalies. In these areas, hyperplastic gingivitis has begun to recur (arrows).

Nevertheless, the clinical situation is remarkably improved in comparison to the initial condition; the gingivae are practically inflammation-free, there are no pseudopockets, no attachment loss. With frequent recall, these improved intraoral conditions can be maintained.

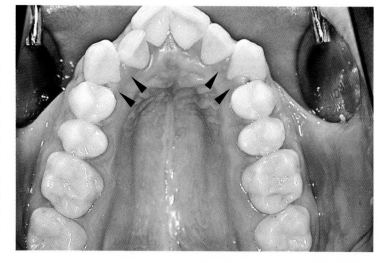 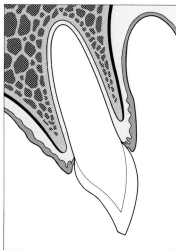

GV/GP – Phenytoin-Induced Gingival Overgrowth

Diphenylhydantoin preparations are frequently employed in the treatment of epilepsy. About half of all individuals who ingest hydantoins (generic: phenytoin) on a chronic regimen develop gingival enlargement (pharmacogenetic factor, Hassell 1981). The development of such gingival lesions is enhanced by microbial plaque. Following initial therapy, gingivectomy is the treatment of choice for phenytoin-induced gingival overgrowth. Plaque control is often difficult, especially in mentally or physically handicapped individuals. In such cases, chemical plaque control (chlorhexidine) is indicated as an adjunct to home care.

The following case is a 20-year-old mildly retarded female who had taken phenytoin for many years and who was incapable of adequate home care.

Initial findings:

HYG 0%	PBI 3.8	TM 2 or less

PD Pseudopockets to 8 mm

Radiographic survey: No bone loss

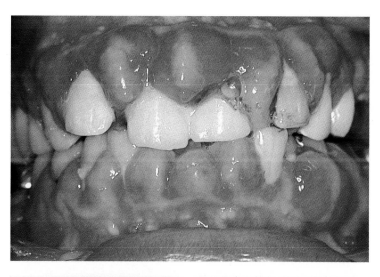

438 Phenytoin-induced gingival overgrowth with severe secondary inflammation
The fibrous gingival overgrowth may have been an etiologic factor in the tooth migration. The treatment plan included gingivectomy after initial therapy, with gingivoplasty to improve gingival contour.

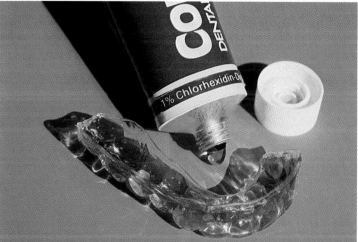

439 Customized acrylic tray used as carrier for chlorhexidine gel
To prevent plaque accumulation and postsurgical recurrence of the gingival enlargement, customized transparent acrylic trays were fabricated for use as medicament carriers in both maxilla and mandible.

The patient, who lacks the dexterity to adequately perform oral hygiene, fills each tray with chlorhexidine gel (1% chlorhexidine gluconate) and wears the tray for one hour each evening.

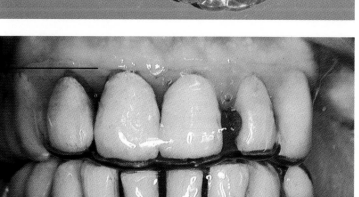

Borders of medicament carriers

440 1 year after GV/GP, with trays in situ
The maxillary incisors have spontaneously regained their proper positions in the dental arch. Recurrence of the gingival overgrowth was completely inhibited by daily chemical plaque control (CHX gel, 1× daily).

The acrylic trays extend to the attached gingiva and are well adapted, thus preventing seepage of the gel into the oral cavity.

GV/GP – Corrective Operations, Minor Procedures

Exposing the margins of restorations and cavity preparations

Gingivectomy and gingivoplasty are particularly useful for minor corrective procedures.

The margins of restorations and crowns should be located supragingivally to avoid irritation of the periodontal tissues. Exceptions to this rule may be considered in anterior regions, for reasons of esthetics. It is nevertheless a fact that tooth preparation and impression taking is technically difficult if the margin is located subgingivally. Also it is considerably easier to place a rubber dam if the preparation margin is supragingival. In the case presented here, carious lesions that extend into the subgingival area are exposed by a labial and palatal gingivectomy procedure. If properly performed, there should be no subsequent esthetic problems.

441 Subgingival caries on teeth 21, 22 and 23
Without a gingivectomy, it would be impossible to create a proper cavity preparation or apply the rubber dam, which is necessary for elimination of moisture when placing a composite resin restoration.

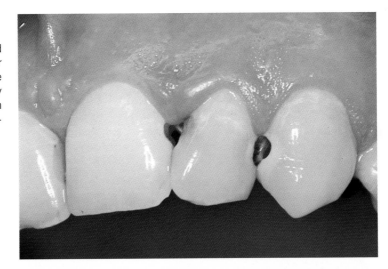

442 GV using the Orban knife
Minor procedures such as this may be conveniently performed with electrosurgery, as well as with the more conventional gingivectomy knives or scapels.

Hemorrhage, depicted here during gingivectomy with a knife, can be avoided for the most part with electrosurgery; moreover, since there is no bleeding, the definitive restorations can often be placed during the same appointment.

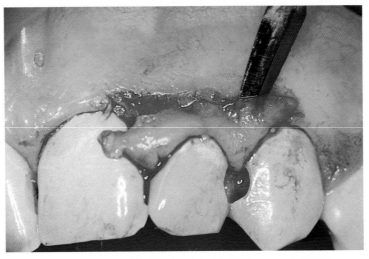

443 After restorative treatment and healing
The apical margins of the 4 scarcely visible composite restorations lie supragingivally and are therefore accessible for oral hygiene by means of toothbrush and dental floss.

This promotes prevention of recurrent caries as well as gingivitis.

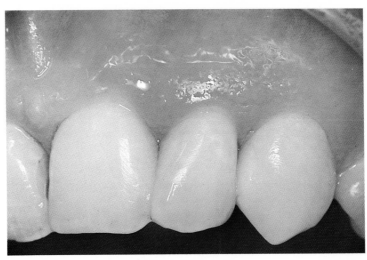

GV/GP for prosthetic, endodontic and esthetic reasons

Minor gingivectomy procedures are often indicated for exposure of preparation margins in endodontically treated, severely broken down teeth that must be restored by means of a core or full crown. The GV is indicated more often in these situations than for routine restorations.

In the case presented here (30-year-old male), a gingivectomy on the labial aspect had to be performed to expose a perforation that had occurred subsequent to a previous endodontic procedure. The GV not only revealed the margins of the post-and-core and the metal/ceramic crown, but also effectively adjusted the length of tooth 11 to correspond to 21. The same procedure also improved the gingival contour.

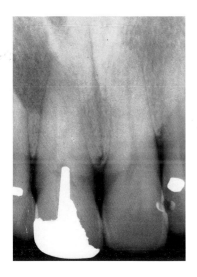 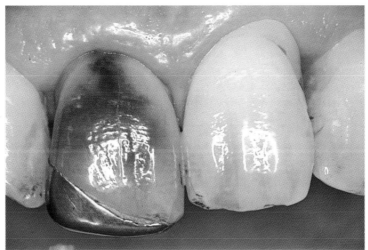

444 Perforation, corrosion
The old post-inlay covering the incisal edge must be replaced. The clinical crown had discolored excessively due to metal corrosion. A perforation was detected about 2 mm subgingivally.

The adjacent tooth, 21, exhibits recession of some 2 mm.

The radiograph reveals the short, corroding post, but no bone loss.

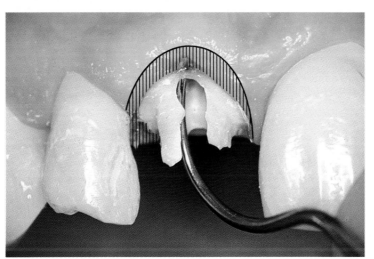

445 Exposure of the perforation via GV
The procedure of choice is a half moon-shaped gingivectomy (indicated by lines) using electrosurgery to expose the perforation site, demonstrated by the explorer tip. The GV procedure can equalize the clinical crown length of 11 and 21.

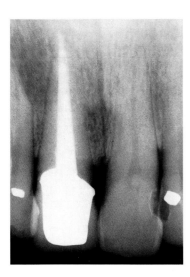 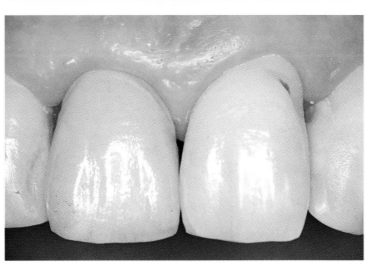

446 Definitive restoration with a metal/ceramic crown
The labial porcelain crown margin covers the perforation site and lies slightly subgingivally (for esthetic reasons). Both central incisors are now approximately the same length.

Left: The radiograph reveals the revised root canal filling, the post, and the new crown.

Gingivoplasty

The gingivectomy procedure can be used purely to correct tissue morphology, for example to recontour bulbous papillae. This can reduce plaque retention and render oral hygiene easier.

The 28-year-old female described below complained of gingival bleeding. In terms of home care, she had never received any professional instruction, motivation or treatment. Her gingivitis was of long duration.

Initial findings:
HYG 40%   PBI 3.7   TM 0–1
PD 5 mm in interproximal areas; pseudopockets

Initial therapy and proper home care essentially eliminated her gingival inflammation; however, some interdental papillae remained bulbously enlarged and appeared morphologically unfavorable. This residual situation was corrected by means of electrosurgery.

447 Gingivitis
Before initial therapy, the inflammatory hyperplastic enlargement of the interdental papillae was especially pronounced in the mandibular anterior segment. Pseudopockets were shallow. The malocclusion was obvious, with a partial anterior open bite.

Poor home care was demonstrated by application of a plaque disclosing agent.

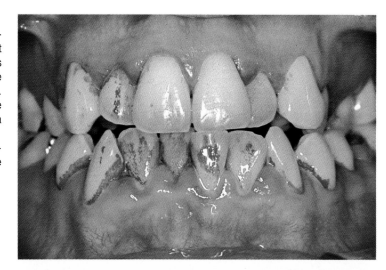

448 Gingivoplasty
After completion of initial therapy, several hyperplastic papillae persisted. These were removed using the rhomboid-shaped electrosurgery tip, which also created a more normal gingival contour interdentally (see schematic occlusal view at cervical level, right).

This procedure reduces plaque accumulation, enhances self-cleansing and makes home care easier for the patient.

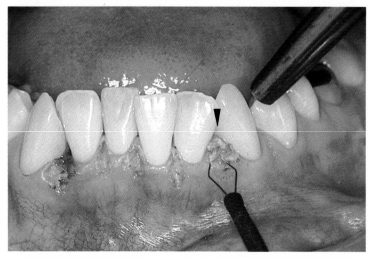
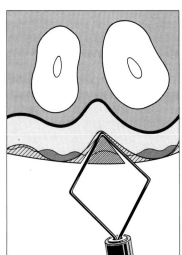

449 10 weeks after gingivoplasty
Bulbous gingival papillae are absent. The re-creation of physiologic morphology simplifies oral hygiene, as evidenced by the 10-week postoperative clinical data:

HYG   90%
PBI   0.8
TM   0–1
PD   max. 2 mm

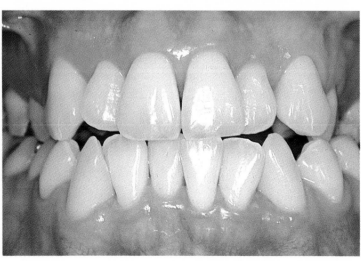

Flap Procedures

Flap procedures are the most universal and most commonly employed of all periodontal surgical techniques. *The reflection of a soft tissue is nothing more than a method for gaining access to deeper periodontal structures,* which can then be treated with direct vision (see Indications).

In order to ensure adequate vascular supply and regeneration, the full thickness (mucoperiosteal) flap is almost always used. The entire soft tissue complex (gingiva, mucosa, periosteum) is separated and reflected from the root and alveolar bone surfaces. Less often, "split thickness" flaps are reflected in which the mucosa and connective tissue are separated from the subjacent periosteum. An example of the split flap may be found in mucogingival surgery (p.228).

Among the different techniques, the modified Widman flap procedure (Ramfjord technique) is the most often selected, particularly in cases manifesting mild to moderate periodontitis.

Indications

Flap procedures are indicated in cases of periodontitis with active pockets (bleeding, suppuration) over 4 mm deep that do not respond sufficiently to initial therapy.

Special indications include:

- Pockets with bases located beyond the mucogingival line
- Pronounced thickening of the marginal bone
- Infrabony pockets
- Osseous transplants and implants in infrabony pockets
- Hemisection of a tooth, or root resection
- Tooth extraction with immediate periodontal treatment of remaining adjacent periodontal structures.

Advantages

Flap procedures have the following advantages over closed curettage / root planing or GV/GP:

- Optimum subgingival scaling and root planing to the base of the pocket can be performed with direct vision
- Pocket epithelium is entirely removed by the internal bevel incision
- At the end of the surgery, the flaps can be replaced at the original location, or repositioned apically, coronally or laterally
- The interdental bone or infrabony defects can be covered by the flaps
- No open wound persists postoperatively
- Little periodontal tissue is actually lost.

Contraindications

- Pronounced gingival enlargement/overgrowth, which is handled more efficiently by means of GV/GP
- Crown lengthening procedures to expose restoration margins (GV/GP usually indicated)
- Difficult access (technical surgical problems).

Disadvantages

- If flaps are repositioned apically, more of the tooth and root structure is exposed, which may be a problem in terms of postoperative sensitivity as well as esthetics (p.194).

Instruments for Flap Procedures...

In general, the instruments used for periodontal flap procedures are the same as those employed for other oral surgical procedures. These include scalpels, elevators and needle holders. The instruments should be as fine as possible, to promote sensitive handling of the delicate tissues.

The various instruments depicted and described below have proven useful in practice. Many other types and manufacturers are available that will yield satisfactory results if used correctly.

If the flap procedure is to be combined with a GV/GP, the gingivectomy knives described earlier may also be required. The flap surgery "kit" also contains various forceps, explorers, periodontal probes, surgical scissors and clamps, and most importantly curettes for scaling and root planing. In addition, bone burs or bone files (osteoplasty) as well as fissure burs or diamond stones may be required for hemisection or root resection etc.

450 Scalpel blades

- **11** (Martin)
- **12 B** (Bard-Parker)
- **15** (Martin)
- **15 C** (Bard-Parker)

To ensure sharpness, only disposable blades are utilized, providing a minimum of tissue trauma and enhanced healing.

Only the most delicate scalpels are indicated for periodontal surgery, where precision is demanded and access often limited.

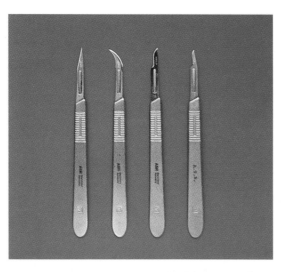
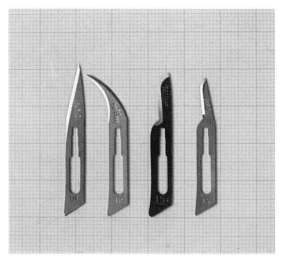

451 Elevators

- **FK 300,** 6 mm (Aesculap; *white*)
- **VT 24, 22, 23,** 5 mm (Deppeler; *red*)
- **VT 27,** 4 mm (Deppeler; *yellow*)
- **Special manufacture** 2.5 mm (Zabona; *blue*)

Small, narrow elevators (2–6 mm wide) are used to reflect the flaps.

These instruments may also be used during root planing or osseous recontouring to deflect the flaps from the field of operation to improve visibility.

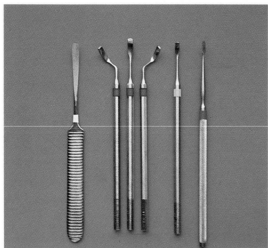
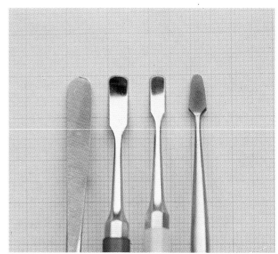

452 Needle holder – Elasticitiy (in gm) of the closure

- **BM 150** (Aesculap; 1500 gm)
- **Special manufacture,** wide (Zabona; 1800 gm)
- **Special manufacture,** narrow (Zabona; 600 gm)
- **BM 563,** Castroviejo needle holder for eye surgery (Aesculap; 500 gm)

Needle holders must fulfill opposing demands: They must hold the needle securely, while allowing the surgeon to release the locking mechanism easily.

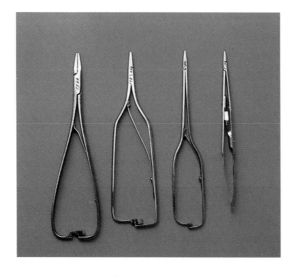
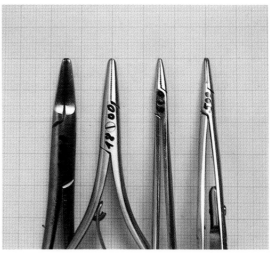

...and Their Use

The use of surgical instruments is depicted in the three clinical photographs below. Widely used routine components of a flap procedure are shown: The initial incision using the 12B scalpel (in this case, an internal bevel incision), the reflection of the flap using the narrow, rounded elevator, and repositioning and adapting the flap using interrupted interdental sutures.

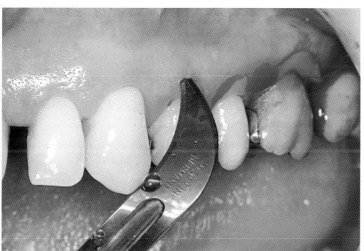

453 Scalloped internal bevel incision
The first incision made during a modified Widman operation (Ramfjord technique) is a scalloped, internal bevel incision.

The preferred instrument for this procedure is the 12B scalpel, which is sharp on both edges of the sickle-shaped blade.

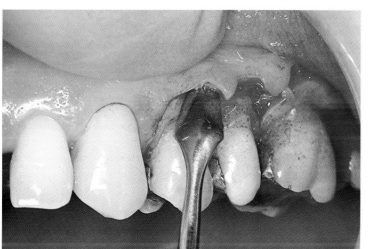

454 Flap reflection
In the region of tooth 24, a small elevator is used to raise a concise tissue flap, following the scalloped line of incision.

Narrow elevators can follow the scalloped incision better than wide elevators, thus preventing tissue trauma and tears.

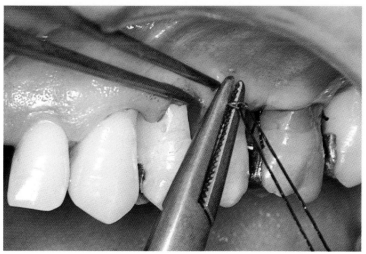

455 Flap fixation with interrupted sutures
Fine needle holders and fine needles are required for atraumatic periodontal flap surgery. Thin papillae and mucosal flaps can easily be torn by thick needles and large needle holders that are clumsy and difficult to open.

Needles, Sutures and Suture Knots

Adaptation of periodontal flaps may be accomplished using a variety of suture materials available in varying thicknesses with curved or straight needles. The needles are also available in various sizes, degrees of curvature, and cross-sectional profiles. Needles may have an "eye," or may have the suture incorporated into the blunt end of the needle ("atraumatic needles").

Periodontal surgeons normally use interrupted sutures but may occasionally employ continuous sutures and mattress sutures. Although there are numerous "surgeon's knots" known, a few will serve adequately in the majority of periodontal surgery situations. The most important considerations in flap repositioning are close adaptation to the alveolar bone and around the teeth, and complete coverage of the interdental area.

456 Needles and sutures
The needle, suture material and needle holder should be synchronized to each other. Atraumatic suturing requires a pointed needle, which cuts as it penetrates.

The suture material should be supple and should permit knots that hold well. The type of suture material (catgut, nylon, silk) determines the type of knot used.

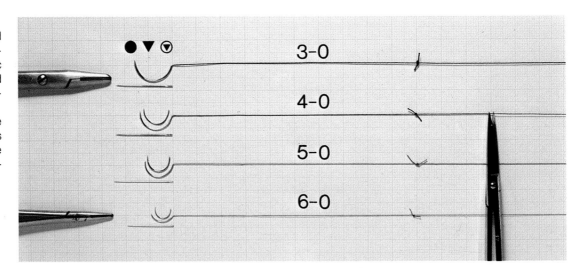

457 The "2–1" surgeon's knot
A double and a single loop are used together in a simple surgeon's knot.

The first double loop prevents any loosening of the suture tension while the second (single) loop is being added.

Right: The "2–1" knot pulled tight. This simple knot is used primarily with braided suture, whether synthetic or natural (silk).

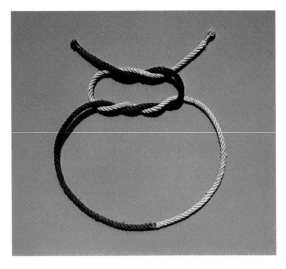
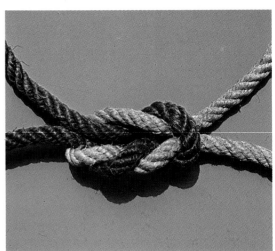

458 The "2–2" double surgeon's knot
Knots placed in catgut or in monofilament synthetic suture loosen easily. When these materials are used, it is wise to employ two double loops when tying sutures.

Right: The "2–2" knot pulled tight. Caution: Large knots such as the 2–2 surgeon's knot may lead to formation of aphthous ulcers on the vestibular mucosa due to irritation. If the patient is particularly susceptible to such ulcer formation, suture knots should be covered with a soft periodontal dressing.

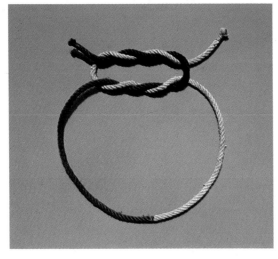
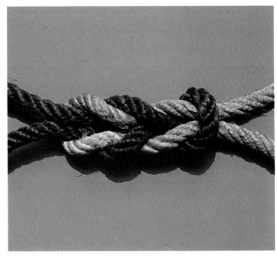

Partially Reflected Mucoperiosteal Flap
Modified Widman Procedure (Ramfjord Technique)

The modified Widman flap is the most frequently used surgical technique, because it provides the most favorable long-term results. The original technique (Widman 1918) was modified (Ramfjord & Nissle 1974; Ramfjord 1977) and improved by means of defined incisions, conservative flap reflection and an atraumatic approach.

The goal of the procedure is "healing" of the periodontal pocket with minimal tissue loss, and not pocket elimination *per se*. Postoperative pain and swelling almost never occur.

The most important aspect of the Ramfjord technique is total removal of subgingival plaque and calculus with direct vision, as well as subsequent smoothing and planing of the root surface to remove layers of cememtum that contain endotoxin. No ostectomy is performed. Corrective osteo*plasty* may be performed to improve the facial or palatal (lingual) bony architecture, and can be especially important in obtaining complete closure over interdental bony defects when repositioning the flaps.

Indications

- Mild to moderate periodontitis, with pocket depths between 4 to 6 mm (the procedure can also be employed in cases with deeper interdental defects).
- Depending upon the particular pathology in an area, the Ramfjord technique can be combined with larger, fully reflected flaps. Less frequently, the procedure may be combined with gingivectomy and with special operations such as wedge excisions, root resection, hemisection etc.

Contraindications

There are practically *no* contraindications:
- Very narrow attached gingiva can render the Ramfjord technique difficult because there is insufficient area to permit a scalloped internal bevel incision. This is often the case in the mandibular area.
- The Ramfjord technique may also be difficult in cases where the planned procedure involves osseous recontouring in the face of extremely deep defects and an irregular pattern of bone loss on the facial and oral aspects. If the bony crest is particularly protuberant in some areas, the Ramfjord technique may be difficult. In such cases, complete reflection of the flaps is indicated, rather than partial/conservative reflection. However, the principles of the Ramfjord technique, especially the incisions, can also be followed during more complex operations.

Advantages

- Root planing is accomplished with direct vision
- The procedure is reparative, not destructive to tissue
- Healing by primary intention
- Reduced postoperative discomfort.

Disadvantages

- see Contraindications.

Principles of the Ramfjord Technique

1. Scalloped inverse bevel incision, along the long axis of the root, down to the alveolar crest
2. Reflection of a mucoperiosteal flap within the attached gingiva, but only to the crest of the alveolar bone
3. Marginal incision (crevicular)
4. Horizontal incision
5. Root planing with direct vision; removal of granulation tissue from osseous defects
6. Thorough adaptation of the flaps using interrupted sutures; complete coverage of interdental craters.

The first incision serves to demarcate the pocket epithelium and the subepithelial infiltrate from adjacent healthy tissue and to preform "new papillae."

An elevator then is used to raise and mobilize the flap, but only far enough to expose the crest of the alveolar bone.

459 First incision – Scalloping
The scalloped incision is performed on both labial and palatal aspects, using the double-edge 12 B scalpel. It is an inverse bevel incision, extending to the alveolar crest. This incision thins the gingival tissue and permits complete closure of the interdental osseous defects postoperatively. The distance of the incision from the gingival margin may vary from 0.5 to 2 mm. In this case, the incision is rather far from the gingival margin; in most cases, this incision is made much closer to the free gingival margin (see schematic).

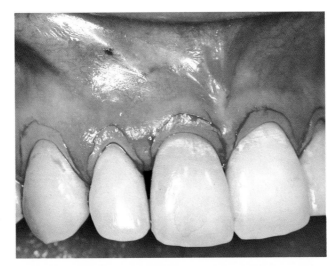 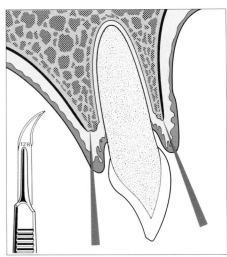

460 Flap reflection
An elevator is used to raise a full thickness mucoperiosteal flap as atraumatically as possible. The flap is reflected only to permit direct visualization of the root surface and the alveolar crest.

In most cases it is possible to stay within the boundaries of the attached gingiva, without extending beyond the mucogingival line (arrow in schematic; conservative flap reflection).

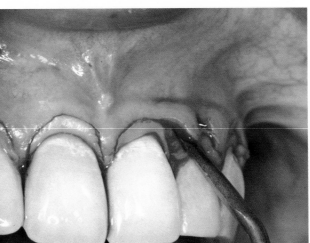 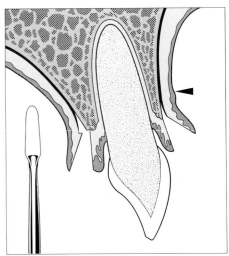

461 Second incision – Crevicular
This incision is carried around each tooth, between the hard tooth structure and the diseased pocket epithelium, to the depth of the junctional epithelium.

The 12 B scalpel is used to advantage.

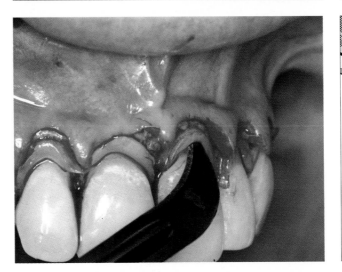 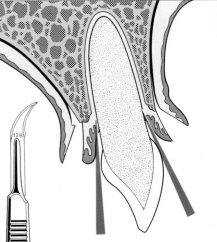

The second incision is made intracreviculary around the tooth to the depth of the pocket, freeing pocket epithelium from healthy connective tissue.

Ramfjord suggests a third horizontal incision, which ensures sharp and atraumatic removal of diseased pocket tissue, especially in the interdental area.

The most important aspect of the Ramfjord procedure now follows: Systematic planing and smoothing of the root surfaces, using fine curettes with direct vision. This phase of the procedure is very time-consuming.

Bone is not removed, but light osteoplasty for flap closure may be carried out on facial and oral surfaces.

Finally, the flaps are repositioned. Because of the shape created by the initial scalloped incision, tight and complete coverage of the interdental bone is possible. This enhances healing by primary intention.

This surgical procedure is routinely associated with excellent long-term results in terms of maintenance or even true gain in periodontal attachment (Knowles et al. 1979; Figs. 383, 396).

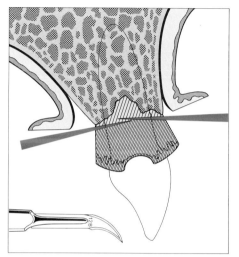
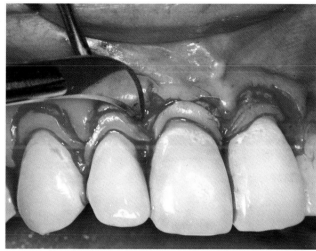

462   Third incision – Horizontal

The horizontal incision is carried along the alveolar crest, thus separating the infiltrated tissue from healthy supporting connective tissue, especially in the interdental area.

The incision also permits atraumatic removal of the diseased tissue.

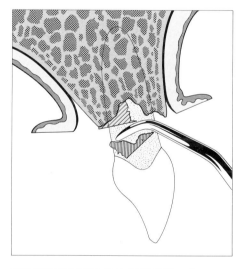
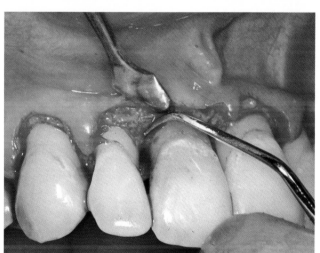

463   Root planing with direct vision

Fine curettes are used to remove remnants of pocket epithelium and granulation tissue.

Systematic root planing is performed with repeated rinsing. Root planing is the most important part of both the modified Widman procedure, and all other periodontal surgical procedures.

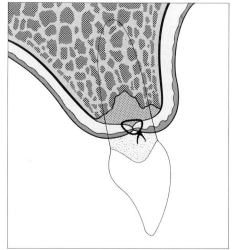
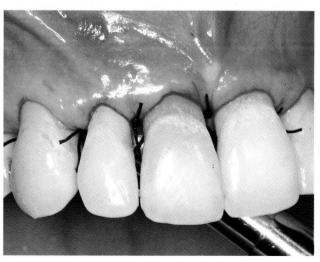

464   Complete coverage of interdental defects

The labial and palatal flaps are closed over the interdental areas without tension, using interrupted sutures. The flaps should be adapted to the underlying bone and the necks of the teeth. New "papillae" were created by the scalloped form of the initial incision. These make it possible to cover interdental defects (e.g., bony defects) even when the interdental space is wide.

For this reason, placement of a periodontal dressing is not absolutely necessary.

The surgical principles described above for the anterior area and illustrated from the frontal view also hold for the posterior segments. The anatomy of flap creation and flap repositioning can be appreciated particularly well when viewed from the occlusal aspect. The posterior segment operation described below is depicted from an occlusal view, at the level of the CEJ.

The first incision (buccal & palatal) is a scalloped one, approximately 0.5 to 2 mm from the free gingival margin. This scalloping creates new papillae for sub-sequently covering interdental defects. At the distal end of the arch, this first incision may end in a wedge. If there are pockets or furcation involvement at this distal site, the appropriate therapy can be performed simultaneously (see Wedge Excision, p. 211). The scalloped margin of tissue will permit complete closure of the interdental osseous septa and curetted bony defects (2-wall defects). In the diagrams below, the second (crevicular) and third (horizontal) incisions are not shown.

465 Initial incision
The first incision is a scalloped inverse bevel incision (internal gingivectomy) in the maxillary posterior segment (compare also Fig. 459). The incision is combined with a wedge excision distal to the last tooth in the arch.

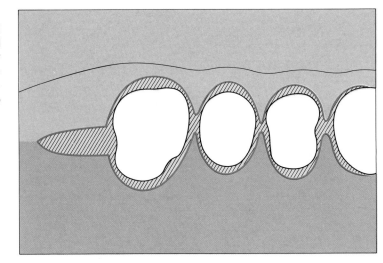

466 Flap reflection
After raising mucoperiosteal flaps, the second (crevicular) and third (horizontal) incisions (see also Figs. 461 & 462) enhance clean removal of diseased soft tissue from the pocket. This is followed by careful debridement of the bony defects and root planing of all teeth, with direct vision.

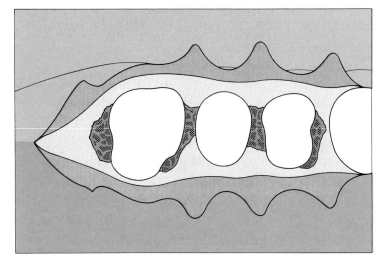

467 Adaptation of flaps and suturing
Complete coverage of the interdental bone is accomplished by fixation of the papilla tips with interrupted sutures. Extremely wide interdental spaces can be filled by lateral repositioning and suturing two papillae into a single space.

If the initial incision results in remaining tissue that is insufficient for complete coverage in the interdental area, small craterlike soft tissue defects may persist after healing. A subsequent minor gingivoplasty can correct such defects.

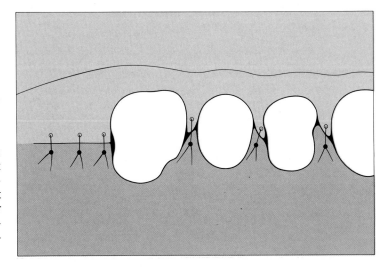

Ramfjord Technique

Operative Procedure

The systematic steps of a modified Widman procedure (Ramfjord technique) are depicted below in the anterior area of a 33-year-old female.

The diagnosis was moderate, rapidly progressive periodontitis (RPP). The patient was well motivated throughout the initial phases of treatment and his co-operation was above average.

Status after initial therapy:
HYG 82%
PBI 1.2
TM   2–3

The clinical picture, probing depths, gingival contour and radiographic findings are shown in the Figures below.

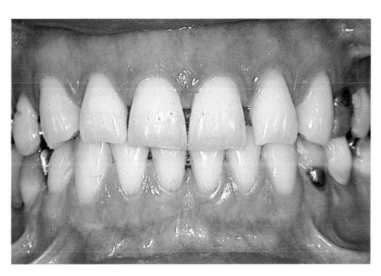

468 After initial therapy
From this view, the gingiva appears to be generally healthy. This is frequently the case after initial therapy, especially in RPP.

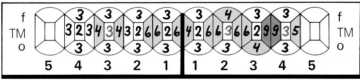

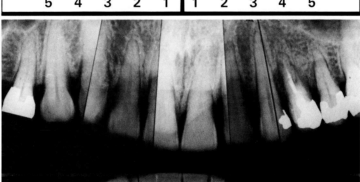

469 Probing depths and tooth mobility (TM) after initial therapy
In the interproximal areas, 4–6 mm pockets remain. Between 23 and 24, a 9 mm pocket with a class F3 furcation involvement of the premolar is observed.

Radiographic survey
Generalized, advanced interdental bone loss with areas of severe defects.

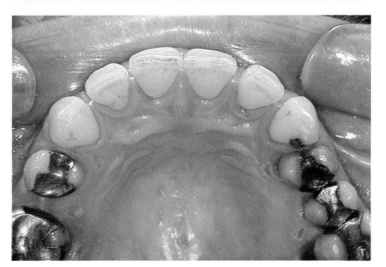

470 Occlusal view
Excessively vigorous oral hygiene has caused traumatic lesions on the palatal tissue. These wounds are clearly visible near 14; 24 and 25.

Tooth 24 will be extracted during the course of the planned periodontal surgery. When periodontal therapy is complete, all posterior restorations will be replaced.

471 Planning the surgery
The planned scalloped incision and the zone of flap reflection are indicated.

Solid line: Initial incision.

Hatched area: The reflection of the flap never approaches the muco-gingival line (conservative flap reflection.

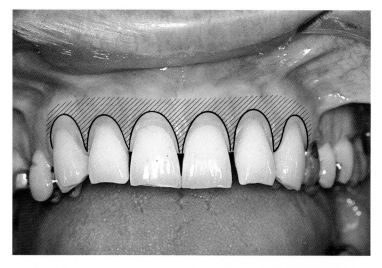

First incision

472 Scalloped initial incision
The goal of this incision is to separate diseased from healthy tissue.
    The tip of the blade is targeted toward the crest of the alveolar process.

Schematic: The tip of the scalpel should approach the crest of the alveolar process. The No. 12 B scalpel is ideal.

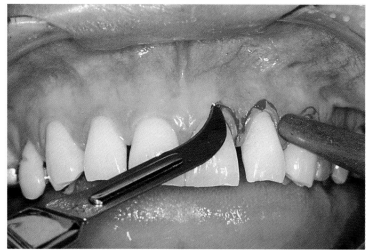
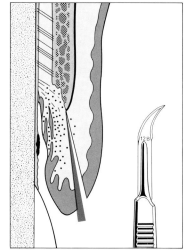

473 Initial incision completed on the labial aspect
The initial incisions in this case are somewhat extensive because of the facial pockets, but normally are kept only ca. 0.5 mm from the gingival margin (see schematic in Fig. 472).

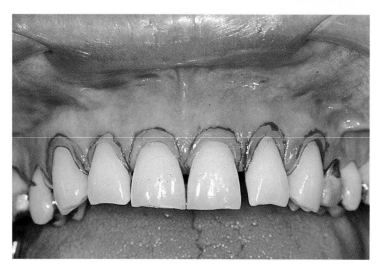

474 Initial incision on the palatal aspect
As on the labial aspect, this incision is scalloped. No special effort is exerted to avoid the incisive papilla.

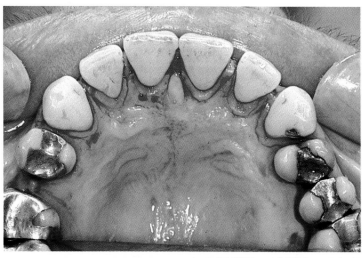

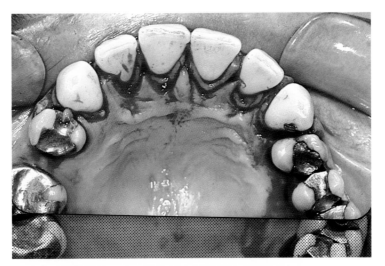

475 Reflection of the palatal flap
Occlusal view of the palatal flap, reflected only a few millimeters.

While making the initial incision, care is taken to create a thin and uniform palatal flap. This will make subsequent flap adaptation without tension much easier to achieve.

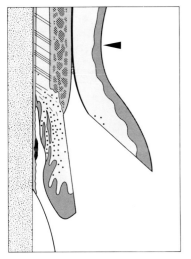
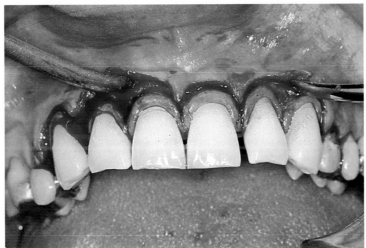

476 Reflection of the facial gingival flap
Here also, the gingiva is reflected until the crest of the alveolar bone is visible.

Schematic: Because the flap is not reflected beyond the mucogingival line (arrow) into the movable oral mucosa, the Widman flap cannot be repositioned apically or coronally. However, such a design does permit secure interdental repositioning.

Second incision

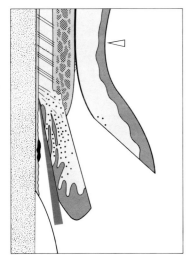
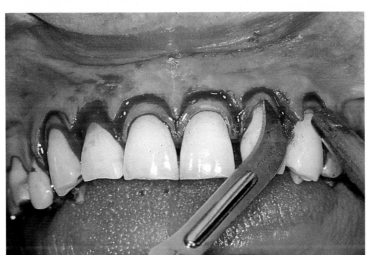

477 Crevicular incision
The 12 B scalpel is used for the second incision between the tooth and the diseased tissue, extending to the base of the pocket.

Third incision

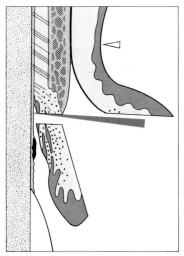
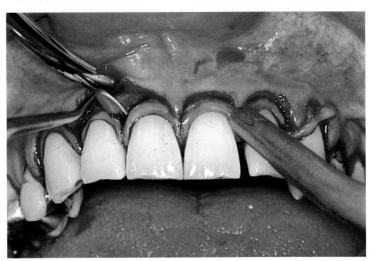

478 Horizontal incision
The Orban knife or scalpel is used to cleave the diseased tissue portion at its base.

This procedure, which dissects the tissue sharply, is likely to be less traumatic than tissue removal using the curette alone. Wound healing may therefore be enhanced.

479 Removal of the excised tissue

It is now a simple matter, using curettes, to remove the diseased tissue that has been delineated by the incisions.

During the procedure, the flaps cover the alveolar bone in all areas except the region being root planed. This undoubtedly reduces postoperative bone resorption.

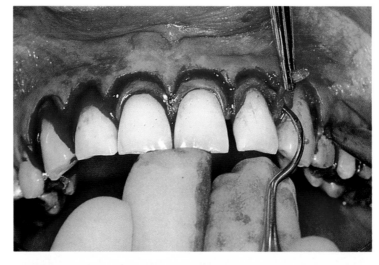

480 Continued removal of the excised tissue

If the incisions were clean and precise, the pathologically involved tissue can be removed in *toto*.

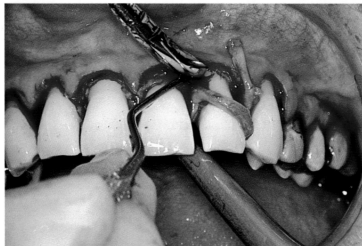

481 Curettage and root planing

After removal of the soft pocket epithelium and debridement of the bony defects, the root surfaces are systematically cleaned and smoothed using curettes.

Schematic: The best angle for the instrument tip is about 80° for calculus removal and root planing.

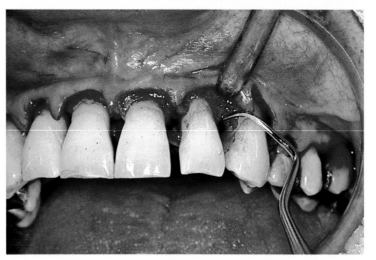 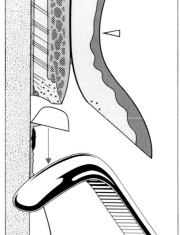

482 Clinical view following curettage and root planing

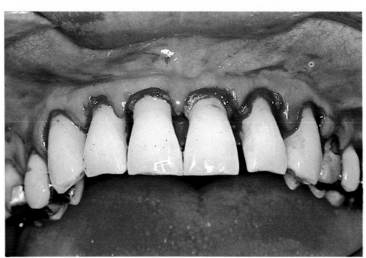

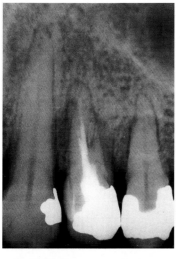

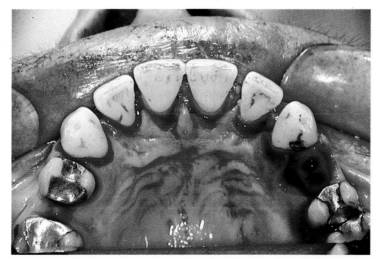

483 Extraction of 24
During the operation the open and untreatable trifurcation of the 3-rooted first bicuspid was discovered. Mesial probing depth was 9 mm. The decision was made to extract the tooth.

Radiograph: After the removal of 24, the gross amalgam overhang on the distal of the cuspid could be corrected.

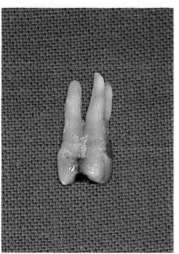

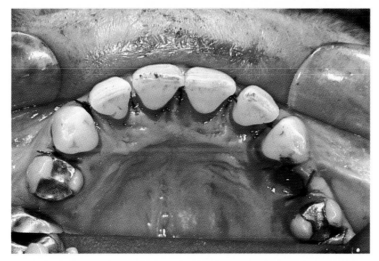

484 Flap adaptation and suturing
The interrupted sutures ensure tight adaptation of facial and oral flaps to the alveolar bone and tooth surfaces. The papilla tips are in contact or immediately adjacent to each other, thereby covering the interdental defects. In this case, a periodontal dressing (Coe-pak) was placed.

Left: The 3-rooted bicuspid after extraction.

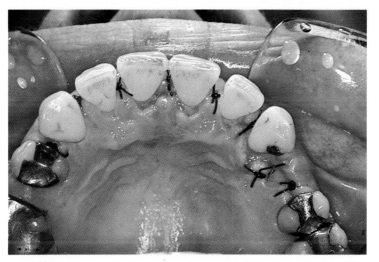

485 10 days postoperatively
Following removal of the periodontal dressing, the interdental sutures are visible in this occlusal view. The interdental spaces are already epithelialized; healing is progressing by primary intention without complications.

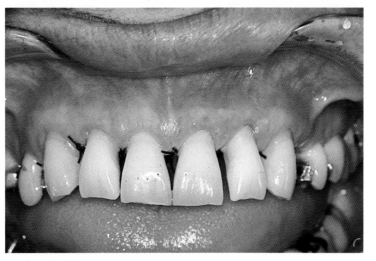

486 Postoperative plaque control
Since the surgery 10 days earlier, the patient practiced no oral hygiene in the maxillary arch, but rinsed twice daily with 0.2% chlorhexidine solution. In the area that was covered by periodontal dressing, neither plaque nor inflammation are detectable.

487 Removal of sutures
Sutures are carefully removed 10 days after surgery. Although the wound margins are well closed by this time, gross manipulation of the suture knots can completely undo the healing that has occurred thus far. Suture removal demands extreme care and tenderness.

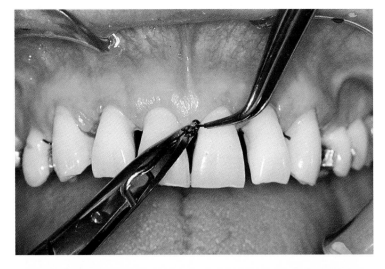

488 Prophylaxis
Following suture removal, exposed crown and root surfaces are thoroughly polished using a soft rubber cup and mild prophy paste or dentifrice.

It is important to remember that the wound healing processes (regeneration, formation of the junctional epithelium) are not yet complete, and that the prophy paste and rubber cup should not be forced into the sulcular area.

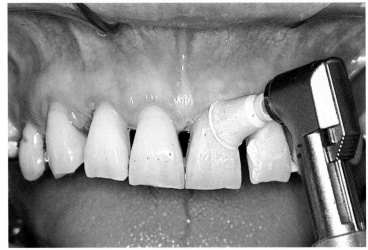

489 Clinical view after suture removal and cleaning
The patient must now begin to carefully perform routine home care. Because the interdental spaces are now more open than they were prior to surgery, the patient will have to use different interdental hygiene aids. In this case, interdental brushes (see Fig. 287) are indicated. The technique should be demonstrated to the patient at this appointment, and evaluated at the first recall visit.

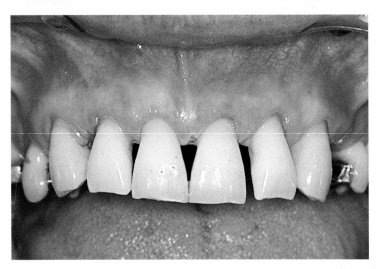

490 Occlusal view 1 year later
Teeth 16 and 18 were also extracted during subsequent periodontal therapy in the posterior segments (the maxilla was treated in sextants).

The resulting spaces were closed by means of fixed temporary acrylic bridges until healing was complete.

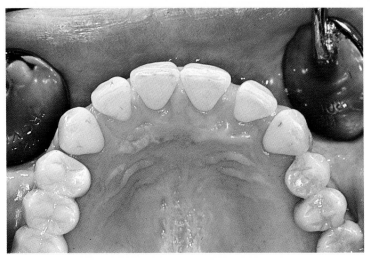

Ramfjord Technique

Summary

Initial therapy, excellent cooperation (home care) by this 33-year-old female, and the surgical procedures resulted in freedom from inflammation (PBI 0.5) and pocket-free periodontal conditions in the anterior and posterior segments.

The esthetic situation in terms of "elongation" of the anterior teeth is acceptable. The patient complained of sensitivity in cervical areas only during the first postoperative weeks.

The healing phase in posterior areas lasts somewhat longer. During this time, the spaces created by extractions are closed temporarily by means of customized long-term fixed temporary bridges (heat-cured acrylic over a metal framework).

After completion of periodontal therapy, a regular 3-month recall was instituted because this was a case of rapidly progressive periodontitis (RPP), where recurrence is not uncommon.

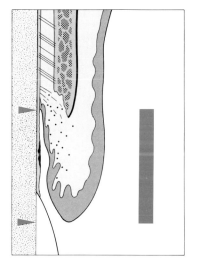

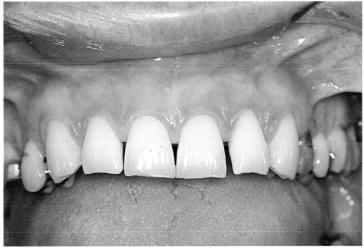

491 Before surgery
Initial therapy has almost completely eliminated inflammation, but some active pockets of up to 9 mm remain in interdental areas.

The schematic depicts an untreated pocket with probing depth noted in red.

Before

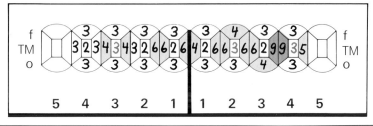

492 Probing depths and tooth mobility (TM) after initial therapy
The cuspid (23) must be maintained, despite a probing depth of 9 mm distally; 24 is destined for extraction.

After

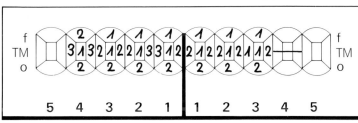

Probing depths and TM after modified Widman operation
Two months after surgery, no probing depths in excess of 3 mm are detected.

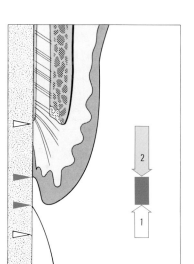

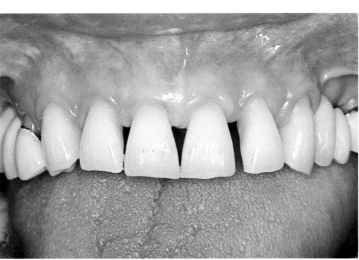

493 1 year postsurgically
While the modified Widman operation is a conservative procedure, in this case "elongated" teeth and open interdental spaces resulted because the primary incision had to be "scalloped" excessively (Figs. 411–413). Interdental hygiene must be modified to fit the postoperative situation.

Schematic: Residual sulcus depth is indicated as the distance between arrows 1 & 2. The original probing depth was significantly reduced due to gingival shrinkage (1) and periodontal regeneration (2).

Fully Reflected Mucoperiosteal Flaps

A surgical procedure in which mucoperiosteal flaps are reflected beyond the mucogingival junction exposes a large expanse of the alveolar bone. Periodontal tissues, particularly the alveolar bone should be treated as conservatively and atraumatically as possible.

Radical ostectomy for complete elimination of infrabony pockets is no longer an accepted therapeutic modality. In advanced cases of periodontal destruction, however, fully reflected flaps are necessary in order to provide a direct view of the pocket for scaling and planing of involved root surfaces, furcations and osseous defects.

Only the visual access provided by fully reflected flaps can provide the surgeon with sufficient information to decide whether to recontour bone, extract a tooth, resect a root, or perhaps use an implant in an infrabony pocket.

Indications

Surgery involving fully reflected flaps is indicated when:

- Buccal and lingual pockets extend apically beyond the attached gingiva, i.e., beyond the mucogingival line
- Pronounced bone loss with reverse architecture is present throughout an arch segment (sextant, quadrant) to be operated
- Osteoplasty or minimal ostectomy must be performed to treat deep infrabony pockets or thickened bony margins. (The principle remains, however, that bone must be preserved; tooth supportive bone is seldom removed).
- A tooth must be hemisected or roots resected
- Infrabony pockets are to be treated with implants
- Flaps must be repositioned other than at the original location (e.g., apically, coronally, laterally).

Contraindications

- Mild to moderate periodontitis
- Uniform, mostly horizontal bone loss throughout the arch
- All areas where the modified Widman operation can be employed successfully.

Advantages

- Direct vision of defects, good access to all root surfaces including furcations, depressions, irregularities etc.
- The coronal portion of the alveolar process is revealed for direct examination.

Disadvantages

- Postoperative edema and pain
- Superficial resorption of exposed bone (bone loss)
- "Elongation" of teeth postoperatively, with the attendant problems of sensitivity, esthetics, and phonetics.

Instruments for Osteoplasty...   # ...and Their Use

Removal of bone must be limited to that which is absolutely necessary. Osteoplasty refers to reshaping the bone without removing supporting bone, while ostectomy includes the elimination of infrabony pockets.

The *bone bur* is the indicated instrument for these procedures. Such burs are round, coarse and made of steel. Any use of rotating instruments, including coarse diamonds, must be performed using sterile saline for cooling. Use of low rpm reduces the chances of thermal damage to the bone.

Bone files are used to advantage for minor osteoplasty.

The rongeur is indicated only for removal of bony margins. Most commonly it is used for the removal of sharp alveolar marginal bone after tooth extraction.

Bone removed during osteoplasty or ostectomy may be used as implant/transplant material in infrabony pockets (see p.216).

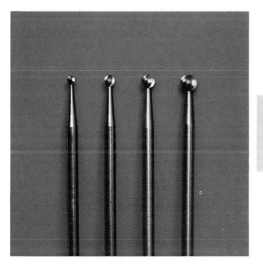 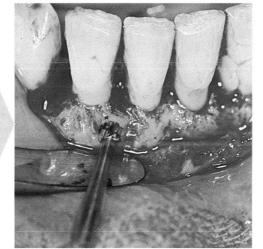

494 Bone bur
Osseous recontouring is best accomplished using low speed round burs. Sterile saline must be used for cooling during this destructive procedure, as heat is generated even at low rpm.

Bulbous bony margins are eliminated, especially on the facial surface between the teeth, by narrowing the buccal and lingual cortical plates. This permits subsequent replacement of the soft tissue flaps and generation of physiologic morphology of the gingival margin.

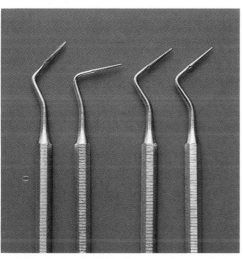 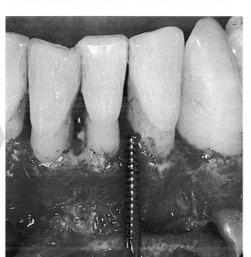

495 Bone file
Hirschfeld or other bone files may be used for minor osteoplasty. These files are available with varying degrees of angulation (left). Files do not generate heat and therefore preserve tissue, but they also remove bone at a slower rate than bone burs.

Patients often find unpleasant the rasping sound generated by bone files.

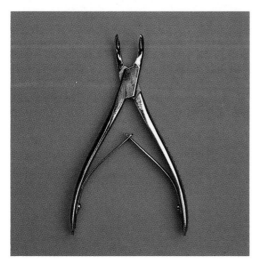 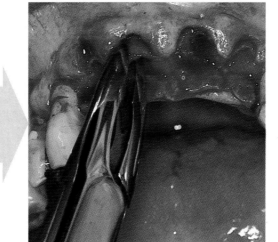

496 Rongeur
This special cutting forceps is indicated primarily for reducing sharp alveolar bone margins that remain following tooth extraction.

Its indication in periodontal surgery is very limited.

Mucoperiosteal Flap without Vertical Incisions
Osteoplasty – Flap Adaptation

In this 21-year-old male the principles of the Ramfjord technique were followed in placing the primary incision. However, the labial flap was subsequently fully reflected beyond the mucogingival line in order to gain access for osteoplasty of the bulbous margin of the alveolar crest.

Following the osseous correction, the flap was repositioned at its approximate original location, for esthetic reasons.

Diagnosis: Rapidly progressive periodontitis of moderate severity, with a localized deep lesion at the mesial of 26. The patient's preoperative home care was only average.

Findings before surgery:

   HYG 78%   PBI 1.4   TM 1–2

The clinical picture, gingival contour, probing depths and radiographic findings are shown in the Figures below.

497   After inital therapy
In the upper left quadrant, active pockets to 8 mm remained after initial therapy (see charting).

   The soft tissue and possibly the bone are thickened, especially on the facial aspect lateral to the interdental craters (arrows).

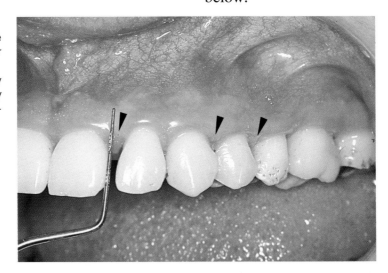

498   Probing depths and tooth mobility (TM) after initial therapy
Periodontal pockets are especially advanced interproximally. The bone loss is not uniform throughout the segment.

Radiographic view
The radiographs reveal a crater-like bony defect mesial of 26.

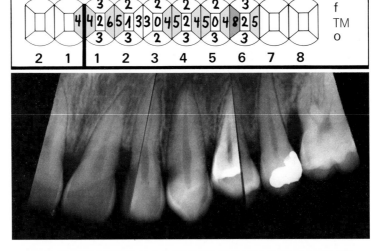

499   Initial incision
When mucoperiosteal flaps are to be fully reflected, the principles of the modified Widman technique should also be followed. The scalloped form provides "papillae" (facial and oral) that can be used to cover interdental defects completely.

   Because the surgery is intended to correct the bulbously thickened buccal bone, the buccal flap had to be reflected apically, beyond the mucogingival line.

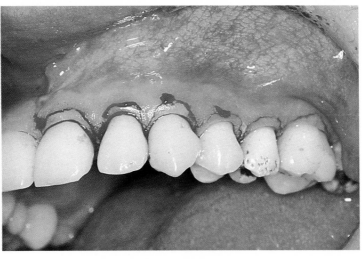

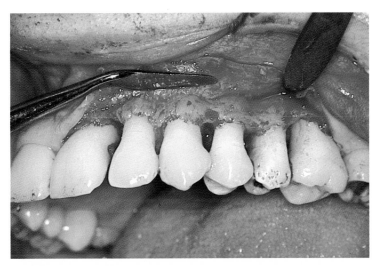

500 Full reflection of the buccal flap
As expected, interdental cratering (2-wall infrabony lesion) and a thickened facial bony margin were observed after flap reflection. Granulation tissue within the pocket was completely removed, and the root surfaces were thoroughly planed and smoothed.

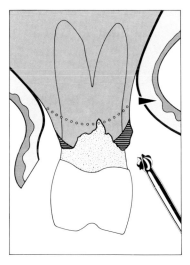

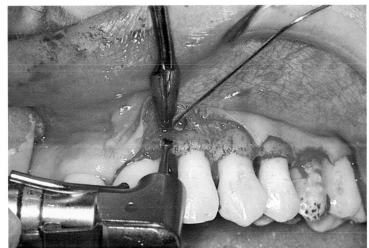

501 Osteoplasty
The mucoperiosteal flap was reflected beyond the mucogingival line (arrow in schematic). A round bur was used under saline coolant to perform a conservative recontouring of the bone (osteoplasty). The craters were slightly opened facially, as depicted by crosshatching in the diagram (ostectomy). The goal was to achieve physiologic gingival contour to simplify plaque control.

Radical ostectomy for complete elimination of the pocket, as indicated by the dotted line in the schematic, is *contraindicated*.

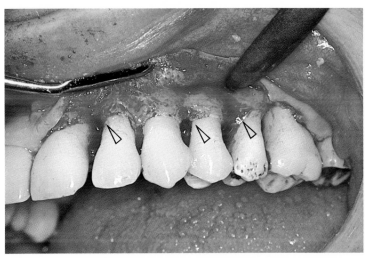

502 Surgical field prior to suture placement
All tooth and root surfaces are clean and smoothed. Pocket epithelium and granulation tissue have been removed completely.

The hemorrhagic sites where osteoplasty was performed are visible (arrows). The facial soft tissue flap can be well adapted interdentally.

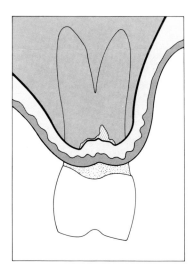

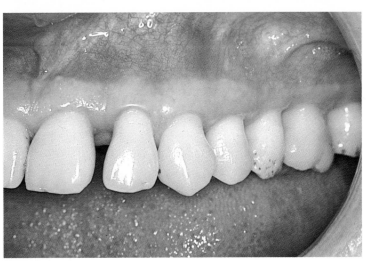

503 3 months postoperatively
Pockets have been eliminated for the most part. It is anticipated that remaining craters will undergo *osseous regeneration* (hatched area in diagram). When this type of osseous surgery is performed, definitive results can be expected no sooner than 3 months postoperatively.

A small depression remains between 21 and 22, indicating that the papillae did not heal together by primary intention.

Mucoperiosteal Flap with Vertical Incisions
Osteoplasty – Apical Repositioning of Flap

The technique for apical repositioning of flaps is demonstrated below in the case of a 34-year-old male with rapidly progressive periodontitis (RPP) manifesting severe osseous defects in the mandibular anterior area. Full reflection of the mucoperiosteal flaps was necessary to gain visual access into the extremely deep lesions, and vertical incisions were required because the planned surgery included apical repositioning of the flaps.

Clinically visible inflammation was almost completely eliminated after initial therapy. However, the hyperplastic gingivae did not shrink appreciably. Several deep pockets continued to show signs of activity.

Findings after initial therapy:
    HYG 80%   PBI 1.3   TM 2–3!
The clinical picture, gingival contour, probing depths and radiographs are depicted in the Figures below.

504   After initial therapy
Probing depths were not significantly reduced by initial therapy, which included subgingival scaling. Pockets to 9 mm persisted, as indicated by the Michigan probe. On the other hand, the *activity* (inflammation) of the pockets was reduced, though not completely eliminated.

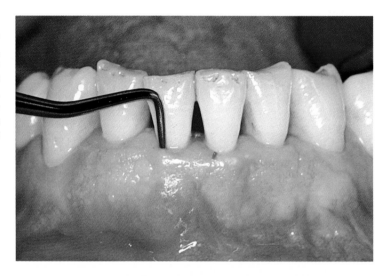

505   Probing depths and tooth mobility (TM) after initial therapy

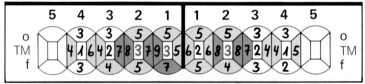

Radiographs
Less than half the root length of the mandibular incisors remains anchored in bone.

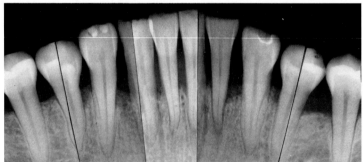

506   Planned incisions

1. Scalloped, internal bevel incision
2. Vertical incisions bilaterally

3. Crevicular incision

The bilateral vertical incisions permit a deep apical repositioning of the labial flap when the procedure is completed.

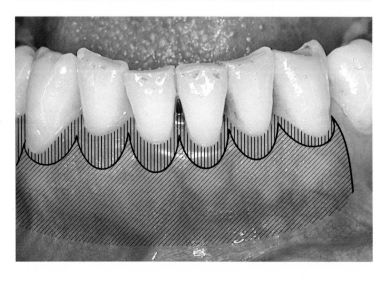

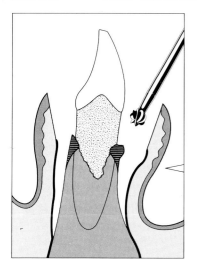

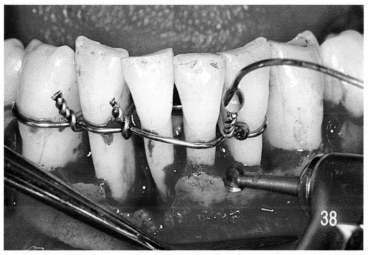

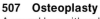

507 Osteoplasty
A round bur with saline irrigation is used to reduce the bulbous, sharp bony edges (osteoplasty). Tooth-supporting bone is not normally removed; however, in this case *ostectomy* is performed to attain more normal architecture (compromise osseous reshaping) of the facial bone level, which is extremely irregular from tooth to tooth. The osteoplasty is shown in cross hatch in the schematic.

The anterior teeth were so mobile that during the surgery it was necessary to fabricate a crude temporary wire splint.

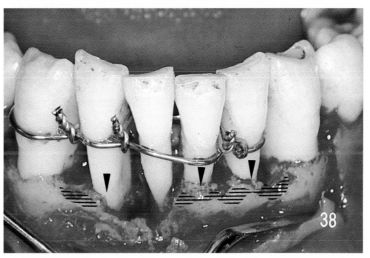

508 Following osseous surgery
The horizontal lines indicate those areas where bone was removed. Note (arrows) that *no* osseous reduction was performed on tooth-supporting bone near the cervix. This case demonstrates that even when reverse architecture is present due to advanced disease, bone removal is still performed most sparingly.

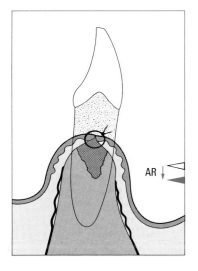

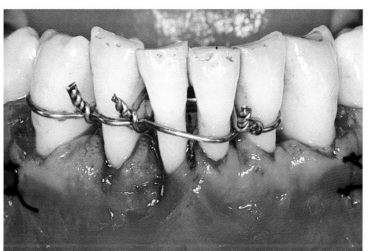

509 Apically repositioned flap
Apical repositioning of the flap (AR, indicated by arrows in diagram) is performed so that the interdental craters, now filled with coagulum, can be tightly covered with the soft tissue when sutured. Clinical elongation of the teeth is pronounced because of the apical repositioning of the flaps.

The wire splint serves a dual purpose since it will also help retain the periodontal dressing material. The dressing provides additional stabilization for the mobile teeth, and should remain in place for 10 days.

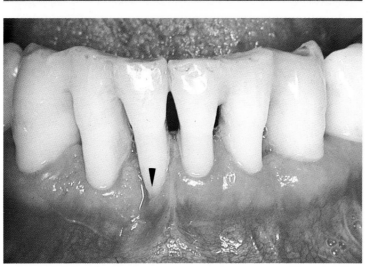

510 6 weeks postoperatively
The teeth appear considerably longer in comparison to the preoperative clinical views. Tooth 41 exhibits no attached gingiva at all.

The extremely mobile anterior teeth were splinted in two groups of three teeth each (43 – 42 – 41 and 31 – 32 – 33), using a semi-permanent composite resin (acid etch technique, p. 293).

Osteoplasty – Apical Repositioning of Flap

Summary

In a 34-year-old male the initial therapy essentially eliminated clinical inflammation. Selective occlusal equilibration was performed due to a parafunctional habit and increasing tooth mobility.

Pocket-free conditions were achieved by means of a relatively radical surgical procedure utilizing fully reflected flaps, osteoplasty and minor ostectomy, as well as apical repositioning of the mucoperiosteal flaps.

Several months later a minor operation (Edlan, p. 245) was performed to create some attached tissue in the region of tooth 41.

The long-term prognosis of such a case is good only if the patient maintains excellent oral hygiene, especially in interdental areas.

This large and complex therapeutic endeavor was justified by the fact that loss of these teeth would reconcile the patient to an expansive 8-unit fixed bridge or a removable partial denture.

511 After initial therapy

Findings before the flap surgery:
– "Short" teeth
– Little visible inflammation
– Very deep pockets (to 9 mm, red in diagram)
– Interdental osseous cratering.

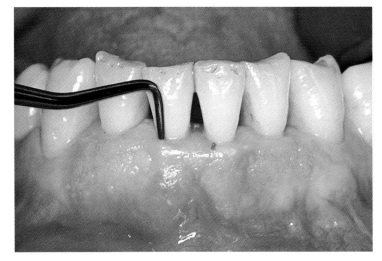
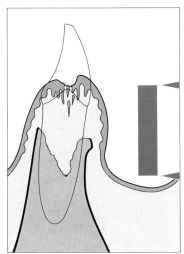

512 Probing depths and tooth mobility (TM) after initial therapy

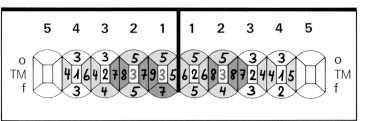

Before

12 months postoperatively
The tooth mobility (TM) values represent the two splinted units (3 teeth each).

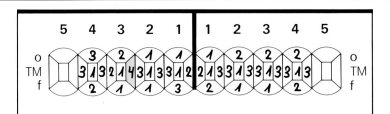

After

513 Clinical picture 1 year later
The former pockets have been eliminated; however, the teeth appear elongated and the cervical areas are still sensitive. A minor vestibular extension procedure ("Edlan") stabilized the mucosa near 41.

Diagram: The residual probing depth is depicted (red bar).
1: Apical repositioning, shrinkage
2: New attachment, bone regeneration.

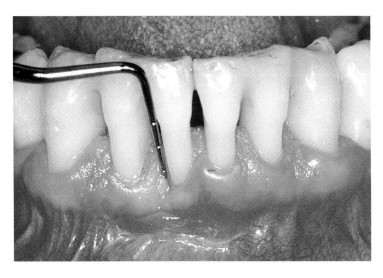
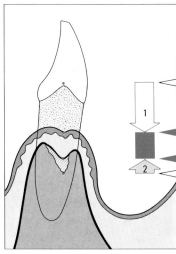

Combined Surgical Techniques

Advanced periodontitis is rarely distributed evenly throughout the entire dental arch. Inflammation, attachment loss and probing depths must be evaluated for each individual tooth. It is not exceptional to find in one patient an area of localized gingivitis, elsewhere severe periodontal destruction, and in a third area localized recession.

Depending upon the localization of attachment loss, the treatment plan may include initial therapy and patient home care as the only treatment necessary in certain areas, while minor surgical procedures such as gingivectomy, gingivoplasty or the modified Widman procedure may be necessary in other areas. In still other segments of the dentition it may be necessary to reflect large mucoperiosteal flaps in order to perform osteoplasty, root resection, hemisection, or intraosseous implants.

Similarly, it is possible for two different surgical procedures to be indicated in the same operative area. Because a palatal flap cannot be repositioned apically due to its lack of elasticity, it is not unusual for a surgical appointment to combine a gingivectomy *(palatal)* and a flap operation *(buccal)* (see Operative procedure, p. 199). Yet another possibility is the performance of a gingivectomy and a flap procedure on the same surface of the same tooth.

These frequently encountered combination techniques are described and depicted below:

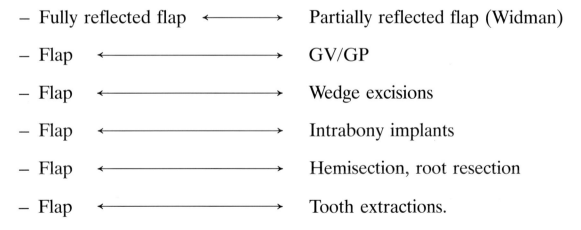

- Fully reflected flap ↔ Partially reflected flap (Widman)

- Flap ↔ GV/GP

- Flap ↔ Wedge excisions

- Flap ↔ Intrabony implants

- Flap ↔ Hemisection, root resection

- Flap ↔ Tooth extractions.

Combining a periodontal flap procedure with removal of an impacted third molar is not recommended, because of the danger of infection in the extraction wound. It is also unwise to perform surgery for periodontitis (flaps, GV/GP) at the same time as mucogingival surgery for recession. In such cases, the periodontitis is generally treated first. Only when the initial surgical site has completely healed should the mucogingival problem be approached surgically.

Combined Surgical Technique, Schematic Presentation
Flap (buccal) – GV and Flap (palatal)

A frequently indicated periodontal surgical technique involves a buccal flap and a palatal gingivectomy with subsequent flap reflection. On the palate, a gingivectomy is often required because flap surgery is technically difficult or impossible.

    The reflection of a palatal flap *after* gingivectomy is indicated when deep pockets are present interproximally and palatally. This procedure permits root planing with direct vision on palatal and interproximal tooth surfaces. It also makes possible adequate coverage of the interdental defects with soft tissue. The palatal gingivectomy wound, which is usually not very expansive, must be covered with a periodontal dressing and permitted to re-epithelialize.

    This procedure is depicted diagramatically below as it would appear in the maxillary bicuspid region.

514   Incision/gingivectomy

Buccal: Flap
A horizontal inverse bevel incision is made to create the flap, according to the Ramfjord principles.

Palatal: Gingivectomy
A standard gingivectomy incision eliminates the palatal pocket to a great degree.

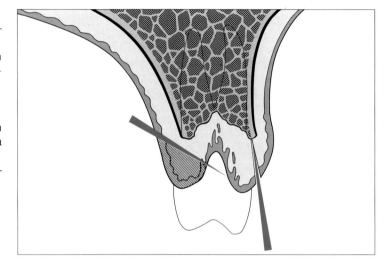

515   Reflection of buccal and palatal flaps – Root planing
After removal of the tissue excised via GV, a crevicular incision is made on the palate and a flap is reflected; thus, this flap is not covered with epithelium. The root surfaces and osseous contour are now exposed. Debridement, root planing and any indicated osteoplasty can now be accomplished with direct vision from both buccal and palatal aspects.

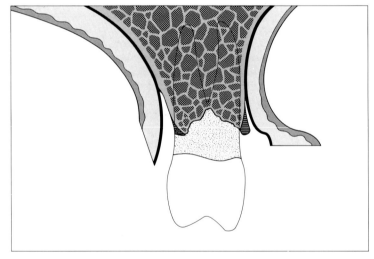

516   Flap adaptation – Wound care
Interrupted sutures serve to closely adapt the buccal and palatal flaps to the bone and tooth surface. Every effort should be made to completely cover interdental craters. This can only be accomplished by sliding the buccal flap into and through the interdental area, causing the mucogingival line to be shifted coronally. Thus the mucobuccal fold becomes shallower.

    The GV wound on the palatal aspect must be covered with a dressing.

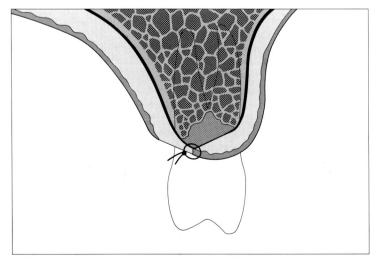

Combined Surgical Technique
Flap (buccal) – GV and Flap (palatal) – Intraosseous Implant

Operative procedure

In the case presented here various periodontal surgical procedures were combined. The primary goal of the surgery was to attempt to accelerate bone regeneration in the 8 mm pocket mesial to the left central incisor by placement of an alloplastic implant (tricalcium phosphate, TCP, see p. 215). This was an esthetic measure as well as a functional one.

The patient was a 27-year-old female manifesting generalized mild to moderate periodontitis. The 8 mm pocket on the mesial of 21 persisted after therapy.

Findings before surgery:

HYG 85%   PBI 1.8

TM   Average of 1, but grade 3 on tooth 21.

Clinical picture, gingival contour, probing depths and radiographs are depicted in the Figures below.

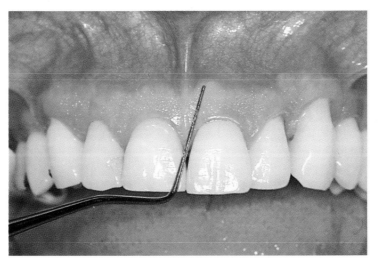

517 After initial therapy
The gingivae are essentially free of clinical signs of inflammation following initial therapy. Several active pockets persist. The deepest, an 8 mm 2- to 3-wall infrabony defect, is mesial to tooth 21. The pocket extent is indicated with the Michigan probe.

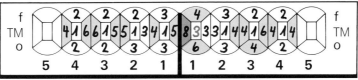

518 Probing depths and tooth mobility (TM) after initial therapy
The highly mobile tooth 21 must be approached surgically.

Radiographic view

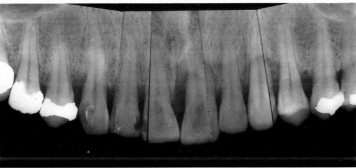

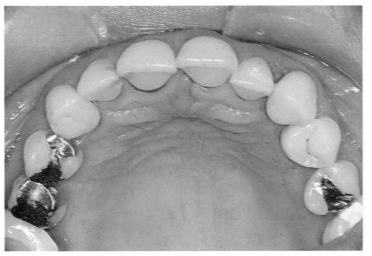

519 Occlusal view after initial therapy
Despite initial therapy, a mild gingivitis persists. The relatively steep anterior palatal vault permits gingivectomy without creation of an expansive wound surface.

Palatal procedure

520 Palatal gingivectomy
The first step is a gingivectomy (oblique incision, see p. 159) without contacting bone.

Using a Kirkland knife with a *double-angled* shank makes access easy and overcomes any technical problems.

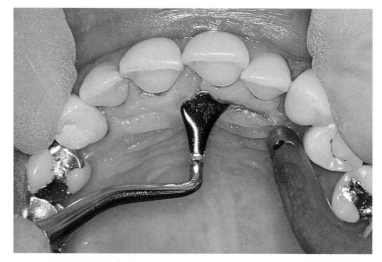
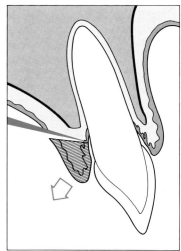

521 Mobilization of the palatal flap
Following the gingivectomy, a crevicular incision (not shown) is made using the scalpel (e.g., No. 12 B).

The flap is reflected with the aid of an elevator, and direct access to the root surfaces, alveolar margin and the osseous craters is gained.

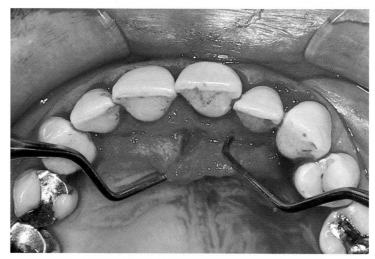

Buccal procedure

522 Buccal flap
The mucoperiosteal flap on the labial aspect is created by means of a special horizontal incision: Around the central incisors a scalloped inverse bevel is used because of the infrabony pockets, while a crevicular incision is made around the other teeth, where no pockets are present.

Schematic: The internal bevel incision for flap elevation has been made. The depicted crevicular incision is the second step.

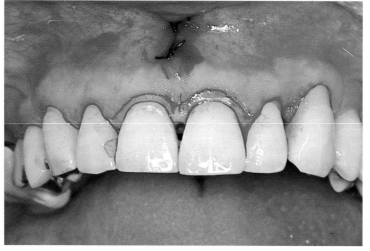
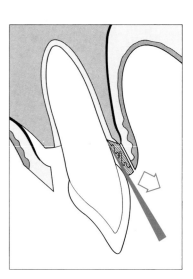

523 Root planing
The deep osseous crater mesial to 21 has filled with blood following thorough but careful debridement and root planing.

Regeneration of new bone in the depth of this crater may be anticipated as a result of the root planing and curettage alone, without the use of an implant of any kind.

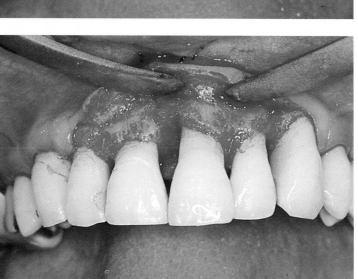

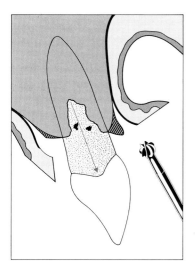

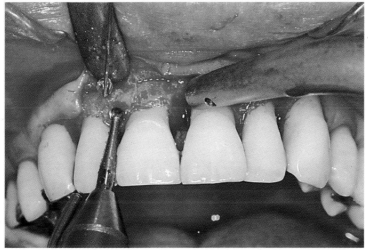

524 Osteoplasty

The bulbous bone margin between 11 and 12 is carefully recontoured without reducing the *height* of the supporting alveolar bone.

The schematic depicts the osteoplasty (cross-hatch) in an orofacial section.

Following the osseous recontouring, the roots are thoroughly planed (red arrow).

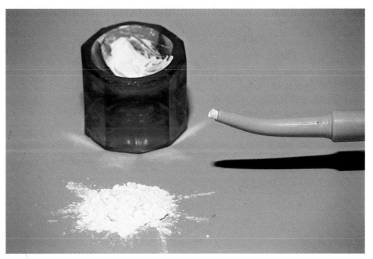

525 Implant material Ca$_3$ (PO$_4$)$_2$ (Tricalcium phosphate, TCP)

The powdered *alloplastic* material is mixed with sterile saline to form a thick paste. A sterile amalgam carrier (Premier Co.) can be conveniently used to transport this implant paste into the osseous crater.

"Synthograft" (Johnson & Johnson) is a commercially available alloplastic (TCP) material.

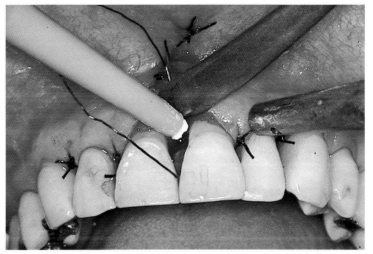

526 Filling the bony defect with tricalcium phosphate

The buccal and palatal flaps have already been adapted and sutured, except in the area of 21 where the suture has been placed but not yet tied. Note that a frenectomy was also performed.

The implant material is forced into the pocket where it must become well mixed with blood. *Immediately* after placement, the remaining flaps are adapted and sutured securely.

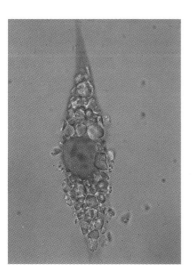

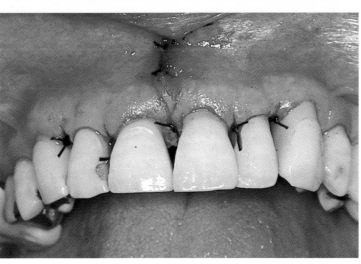

527 Tight flap adaptation

To preclude loss of the implanted material, flaps must be closely adapted and completely closed over the interdental defect.

Phagocytosing fibroblast

Tricalcium phosphate is a resorbable implant material.

The cultured fibroblast shown at left has phagocytosed tricalcium phosphate particles. The biocompatible alloplastic material is slowly resorbed (carbol fuchsin, × 1000).

Wound healing

528 Periodontal dressing
In order to guarantee undisturbed wound healing, the operative site is protected from mechanical trauma by placement of a well adapted periodontal dressing. Coe-pak rolled in chlorhexidine-HCl was employed in this case.

The schematic shows the blood coagulum with tricalcium phosphate particles (blue) completely filling the osseous defect. The suture location (arrow) is protected by the dressing (light blue).

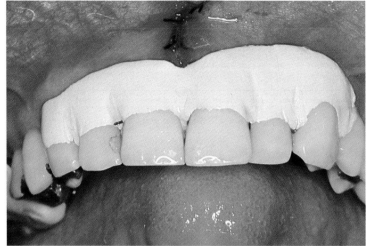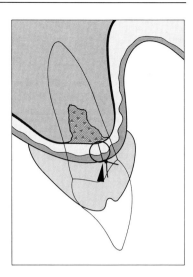

529 2 weeks postoperatively
After dressing removal, whitish patches consisting of desquamated epithelial cells are visible.
   Sutures are removed and the entire area is cleansed gently but thoroughly using hydrogen peroxide (3%) on cotton pledgets. The tooth surfaces are polished with rubber cups and dentifrice.

Caution: Paste must not be rotated into the sulcus as regeneration of the periodontal tissues is not yet complete!

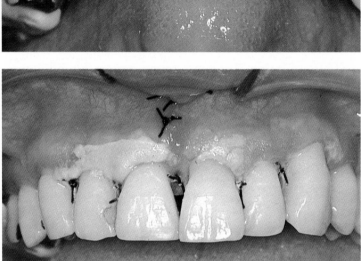

530 Clinical view after suture removal and cleansing
Gingival shrinkage has occurred mesial to 21.

The schematic depicts the expected initial osseous regeneration (cross-hatch) within the crater, as well as resorption of some of the tricalcium phosphate particles (blue).

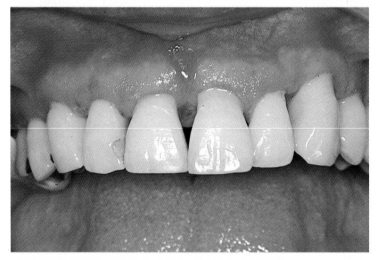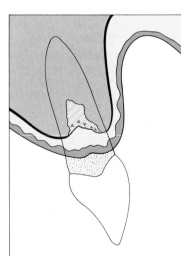

531 6 weeks postoperatively
The palatal view reveals persistent slight gingival erythema. The patient must be encouraged to improve home care in this area.

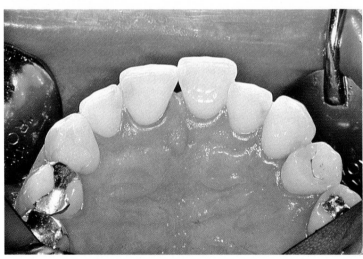

Combined Surgical Technique – Intraosseous Implant

Summary

The young female patient responded positively to initial therapy and demonstrated a high level of motivation before the surgical intervention. Despite this, some active pockets persisted, especially in interdental areas (cratering).

The combined surgical procedure successfully eliminated all periodontal pockets. The 8 mm pocket mesial to 21 was reduced to 3 mm, owing primarily to a significant amount of gingival shrinkage. It is possible that some osseous regeneration occurred in the depth of the pocket, but whether or not the tricalcium phosphate implant accelerated or increased bone regeneration cannot be determined (Scott-Metsger et al. 1982; Strub et al. 1979; see also Transplants and Implants in Bony Pockets, p.215).

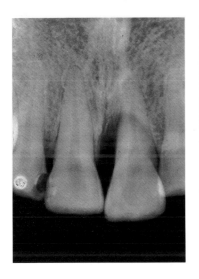
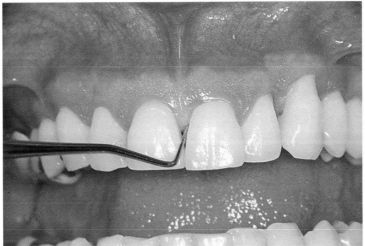

532 After initial therapy
The gingival contour is satisfactory after initial therapy. A deep infrabony pocket (8 mm) is present on the mesial of the left central incisor.

The radiograph reveals a 2- to 3-wall defect on the mesial aspect of 21.

Before

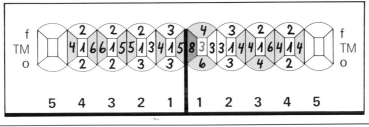

533 Probing depths and tooth mobility (TM) after initial therapy

After

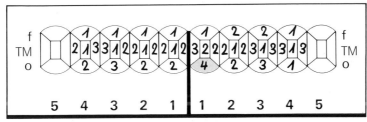

Probing depths and tooth mobility (TM) 1 year after surgery

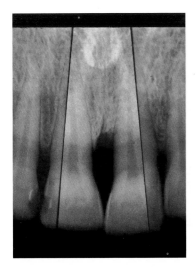
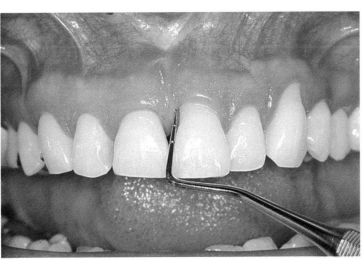

534 1 year postoperatively
The combined surgical procedure led to a reduction of pocket depth from 8 to 3 mm. This reduction could be accounted for by gingival shrinkage as well as some osseous regeneration.

The radiograph reveals what appears to be some filling of the osseous defect mesial to 21 (compare pre-op radiograph, Fig. 532).

Combined Surgical Technique
Flap – Extraction – Revision of Adjacent Periodontal Structures

Operative procedure

In the treatment of advanced periodontal diseases, teeth with poor prognoses often must be extracted. Following initial therapy, this may be accomplished during a flap procedure, at which time the periodontal supporting structures of adjacent maintainable teeth can be revised. This procedure is demonstrated here in the maxilla of a 45-year-old female. The treatment plan was radical because of the patient's desire for a long-term prosthetic solution. Seven teeth (17, 15, 14, 12, 11; 21, 25) were extracted; five (16, 13; 22, 23, 24) were treated periodontally and maintained as abutments.

Findings before initial therapy:

HYG 53 %   PBI 2.2

TM   3 (hopeless teeth)

         2 (maintainable teeth)

The clinical picture, gingival contour, probing depths and radiographs are depicted in the Figures below.

535   Before initial therapy
The severity of the periodontal destruction cannot be totally appreciated from the clinical presentation. Probing depths of up to 10 mm were recorded.

Consideration of the clinical findings led to a diagnosis of rapidly progressive periodontitis (see RPP, Diseases of the Periodontium, p.68). Attachment loss was generally moderate throughout the mouth, with several areas of advanced loss.

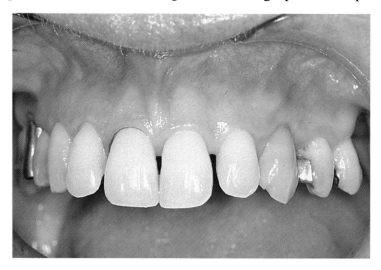

536   Initial findings:

Probing depths and tooth mobility (TM)
Several teeth were highly mobile and some of the periodontal pockets very deep.

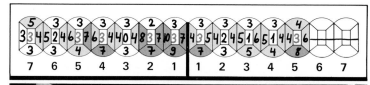

Radiographic findings
Teeth destined for extraction due to the severity of periodontal destruction are marked (✱) on this film and in the clinical photograph below.

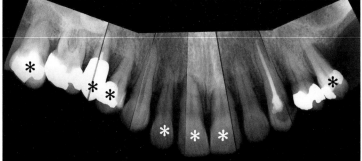

537   Surgical plan

1. Scalloped horizontal internal bevel incision on buccal and palatal aspects (solid line).
2. Flap reflection. The zone of reflection is relatively narrow (oblique hatch).
3. Extractions. The asterisks indicate teeth destined for extraction.
4. Frenotomy of the high labial frenum attachment.

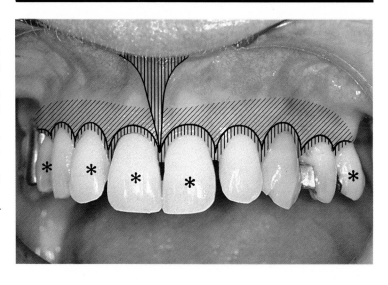

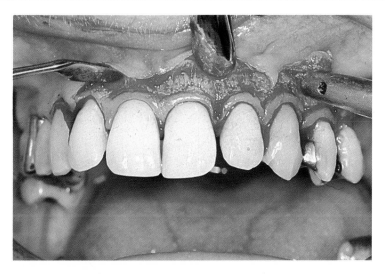

538   Flap reflection
Following a horizontal scalloped internal bevel incision, the buccal and palatal mucoperiosteal flaps are elevated, revealing the alveolar bone.

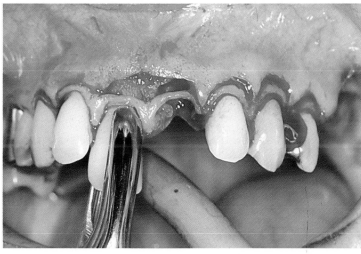

539   Extractions
The hopeless anterior teeth (12, 11; 21) are removed.

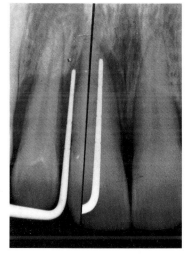

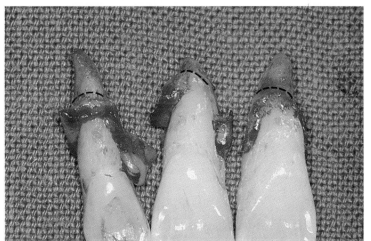

540   Palatal surfaces of the extracted teeth
It is clear how little of the roots of these teeth were still anchored in bone (dashed line indicates remaining periodontal ligament).

The radiograph of the initial condition revealed the minimal osseous support for the extracted teeth.

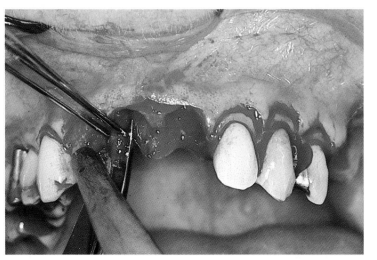

541   Thinning the flap
Granulation tissue not completely removed by the initial incision is excised from the internal surface of the flap using a small, curved scissors.
     This gives the flap a uniform thickness throughout, enhancing repositioning and adaptation.

542 Debridement and root planing
The root surfaces of teeth destined for maintenance (abutment teeth) are systematically planed under direct vision.

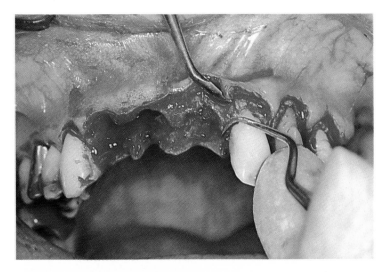

543 Correcting bony marginal contour
Sharp bony edges are removed using rongeurs or bone burs to preclude damage to the tissue of the repositioned flaps.

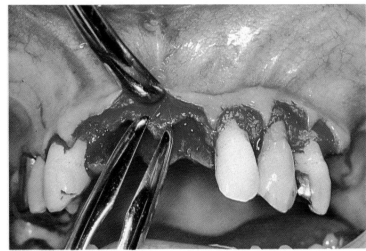

544 Flap adaptation
Flaps are first adapted closely to the remaining teeth.

The extraction wounds can then be completely closed if the papilla tips of one flap are sutured into the depression between the papilla tips of the other flap (see diagram: buccal flap = light blue; palatal flap = darker blue). Closure ensures healing by primary intention (schematic adapted from *Krueger* 1977).

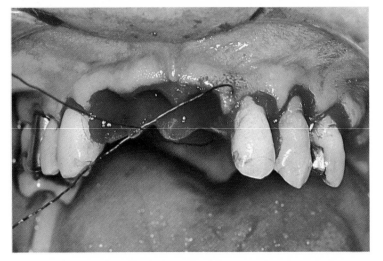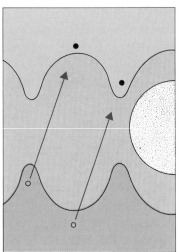

545 Surgical procedure complete
In addition to the extractions and the periodontal treatment, a frenotomy was performed.

The flaps have been closed tightly over the alveolar process. A temporary denture, prepared in advance, can be seated.

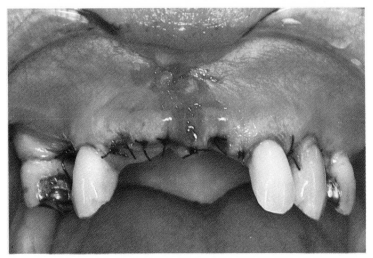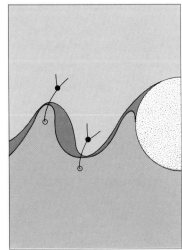

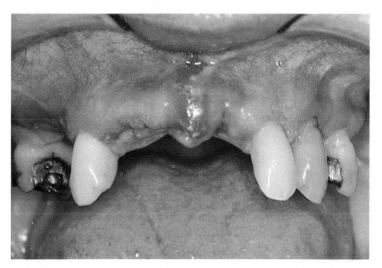

546 Suture removal 10 days postoperatively
Plaque and stains are carefully removed using rubber cup and dentifrice.

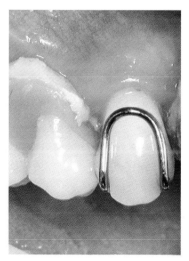

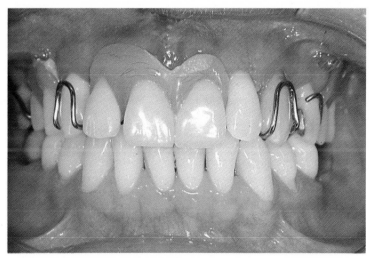

547 Relined temporary denture
Depending upon the severity of the periodontal destruction, an extended healing and consolidation phase of 6 ± 3 months between the periodontal surgery and definitive prosthetic treatment follows.

Detail, left: The temporary denture will be worn for an extended period of time; it must be tooth-born, with clasps that hold each tooth bodily. It is often necessary to reline the temporary denture during the healing period (see Reconstruction, p. 299).

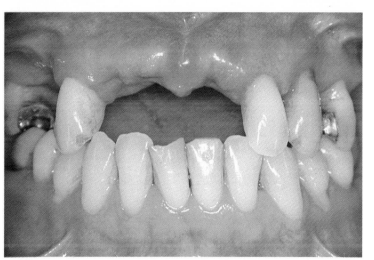

548 4 weeks postoperatively
The recall interval is established at this point, based on the patient's degree of motivation and the clinical re-evaluation.

The light brown stains are from chlorhexidine, which the patient used as a mouthwash.

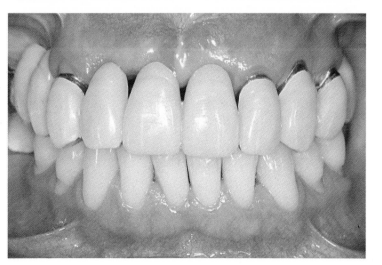

549 Telescoping definitive reconstruction
Nine months after the surgery an 11-unit removable bridge was seated over telescope crowns on all 5 remaining maxillary teeth (see also Reconstruction, p. 301).

Extraction with Revision

Summary

In this female patient manifesting advanced rapidly progressive periodontitis (RPP) in the maxilla, somewhat radical treatment was performed in order to satisfy the patient's wishes in terms of prosthetic rehabilitation. After initial therapy, seven hopeless teeth were extracted and the five remaining maxillary teeth were treated periodontally during the same procedure. Immediately following the surgery, a tooth-born removable temporary denture was seated.

After an extended (9 months) healing and consolidation phase, the definitive removable telescope bridge was seated. Telescoping bridges permit optimal hygiene by the patient, and can be modified later if necessary.

550 Radiographic findings
Advanced periodontal destruction. More than half of the maxillary teeth are hopelessly involved.

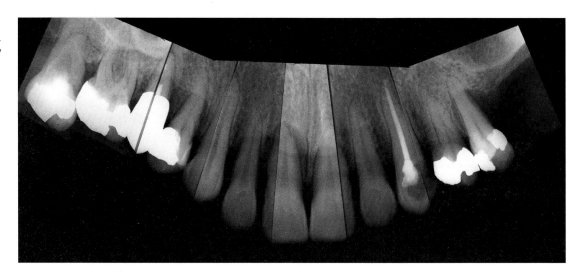

551 Initial probing depths and tooth mobility (TM)
Deep pockets and highly mobile teeth characterize the clinical situation.

Before

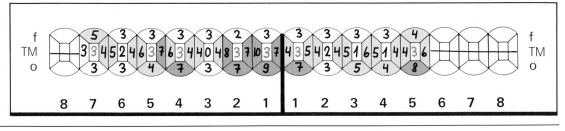

After

Post-treatment probing depths and tooth mobility (TM)
Prior to commencement of the definitive reconstruction phase, physiologic probing depths are found around all five remaining maxillary abutment teeth.

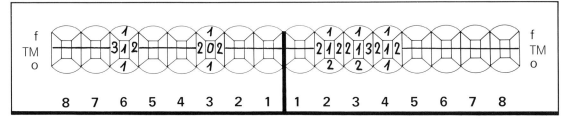

552 Final radiographic picture
This radiographic survey was prepared after completion of the definitive reconstructive phase of therapy, 9 months after periodontal surgery. All five remaining maxillary teeth now bear telescope crowns.

The long-term prognosis is good if the patient is diligent in home care and if regular maintenance therapy is persued.

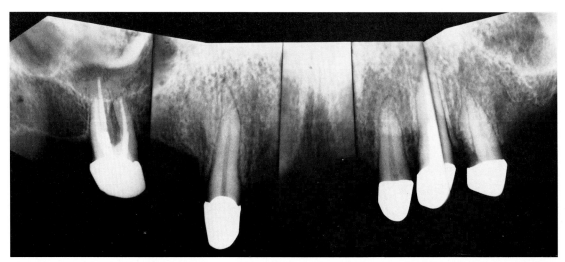

Surgical Removal of Impacted Third Molar – Prevention of a Pocket Distal to Second Molar

Impacted or retained third molars are often associated with an active periodontal pocket on the distal aspect of the second molar. Removal of such third molars should therefore be performed as early as possible, preferably before age 25. The extraction procedure must be as atraumatic as possible in order to protect the periodontal supporting structures of the adjacent second molar. Sectioning the third molar prior to removal is often indicated.

The postoperative results are generally better in young individuals than in older persons, who often manifest a persistent active pocket distal to the second molar. In young persons, third molar root formation may not be complete and the osseous structure is not so compact. The wound healing process is efficient and proceeds at a more rapid rate. For all of these reasons, third molar extraction should be done as early as possible to preclude persistent active pockets distal to the second molar (Eichenberger 1979).

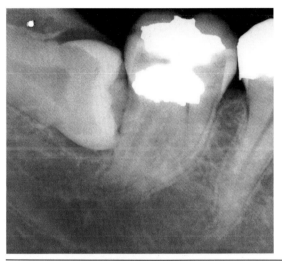
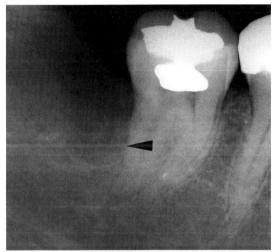

553 Third molar extraction later in life
Nine months after the surgical removal of the wisdom tooth in this "older" (45 y.) patient, no osseous regeneration is detectable distal to the second molar, despite repeated debridement and planing of the root surface. An active pocket of 12 mm can be probed (arrow).

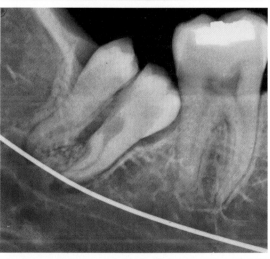
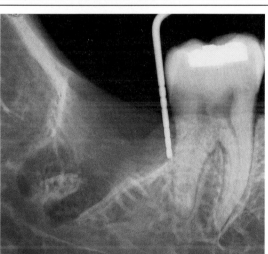

554 Atraumatic third molar extraction – Skull preparation
Injury to the mandibular canal can occur with surgical removal of third molars. Left: Horizontal impaction, wire demonstrates mandibular canal. When such teeth are removed the supporting structures of the adjacent second molar must be preserved.

The distal root of the second molar must be thoroughly planed to remove endotoxin, enhance healing, and preclude recurrence of periodontal pocket.

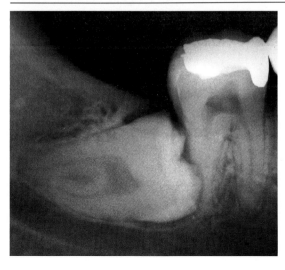
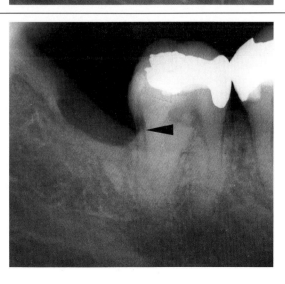

555 Early third molar extraction
In this 24-year-old female, osseous regeneration within 6 months has almost completely filled the defect created by surgical removal of the horizontally impacted third molar. Probing the distal aspect of the second molar reveals only a 3 mm sulcus (arrow).

Wedge Excisions – Surgical Principles

Periodontal pockets distal to the last tooth in an arch, as well as pockets on lone-standing teeth, are often difficult to eliminate. The best surgical solution in such cases is often the wedge excision. This procedure is generally successful only if it can be performed within the region of the attached gingiva.

The danger of recurrence is particularly high in the mandible distal to the second molar, i.e., in the region of movable mucosa at the periphery of the retromolar pad. If surgery in this area is unavoidable, care must be taken to avoid the lingual nerve, which often assumes a more superior position. In many instances, repeated root planing is preferable to surgical intervention, for the aforementioned reasons. Various possibilities for surgical pocket elimination distal to end-standing teeth are depicted diagramatically in the Figures below.

556 "Classic" distal wedge excision
The triangular-shaped wedge excision is generally used for pocket elimination distal to the last tooth in an arch. The initial incisions (red, left) delineate the central excision. These two incisions converge at the base of the pocket.

The second incisions serve to undermine (arrow, right) and thin the buccal and lingual tissue flaps overlying the alveolar ridge. Repositioning the flaps with sutures essentially eliminates the distal pocket.

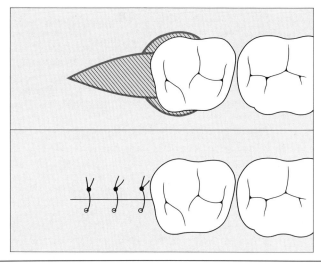 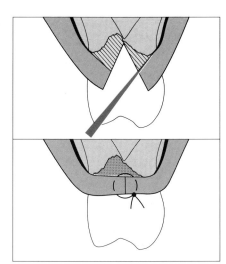

557 Modified incision
If the elimination of a pocket distal to the last tooth in the arch is simply one part of a flap procedure in the region, a modified wedge excision may be employed.

The modified technique considerably simplifies the reflection of facial and oral flaps, and direct vision of the root surface and bone is improved. The procedure is depicted in the clinical situation that follows (p. 211).

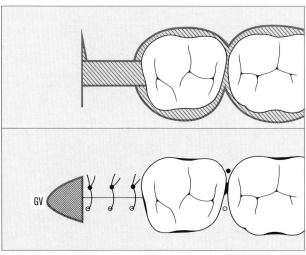 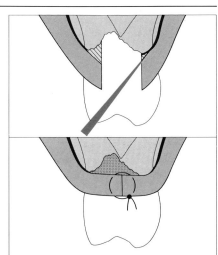

558 Wedge excision according to Chaikin (1977)
After making a curved incision from the buccal around the distal of the tooth (see schematic), a lingual pedicle flap is reflected. Subjacent tissue is excised down to underlying bone, and root planing performed.

The tip of the half-moon shaped flap is shortened somewhat, then sutured to the primary incision site. The slight tension placed on the flap by this repositioning and suturing method serves to adapt the flap well around the distal aspect of the tooth (small arrows).

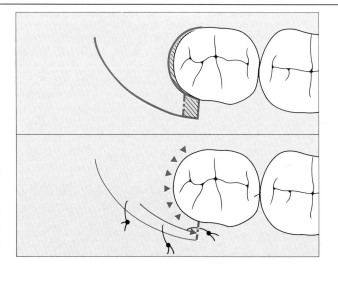 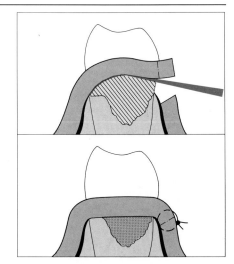

Wedge Excision – Most Distal Tooth

Operative Procedure

In a 38-year-old female, mild inflammation and an active 7 mm pocket persist distal to 26 following initial therapy. The treatment plan calls for elimination of the pocket by means of the modified wedge technique (Fig. 557).

The operation is feasible because there is sufficient attached gingiva distal to the tooth. The distal furcation is involved slightly (Class F 1).

No surgery is indicated for the remainder of the dentition, but repeated scaling will be performed. The composite restorations in 24 and 25 will be replaced with amalgams after conclusion of the periodontal therapy.

Findings after initial therapy:
HYG 60%   PBI 2.2   TM 0–1
Clinical and radiographic findings are depicted in the Figures below.

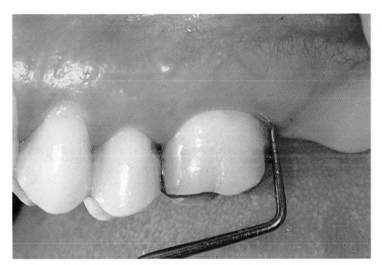

559   Active distal pocket
An active 7 mm pocket distal to 26 persists after initial therapy. The distal furcation could be probed 2 mm horizontally using the Nabors −2 probe, indicating a Class F 1 furcation involvement.

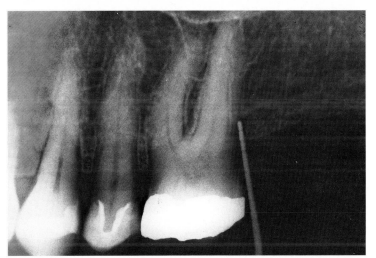

560   Radiograph with probe in situ
The Williams probe encountered no resistance from the inflamed tissue, and penetrated to the alveolar bone.

The markings on this probe are at 1, 2, 3, 5, 7, 8, 9 and 10 mm. The thickness of the alveolar soft tissues can be appreciated in this view.

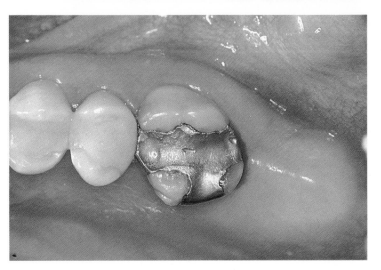

561   Occlusal view of 26
Sufficient attached gingiva is present distal to 26. The old amalgam restoration must be recontoured and polished before surgery.

562 Surgical plan – Incisions

1. Half-moon shaped internal bevel incision from the midbuccal to the midpalatal aspect of 26, then a corresponding pure crevicular incision.
2. Wedge shaped parallel incisions carried ca. 10 mm distally.
3. Perpendicular incision at the distal extent of the parallel incisions.
4. Undermining incisions for flap formation and reflection (oblique hatching).
5. Contouring gingivectomy of redundant tissues.

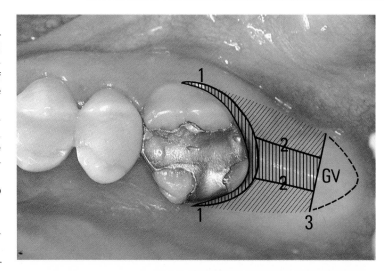

563 Incisions
Clinical view after performing the incisions depicted above. The old amalgam was recontoured and polished before surgery.

Right: The schematic depicts the wedge excision in orofacial section (incision no. 2, see Fig. 562).

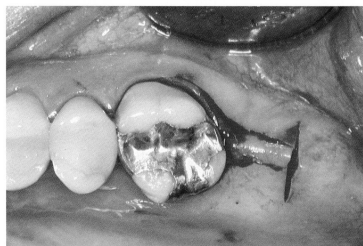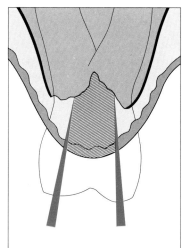

564 Removal of the wedge
A lingual scaler may be used to advantage for freeing the tissue wedge from subjacent bone.

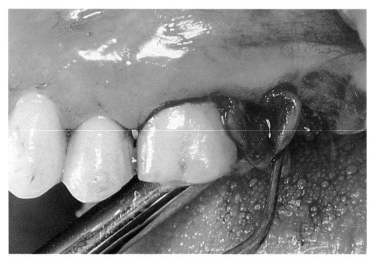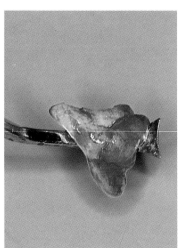

565 Flap reflection – Root planing
The undermining incisions (see schematic) parallel to the gingival surface create flaps of uniform thickness (2–3 mm) both facially and orally.

The exposed root surface is thoroughly planed (right, thin red arrow), especially in the furcation area.

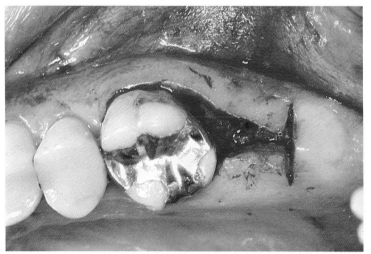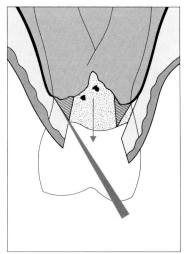

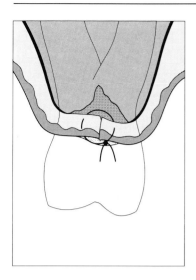

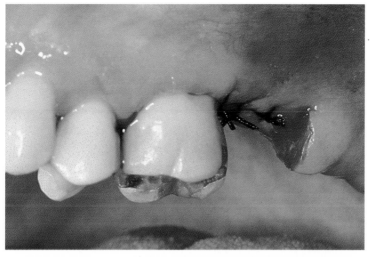

566 Suturing the thin flaps

The technique of wedge excision with modified incisions permits particularly effective adaptation of the flaps and secure closure of the defect.

At the distal end of the operative site there remains redundant tissue in the tuberosity area.

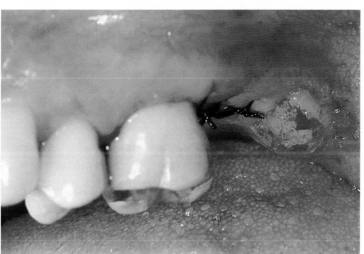

567 Gingivectomy of redundant tissue

The excess tissue distal to the molar may be removed by means of electrosurgery or scalpel. The goal is to recontour the tuberosity. This small open wound is left to epithelialize without any periodontal dressing; the patient may experience some discomfort initially.

Alternatively, the wound may be covered with a cyanoacrylate tissue adhesive.

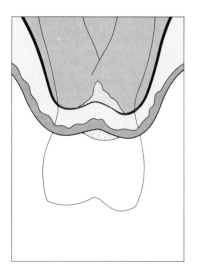

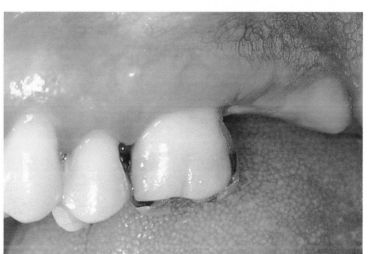

568 2 months postoperatively

Pocket depth has been reduced by about 4 mm (note restoration margin and gingival contour). The sulcus can be probed to a depth of 3 mm, and there are no signs of disease activity.

Schematic: Some degree of osseous regeneration may be expected in the defect. The slight depression in the gingiva distal to the molar (furcation) must be given special attention by the patient during home care procedures. Interdental brushes can be used to keep this area plaque-free.

569 Occlusal view 4 months postoperatively

At the first recall appointment, an inflamed papilla was noted facially between 25 and 26. Treatment including plaque removal, root planing, patient motivation and reinstruction was initiated immediately. Gingival inflammation was eliminated within a few days.

The composite resin restoration in the second bicuspid should be replaced with amalgam.

Wedge Excision – Lone Standing Tooth

The surgical elimination or reduction of periodontal pockets around lone standing teeth requires a modified technique that is similar to the previously described wedge excision.

A 55-year-old female, whose case is depicted below, presented with advanced periodontitis. In the mandible, all hopeless teeth and an old bridge were removed. On the three remaining teeth (47, 43; 33), the probing depths after subgingival scaling were 7 mm mesially and distally, but only 2 mm facially and orally. The treat-

ment plan included surgical elimination of the mesial and distal pockets by means of wedge excisions.

Following healing, an Edlan procedure (p. 245) was performed on teeth 43 and 33 to enhance the narrow band of attached gingiva. The Edlan was done in preparation for definitive prosthetic treatment (removable prosthesis over telescope crowns).

The modified wedge procedure is demonstrated below on tooth 43.

570 Mesial and distal wedges
The pointed gingivectomy knife is used to make mesial and distal incisions outlining the wedge to be excised.

The wedges must be large enough to permit direct vision of the exposed root and the bony margins.

After removal of the tissue wedges, undermining incisions are made to create thin, even flaps.

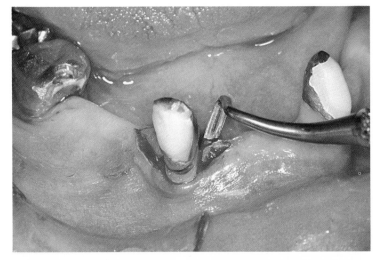 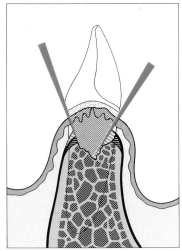

571 Osteoplasty
Following thorough root planing, the sharp bony edges are smoothed, but *no supporting bone* is removed (see schematic above).

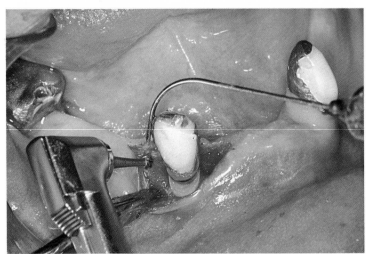

572 Flap adaptation and wound closure
The triangular wounds mesial and distal to 43 are closed using interrupted sutures, without creating tension. Wound closure can be enhanced by application of a tissue adhesive (cyanoacrylate).

The *definitive telescope construction* was completed 6 months after surgery. The margin of the primary abutment lies supragingivally and is thus accessible for oral hygiene procedures by the patient.

At the lower margin of this photograph, the scar from the Edlan procedure is visible.

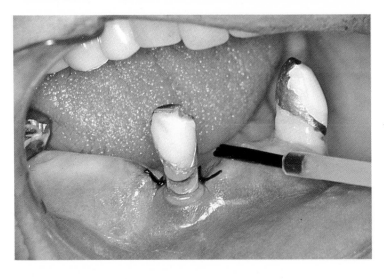 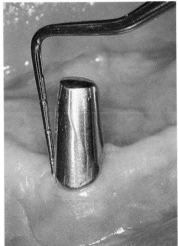

Transplants and Implants in Infrabony Pockets

Transplantation signifies surgical transfer of a *living* tissue or organ to a different site or to a different individual. The tissue must maintain its vitality in the transplant bed of the new location.

The term *implantation* implies surgical insertion of a *nonvital* tissue or material. In discussing osseous replacement techniques, both old and new terminology for transplant and implant materials are used (see table).

Old nomenclature	New nomenclature	Origin of the material	Type of material
autologous ———————— autologous		– Same individual	**Bone**
homologous ⟨	isologous (syngeneic)	– Monozygotic twin or inbred strain	**Bone**
	allogeneic	– Same species (no genetic "matching")	**Bone bank** **Lyophilized bone and cartilage**
heterologous ———————— xenogeneic		– Different species	**Bone (fetal)** **Collagen**
alloplastic ———————— alloplastic		– Inorganic, "foreign body" material (e.g., ceramic, metal etc.)	**Calcium phosphate** as: – **Hydroxyapatite** (HA, *non-resorbable*) e.g., **Periograf, Calcitite, Durapatite** – **Tricalcium phosphate** (TCP, *resorbable*) e.g., **Synthograft, Frialit** **Bioglass** **Calcium sulfate** etc.

The benefit of transplants and implants in periodontal osseous surgery remains a topic of discussion and controversy. The literature contains numerous references to new bone formation in periodontal pockets after transplantation or implantation. However, similar results have been reported following thorough root planing and curettage in infrabony pockets after reflecting flaps for access. A tight postoperative suture closure coupled with perfect plaque control would appear to be more important prerequisites for osseous regeneration than the filling of bony pockets with some "material."

Autologous bone is the most promising material in terms of enhancement of new bone formation. The source for such bone may be the alveolar process, for example between two tooth roots or from an edentulous area (see operative procedure, p. 218).

Bone spicules gathered on a filter during osteoplasty procedures may also be used as a transplant material.

Cancellous bone from the hip, though a successful transplant material, does not represent a realistic solution to the problem of periodontal pockets because of the costs in time, effort, discomfort and money. Removal of hip bone is almost always performed under general anesthesia (Schallhorn et al.1970, 1972). The general surgical effort and risk for the patient far outweigh the potential gain, i.e., the filling in of periodontal bony defects.

Instruments for Removal of Autologous Bone...

Allogeneic, xenogeneic and alloplastic implant materials have the advantage that they can be stored in the dental office (see combined surgical technique, p. 199).

Autologous bone, on the other hand, must be obtained fresh during the surgical procedure. Various instruments are available for this purpose. For example, a filter (Fig. 573) inserted distal to the evacuation tip during osteoplasty can trap particles of bone for subsequent use in infrabony pockets (Robinson 1969; Dayoub 1981).

Additional instruments for harvesting autologous bone include trephine drills. These are available in various sizes for use manually or in the contraangle handpiece. Fine fissure burs or Lindemann drills can also be used to gather bone from the edentulous ridge or from exostoses.

573   Bone filter in-line in the surgical evacuation tip
This sterilizable filter system can be dismantled for cleaning, and is available from Gelman Sciences, Inc. (Ann Arbor, MI 48106, Product No. 4320).

The grid size of the filter is ca. 0.25 × 0.25 mm (*Dayoub* 1981).

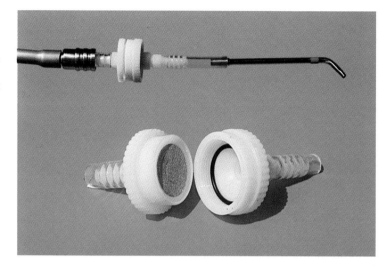

574   Trephine drills

Left: Three trephine drills for use in the handpiece (Jota, Inc.)
Outside diameter: 2.3 mm
                   2.8 mm
                   5.0 mm
Right: Working end of the manual trephine drill (see below), with dispensing attachment.
Outside diameter: 5.0 mm.

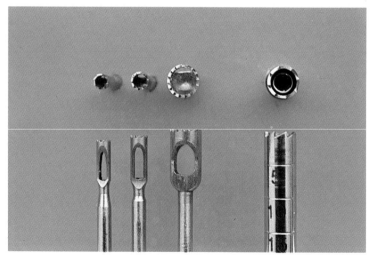
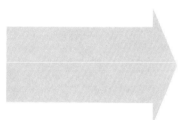

575   Hand trephine
This trephine is engraved every 1/4 inch or 5 mm so that the surgeon can always ascertain how deep the tip has penetrated. (This instrument is available from Maurice Bovard, Fabrique d'Objets de Pansement à l'Ambulance. 16, place des philosophes, CH-1211 Geneva, Switzerland.)

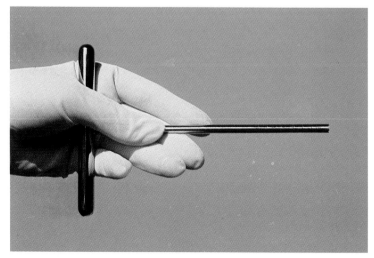

... and Their Use

In order to obtain autologous bone with a trephine, the periodontal surgical site must generally be extended beyond normal limits. Extending the flaps may expose an adjacent edentulous area as a site for harvesting autologous bone for transplantation.

It may be necessary to raise mucoperiosteal flaps in another area of the mouth in order to gain access to an appropriate site for the harvest of autologous bone. The transplant should include spongiosa as well as cortical bone. Before transferring autologous bone to the periodontal defect, it must be split into tiny chips that do not exceed 1 mm³. The rongeurs or scissors can accomplish this.

Extension of the surgical site, or creation of a second site, can be avoided if osteoplasty is planned for the primary site. If this is the case, a sterile filter system (Fig. 573) can be used to collect autogenous bone for transplantation.

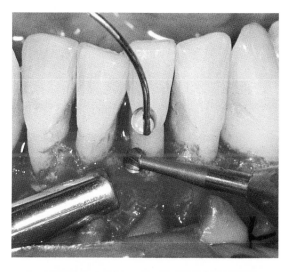
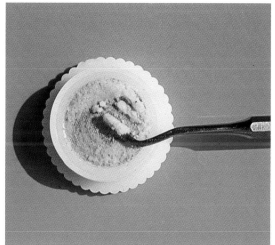

576 Harvesting bone
Considerable amounts of osseous substance can be collected on a sterile filter in the evacuation system when a round bur is used for osteoplasty with copious irrigation using sterile saline.

This material becomes mixed with blood when placed into a debrided defect *("osseous coagulum")*. 2- and 3-wall infrabony defects are easily filled with osseous coagulum.

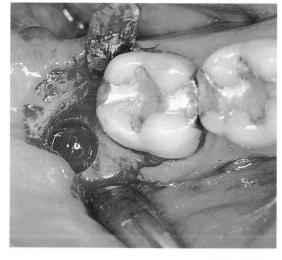
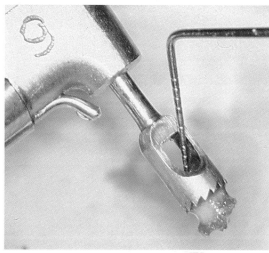

577 Harvesting autologous bone with a handpiece-mounted trephine drill
The retromolar area has been the site for collection of autologous bone, using a 5 mm trephine drill mounted in the contraangle handpiece. Constant irrigation with sterile saline is mandatory during such procedures. The core of bone must be freed using the drill or an elevator.

The durable Williams probe is used to dislodge the bone, which is reduced to chips in saline solution before implantation.

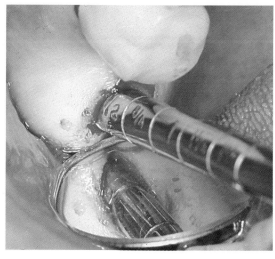
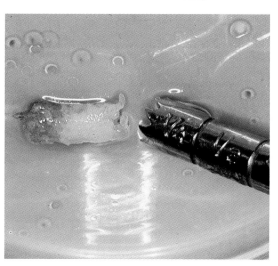

578 Harvesting autologous bone with the manual trephine drill
Access in the oral cavity is difficult with this relatively gross instrument. It is indicated almost exclusively for harvesting bone from the edentulous ridge, especially in the tuberosity region.

A sagittal incision through the mucosa is made to permit entry of the trephine. Soft tissue should be removed from the osseous material before transplantation.

Autologous Bone Transplantation

Operative procedure

A 30-year-old female wished to have the space in her upper left quadrant closed by means of a fixed bridge. Because the mandible was fully dentulous, it was prudent to maintain the lone-standing maxillary second molar (27) as an abutment, but a 7 mm infrabony pocket could be probed on the mesial of this tooth. The examination led the practitioner to suspect a multi-walled defect.

The treatment plan called for filling this defect with autologous bone. The edentulous area between 24 and 27 was available as a site for harvesting the transplant material; however, because of the proximity of the maxillary sinus, this is a "dangerous" donor site.

Findings after initial therapy:
HYG 82%   PBI 1.2
TM   Grade 2 for tooth 27, grade 1 for 23 and 24.
The clinical picture and radiographs are presented in the Figures below.

579   After initial therapy
The persistent 7 mm infrabony pocket mesial to the second molar is depicted clinically and radiographically with a Goldman probe in situ.
  A 5 mm gingival pocket was present on the distal surface of 24.

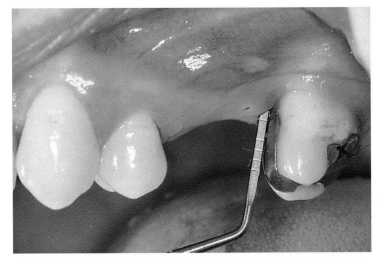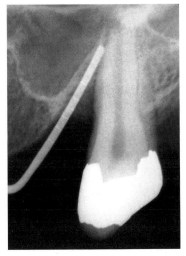

580   Incisions
Facial and oral flap reflection is necessary in order to perform periodontal treatment on 24 and 27 with simultaneous harvest of autologous bone. The primary incision courses parallel to the alveolar crest in the edentulous area between the two teeth. As the incision approaches the teeth, it becomes a crevicular incision on both facial and oral aspects.
  Distal to 27, the incision ends as a modified wedge procedure (compare Fig. 557).

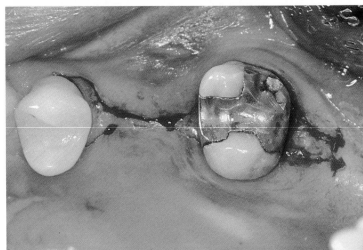

581   Surgical field exposed
Following root planing and debridement of the infrabony pocket, the 3-wall defect mesial to 27 and two of the three donor sites are visible.

Caution: Maxillary sinus!

Instead of a single large (5 mm) explant, several smaller (2.8 mm dia.) pieces were taken, without altering the contour of the alveolar ridge. The three pieces of bone were further reduced in size before transfer to the defect.

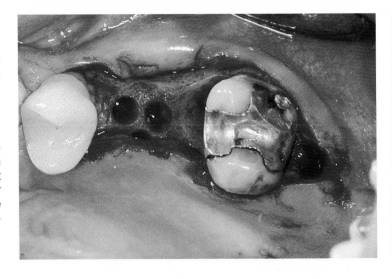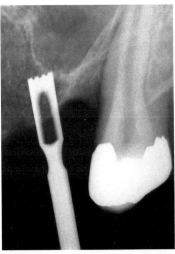

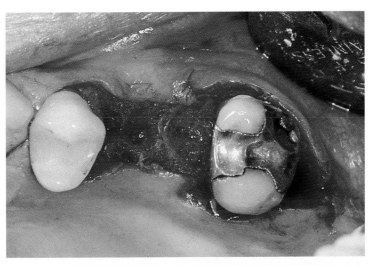

582   After transplantation of the bone
Bony chips with a maximum size of 1 mm³ are tightly wedged into the 3-wall defect.
    The crater is completely filled, and blood clots fill the donor sites.

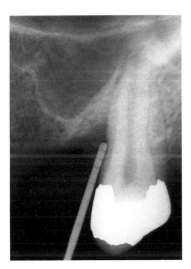
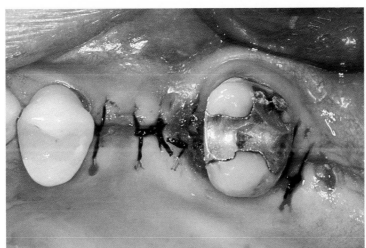

583   Tight closure of the surgical site
Healing of the site can only occur optimally if the flap closure is complete and secure.
    The surgical site should be protected from mechanical trauma by a periodontal dressing.

Radiograph: Filling of the defect is evident.

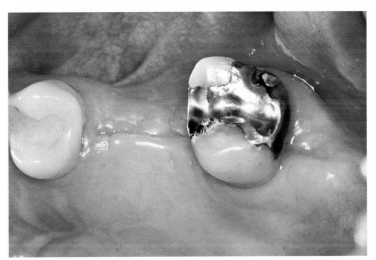

584   3 months postoperatively
Healing proceeded without complication. Fabrication of the fixed bridge can begin in a few more months, after complete consolidation of the site.

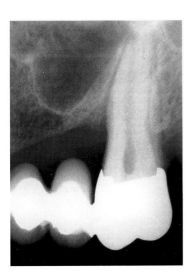
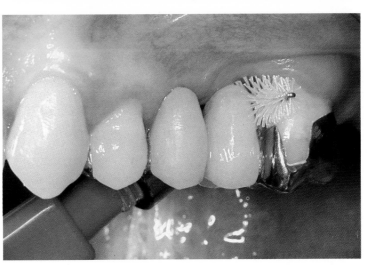

585   7 months postoperatively – Seating the bridge
The 4-unit bridge is first seated temporarily. The bridge abutments were prepared for *3/4 crowns,* with all margins located supragingivally. Interdental hygiene is easy, using spiral brushes. The periodontal pocket mesial of 27 has been eliminated via apical positioning of the gingiva and possible osseous regeneration.

The radiograph reveals that the previous osseous crater has filled with newly regenerated bone.

Bone Regeneration without Transplantation – Case Report

It is not universally accepted that osseous regeneration in periodontal pockets can be initiated, enhanced or accelerated by transplants or implants.

However, it has been demonstrated that significant periodontal regeneration can occur in the absence of any sort of "filling" of an osseous defect. Prerequisites for such regeneration include perfect root planing, curettage and postoperative plaque control (Polson & Heijl 1978).

The radiographs below depict this type of osseous regeneration, which occurred over a 6-month period in a 35-year-old female.

It is imperative to remember, however, that osseous regeneration is no guarantee that the complex periodontal supporting structure has been renewed, with reformation of cementum, connective tissue attachment and periodontal ligament (see Regeneration, p. 261). In many cases, only a long junctional epithelium is present, extending apically beyond the newly formed bone, even to the depth of the original pocket.

586 9 mm infrabony pocket
The pocket distal to tooth 36 was debrided and root planed with direct vision (flap operation).

The *schematic* representation of the radiograph depicts the level of the CEJ (red line), the level of the original bony margin (black line) and the expanse of the osseous defect.

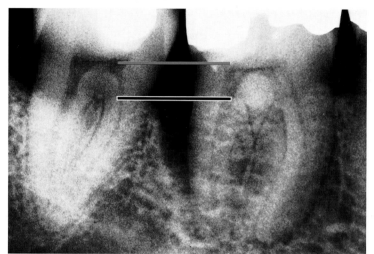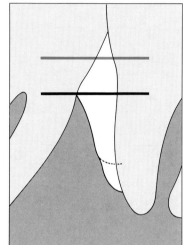

587 Beginning osseous regeneration
Several weeks after the surgery the defect appears to be 1/3 filled (red in diagram).

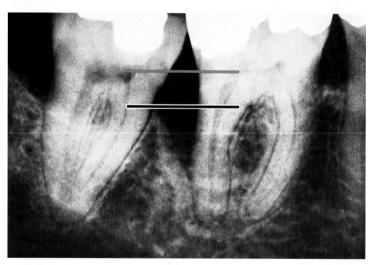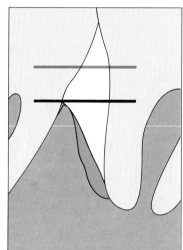

588 Bone regeneration 6 months postoperatively
The original vertical defect has almost completely filled in. The clinical probing depth is 3 mm.

The osseous regeneration visible in the radiograph, however, cannot be taken as a qualitative indication of the degree of new attachment.

Radiographs courtesy of *G. Cimasoni*.

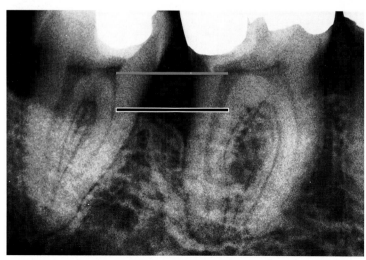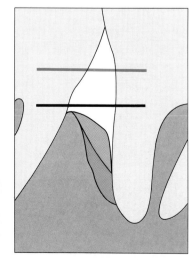

Surgical Treatment of the Furcation

The various degrees of severity of furcation involvement in multirooted teeth were described and portrayed in the chapters dealing with "Diseases of the Periodontium" and "Charting – Diagnosis – Prognosis" (pp.60 & 90). Furcation involvements of Classes F1 to F3 are based on horizontal probing. A Class F1 furcation involvement can be probed less than 3 mm horizontally, while a Class F2 involvement can be probed more than 3 mm. A Class F3 furcation involvement is the "through-and-through" situation, where the degree of severity can vary (subclasses A, B and C; Tarnow & Fletcher 1983), and is frequently combined with deep "moat-like" infrabony pockets.

Treatment of an involved furcation is usually carried out during the course of comprehensive periodontal therapy, but furcations are always particularly problematic. For this reason, this entire chapter is dedicated to the discussion of furcation treatment (Ramfjord & Ash 1979; Mutschelknauss & von der Ohe 1982; Lindhe 1983).

Indications for various treatment modalities

Class F1 furcation involvement and shallow pocketing: Subgingival scaling, root planing and curettage (cf. p.146) are usually successful treatments, sometimes in conjunction with a furcation-plasty (odontoplasty). Treatment may also be combined with a gingivectomy or a modified Widman flap depending on comprehensive findings and the overall treatment plan.

Class F2 furcation involvement: The treatment of choice is surgical (e.g., modified Widman flap), in order to reveal the morphology of the furcation entrance and to permit scaling and root planing with direct vision. The plaque-retentive area represented by the furcation entrance can be reduced by odontoplasty at the gingival margin (cf. p.147).

Class F3 furcation involvement: The prognosis is poor if untreated, especially in advanced cases, and hopeless without extraordinary patient motivation. Tooth extraction is indicated in many instances. However, if the tooth is important, for example for masticatory function or as a prosthetic abutment, various treatment possibilities are available, with various prognoses:

1. *Maintenance of the tooth,* including all roots, by means of flap operation and scaling, root planing and curettage in the furcation area.

With apical repositioning of the flap, the furcation can be kept completely open and accessible for cleaning *(tunneling).* If oral hygiene is not optimal in the area, caries frequently occurs. For this reason, tunneling therapy is seldom indicated.

2. *Hemisection* of mandibular molars or *resection* of one or two roots of maxillary molars. These surgical procedures essentially eliminate the furcation *per se,* and the prognosis is thereby improved.

Hemisection of mandibular molars with maintenance of both halves of the tooth *("premolarization")* is indicated only if the two roots are widely separated. If the furcation is narrow, a plaque-retentive area remains after hemisection of the tooth and crowning of the two halves.

Hemisection in the Mandible – Reconstruction

In this 45-year-old female, the furcation of tooth 46 was involved in a through-and-through manner (Class F3), and the radiograph revealed a massive periapical radio-lucency. The treatment plan included hemisection of the tooth and extraction of the mesial root. This procedure was chosen in order to preclude a free-end saddle situation against the natural dentition of the maxillary arch (see Fig. 595).

The hemisection was performed with a conservative flap. A temporary bridge was required during the heal-ing and consolidation phase, to prevent drifting of teeth. Definitive restorative therapy was accomplished 7 months after the periodontal surgery. The patient exer-cised excellent home care.

Findings before surgery:

    HYG 92%   PBI 1.3
    TM   1

The clinical picture and radiographs are depicted in the Figures below.

589   Molar tooth 46 with Class F3 furcation involvement
The crown of 46 is severely broken down, and the furcation involve-ment is through-and-through (Class F3).

The radiograph reveals a massive apical radiolucency on the mesial root of 46. Primarily for endodontic reasons, hemisection of the tooth and extraction of the mesial root are indicated. The root canal of the retained distal root must be filled endodontically *before* the hemi-section procedure.

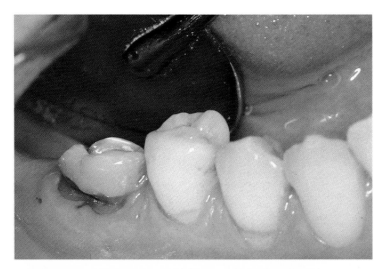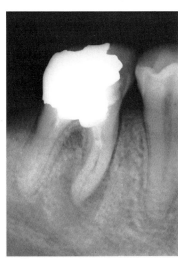

590   Flap procedure and hemisection
The crown is halved using dia-mond and carbide burs.

Right: On an extracted tooth, the line of hemisection is shown to be toward the mesial root. This pre-vents any damage to the distal root, which will be retained; how-ever, this precautionary measure often leads to a detectable over-hang (plaque retention) in the fur-cation region. This must be re-moved during tooth preparation, at which time the root surface can also be thoroughly planed.

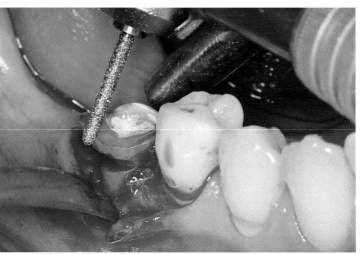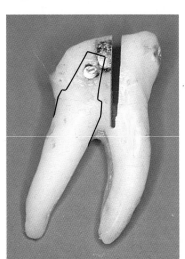

591   After extraction of the mesial root
All sharp edges on the remaining portion of the tooth should be smoothed before terminating the procedure. This may be consider-ed as "initial tooth preparation."

In the radiograph the distal root of 46 appears similar to a single-rooted bicuspid.

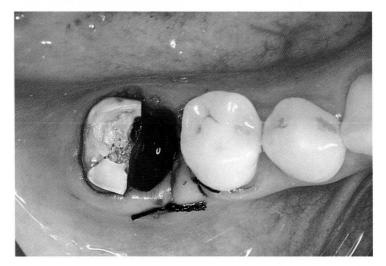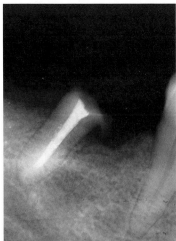

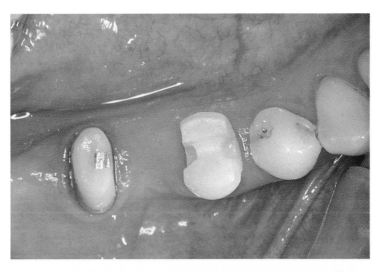

592   6 weeks after hemisection
After primary healing of the extraction wound, the distal portion of 46 was prepared to receive a full cast crown using a screw-type post and a composite resin build-up.

The mesial abutment, 45, was prepared for a 3/4 crown.

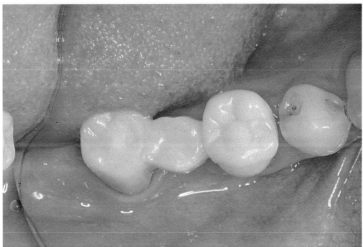

593   Temporary resin bridge
The temporary bridge should be seated as soon as possible because lone-standing roots of hemisected teeth tend to drift. The shape and occlusal form of the temporary bridge should anticipate that of the planned definitive restoration.

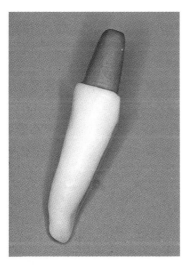

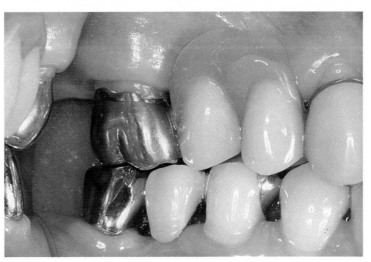

594   7 months after hemisection – Definitive bridge in situ
Right: Occlusal view demonstrates that the bridge extends from the bicuspid to the distal root of the first molar.

Left: This model demonstrates the bicuspid-like form of a prepared distal molar root.

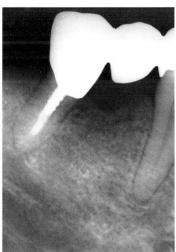

595   Final documentation – Prognosis
The teardrop-shaped pontic lightly contacts the ridge. The interdental spaces are contoured such that hygiene can be accomplished with spiral brushes.

The maxillary antagonist is a removable partial denture over telescope crowns (cf. p. 301).

The radiograph shows the cemented bridge with the single-rooted molar 46 as the distal abutment. The prognosis for the molar is the same as for any single-rooted tooth.

Root Resection in the Maxilla – Reconstruction

Depending on the degree of trifurcation involvement, it may be necessary to resect one or two roots from 3-rooted maxillary molars.

The case presented here is a 39-year-old female, who presented with severe mobility and Class F3 furcation involvements of both upper left molars.

Tooth 27 was hopelessly involved, and was extracted. Both buccal roots and the buccal portion of the crown of 26 were resected. After healing of the surgical site, the remaining palatal root of 26 and the two bicuspids (24, 25) were prepared for full coverage restora-

tions. The two bicuspid crowns were soldered to serve as a firm anchor for the palatal root of 26, which remained highly mobile (permanent splint, see p. 291).

Findings after initial therapy:
    HYG   78%
    PBI   2
    TM   3 for teeth 26 & 27
The clinical view and radiographs are shown in the Figures below.

596 Initial clinical situation
Interproximal probing depths of 7 mm were detected around teeth 26 and 27. Both molars exhibited Class F3 (through-and-through) involvement of the trifurcation.
    Both teeth were highly mobile (TM = 3).

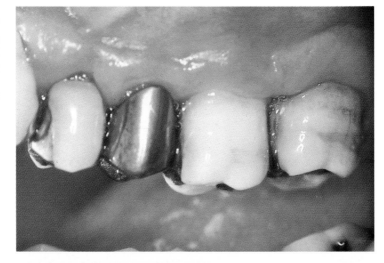

597 Radiographic view
The furcation involvements are obvious, as is the especially pronounced loss of support on the buccal roots of the molars.

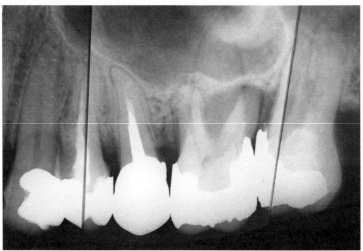

Before

598 Periodontal surgery
After initial therapy, the first molar (26) was treated endodontically, but it was found that none of the 3 roots of the second molar (27) could be maintained. Reflection of a mucoperiosteal flap revealed the wide open furcations; 27 was extracted and both buccal roots of 26 were resected.
    Only the palatal root of the first molar could be maintained as a participant in a cast splint reconstruction.

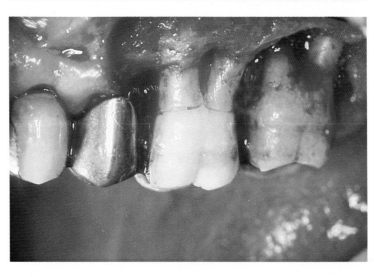

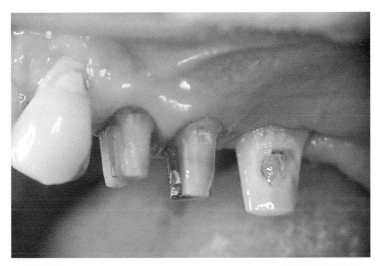

599   6 weeks after the resection
Teeth 24, 25 and the palatal portion of 26 have been prepared to receive temporary full coverage restorations. The buccal surface of 26 reveals the former pulp chamber, now filled with AH-26.

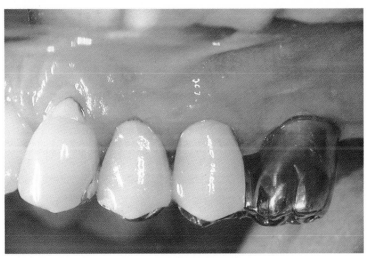

600   Definitive reconstruction
Eight months postsurgically, the teeth were definitively prepared and the palatal root of 26 received a post. Cast gold crowns with porcelain facings were fabricated. The two bicuspid crowns were soldered and the molar crown incorporated into an intracoronal precision attachment; this splinting was done to enhance patient comfort, as the palatal root of 26 remained highly mobile and was palatally positioned. The interdental areas were left wide open to facilitate hygiene.

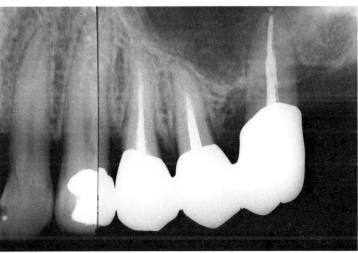
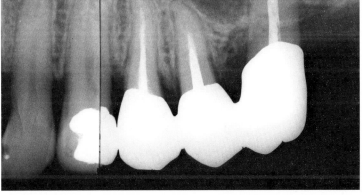

After

601   Radiographic view 8 months after surgery
The 3-unit splint consists of two soldered crowns and a precision attachment from the molar, the latter necessitated by the tipped, palatal position of 26.

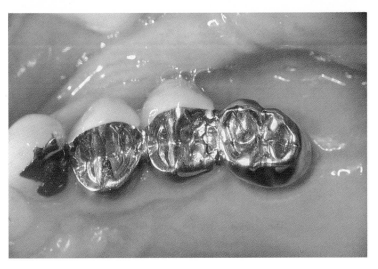

602 Occlusal view 6 years later
Despite the palatal location of the remaining root of 26, it was possible to achieve a harmonious dental arch form. The intracoronal precision attachment effects a stable splinting of 26 to the soldered crowns on 24 and 25.
   The long-term prognosis for this segment of the dental arch remains good.

Root Resection in the Maxilla – No Reconstruction

An alternative method for treating a Class F3 furcation in a maxillary molar involves resection of one root with maintenance of the entire crown. An advantage of this procedure is that it eliminates the inaccessible plaque-retentive area. This procedure can be employed only if the furcation between the two remaining roots is not involved.

The case presented below is a 54-year-old male with excellent oral hygiene. The last remaining upper right molar had a Class F3 involvement between the buccal and distal furcations. The furcation between the palatal and mesiobuccal roots was not involved. Resection of the distobuccal root was indicated, with concommitant recontouring of the tooth crown via odontoplasty, to facilitate home care.

Findings after initial therapy:

HYG	83%
PBI	1.1
TM	0–1

The clinical situation and radiographs are depicted in the Figures below.

603 Probing prior to root resection
Vertical probing depth of 5–6 mm is noted between the buccal roots of the first molar.

The radiograph reveals considerable bone loss, arousing suspicion of furcation involvement. Careful horizontal probing detected a through-and-through (Class F3) involvement between the distobuccal and palatal roots.

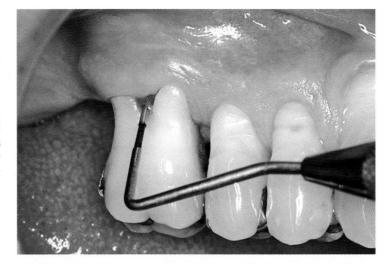 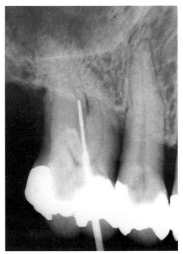

604 Separation of the distobuccal root, and odontoplasty
Prior to root resection, the tooth was treated endodontically and the coronal portion of the distobuccal root canal was filled with amalgam.

Right: Lines on an extracted tooth depict the resection area and the degree of odontoplastic recontouring.

Because the resection site is located supragingivally, root extraction can be accomplished without reflecting a mucoperiosteal flap.

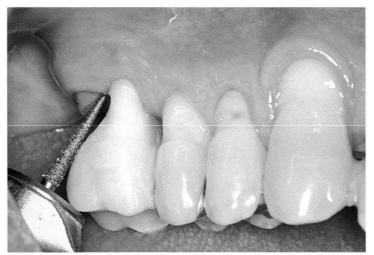 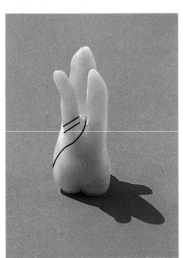

605 Extraction of the distobuccal root using an elevator
The odontoplasty is performed and the site is completey smoothed and polished *before* extracting the distal root. This prevents the introduction of amalgam dust or debris into the extraction site.

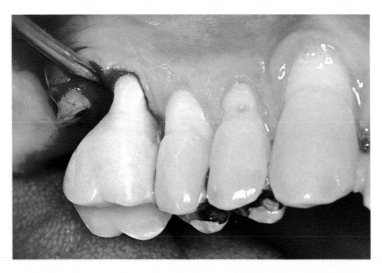

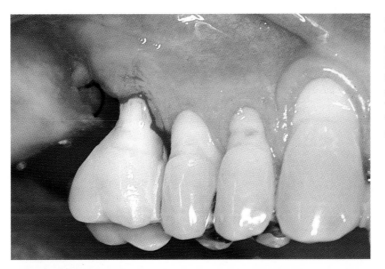

606 Suture closure
The thin buccal osseous plates are depressed toward the open alveolus. After thorough planing and smoothing of the resection site and the remaining tooth roots, sutures are placed to close the extraction site and adapt the gingiva around the tooth.

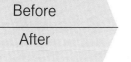

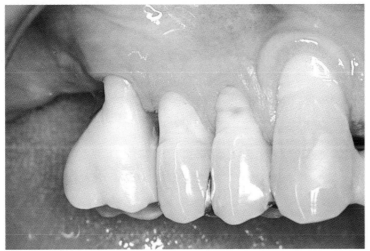

607 6 weeks postoperatively
The tooth is retained without any type of splint or reconstruction.

The occlusal surface of the tooth is essentially unchanged, but makes contact with its antagonist *only* in centric occlusion. The tooth should not serve any guidance function during lateral or protrusive mandibular excursions.

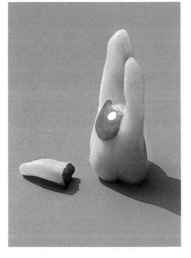

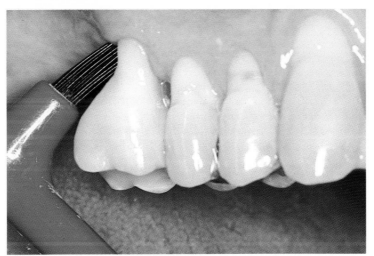

608 Hygiene for the resection site
The patient must be made aware of the particular home care technique demanded by the new tooth form. Marginal/interdental brushes are indicated (e. g., Jordan or Lactona no. 27). The resection site receives regular topical applications of fluoride.

Left: The model demonstrates the recontoured resection site (red) and the root canal closure (amalgam).

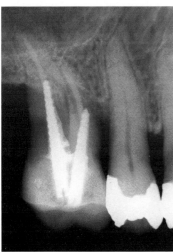

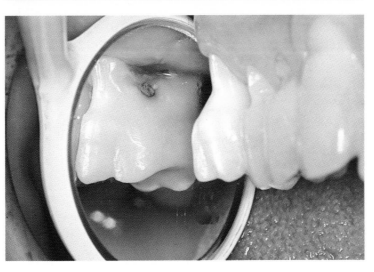

609 Findings after 6 weeks
The entrance to the pulp chamber of the former distobuccal root canal was filled with amalgam. The gingiva is mildly inflamed because the patient's home care in the area is not yet optimal.

The radiograph reveals the metal posts used in the endodontic treatment; these obscure the amalgam closure of the root canal.

Mucogingival Surgery
Halting Recession – Covering Denuded Areas

The indications for mucogingival surgery as a treatment modality for recession have been sharply reduced in scope in recent years. Numerous studies have demonstrated that periodontal health (freedom from inflammation) can be maintained regardless of the finite width of attached gingiva. This realization has reduced the indications for mucogingival surgery to attempting 1) to halt *progressive* recession or 2) to achieve a creeping attachment (Rateitschak et al. 1979; Marxer et al. 1982; Matter 1979, 1980; Dorfman et al. 1982).

If such mucogingival surgery is performed, an additional benefit may be a widened band of attached gingiva and a slight deepening of the buccal vestibule, both of which may enhance plaque control (Lang & Löe 1972). In rare instances, mucogingival surgery may be employed in an attempt to cover a denuded area for esthetic reasons.

The term mucogingival surgery includes the following:

- Gingival extension without free gingival graft (FGG)
- Gingival extension using a FGG
- Frenotomy/frenectomy
- Extension operation of Edlan-Mejchar (1963)

- Covering a denuded root surface by means of:
  - Sliding flap (Grupe & Warren 1956)
  - Direct free gingival graft (one-step procedure)
  - Coronal flap repositioning after FGG (two-step procedure).

General consideration concerning indication

In many cases, recession can be halted by changing the patients brushing method to improve plaque control. After re-evaluation, no surgery may be indicated in such cases. The following steps may spare the patient with recession a surgical procedure:

---

1. Thorough oral prophylaxis: Scaling, root planing, and polishing.
2. Modification of the patient's home care technique. The vertical-rotatory method (modified Stillman) in which the toothbrush moves from the gingiva onto the tooth surface has been shown to be beneficial in patients with recession.
3. Photographs or study models for later comparison (progressive recession).
4. Initially, short-interval recall.

If recession *continues to progress* after this "observation phase," mucogingival surgery is indicated.

Exceptions to this rule include frena that radiate directly into the marginal gingiva and elicit pronounced localized recession. In these cases, surgery should be performed immediately after initial therapy.

Some surgical procedures that were common in the past are performed only infrequently today, e.g., extension operation *without* a FGG, sliding flap procedure, and direct coverage of a denuded area with a free gingival graft.

Gingival Extension with a Free Gingival Graft (FGG)

The most common mucogingival surgical procedure is the gingival extension operation employing a free gingival graft (FGG). The technique was first reported by Björn (1963) and was later systematized by Sullivan and Atkins (1968 a, b). The procedure leads to creation of true keratinized gingiva. This makes the FGG superior to the Edlan-Mejchar procedure (p. 245), since the latter results only in stabilized but not keratinized mucosa.

Indications

Free gingival grafting is indicated in cases of *progressive* recession on single teeth or small groups of teeth in the arch. If *localized* recession extends to the mucogingival line or beyond, home care is rendered very difficult, leading in some cases to extremely persistent inflammation (p. 255). Free gingival grafting is often the only possible treatment.

The treatment of *generalized* recession by means of free gingival grafting is possible, but often requires repeated operations because the quantity of palatal donor tissue is limited. Free gingival grafting is a prerequisite for success in coronal repositioning of tissue to cover denuded root surfaces.

Contraindications

The FGG procedure is not indicated in cases of *stationary* recession that poses neither esthetic concerns nor plaque control problems. Areas of recession exhibiting pronounced McCall's festoons are usually stationary and require no therapy.

A free gingival graft often retains the whitish color of the highly keratinized palatal mucosa. This may be an esthetic concern in the maxillary anterior and cuspid area if the patient has a high smile line.

Surgical principles

The procedure is performed using a local anesthetic that contains a vasoconstrictor to prevent excess hemorrhage.

The *first phase* of the surgery involves preparing the recipient bed apical to the recession area. An initial horizontal incision is made along the mucogingival line. If attached gingiva is completely absent, the incision is made 1–2 mm apical to the gingival margin. The incision is through the mucosa and submucosal tissues, but does not encroach upon the periosteum.

The horizontal incision assumes an arcuate shape as both ends turn toward the vestibular fold; this permits subsequent apical repositioning of the mucosal flaps without tension. Mucosa, submucosal connective tissue and muscle fibers are carefully separated from the underlying periosteum. In this way, a *recipient bed covered with periosteum* is prepared to receive the free gingival graft.

The *second phase* of surgery is the removal of a 1 mm thick graft, usually from the palate. Patient comfort is enhanced if the graft is taken from the same side of the mouth as the recipient site, so that function can be maintained on one side of the mouth during the healing phase.

The *third phase of surgery* involves fixation of the graft to the recipient site.

Instruments for Harvesting a Graft...

The mucosa for a free gingival graft is usually taken from the palate. Several special and easy-to-use surgical instruments are available for this procedure.

The *hand mucotome* may be used to harvest graft tissue of varying width and thickness.

The *motor-driven mucotome,* on the other hand, always provides a strip of graft tissue of identical width and thickness. The connective tissue undersurface of such a strip is so smooth that it may be confused with the epithelial surface. For this reason, the epithelial surface should be marked before the operation, using a nontoxic, waterproof felt-tipped pen. A graft implanted with the wrong side up will not take!

For harvesting graft tissue with individual shapes, *scalpels or gingivectomy knives* may be used.

610 Hand mucotomes
These instruments (Deppeler Co.) consist of a handle and cutting head onto which disposable blades are affixed. The Deppeler mucotomes are available straight (as shown here) or with an angled handle.

PR 1: 7 mm wide
PR 4: 9 mm wide
PR 2: 11 mm wide
PR M: 16 mm wide

Right: Disposable blades fabricated from razor blade steel.

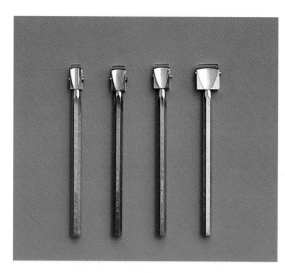
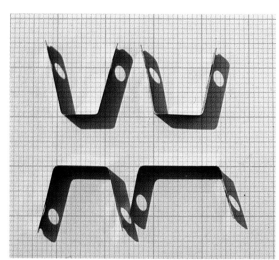

611 Motor-driven mucotome blades by Mörmann
This instrument (Aesculap Co.) permits removal of uniform grafts, 6.5 mm wide and ca. 0.75 mm thick. The apparatus resembles a contraangle handpiece, and is driven by the micromotor. The cutting head can be positioned as desired.

Right: The blades are removed from the cutting head using a special plunger, and can be sharpened.

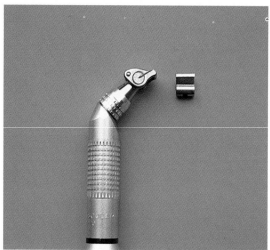
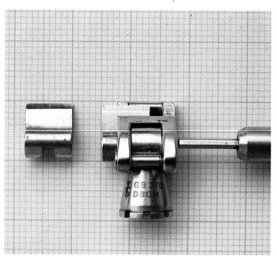

612 Scalpel, gingivectomy knife, surgical forceps, minihook
An individualized free graft can be obtained using fine scalpels (no. 15 or 15 C) or the gingivectomy knife.
    For lifting the graft out of the palate, the mini-hook (Gillis) can be less traumatic to the tissue than a forceps, which can crush tissue. A suture can also be used to lift the graft.

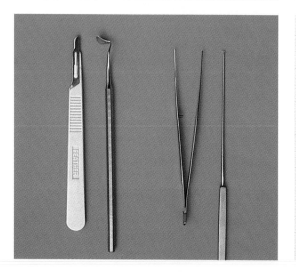
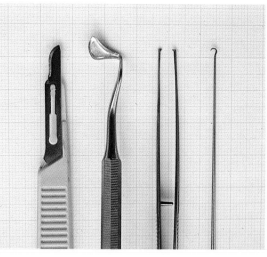

...and Their Use

The mucotome provides rectangular strips of graft tissue that must be trimmed to fit the prepared recipient bed.

If the operator desires a perfectly fitting graft of specific shape, it must be obtained using the scalpel or GV knife plus a pattern or template made of aluminum foil or wax. The individual method for harvesting a graft is indicated especially when the recession to be treated is severe and must be covered with arcuate grafts. This is also true when a graft is to be placed around a lone standing tooth or a tooth at the distal end of the arch. In these instances the graft itself must be adapted around the tooth toward the alveolar ridge.

Removal of palatal tissue is accomplished with terminal anesthesia. If the anesthetic solution is injected with elevated pressure, the palatal mucosa will be lifted somewhat and may prove easier to remove after the incisions are complete.

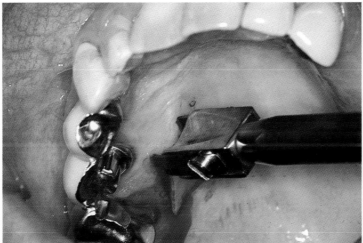

613 Removing a graft from the palate using a hand mucotome PR 1 (7 mm)
The cutting head is moved slightly back and forth as the cut is made. To provide a precise cut, the index finger of the left hand is used for guidance and application of pressure. The ideal graft is uniform and less than 1 mm thick.

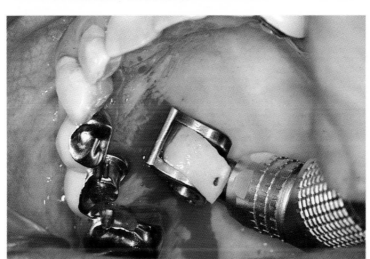

614 Graft harvesting with the motor-driven mucotome
The head of the instrument must be pressed tightly against the palatal mucosa so that the blade engages the tissue fully and a uniformly thick graft is achieved. Marking the epithelial surface precludes suturing the graft incorrectly into the recipient bed.

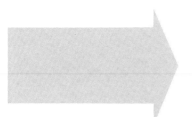
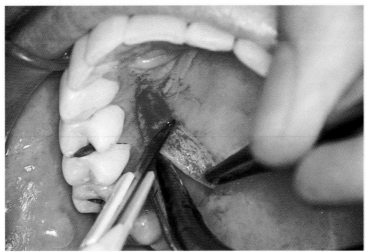

615 Harvesting an individual graft
Using a pattern prepared at the recipient site, palatal tissue is harvested using a scalpel. The first incision is made around the periphery of the graft, to a depth of 1 mm. The GV knife can then be used (without the pattern) to undermine the graft margins, before teasing out the graft with forceps and scalpel.

Free Graft
Thickness and Shape

The structure of the epithelium (keratinization pattern, cell layers) is determined by its *subjacent connective tissue*. It is for this reason that a free graft must contain subepithelial connective tissue, and this is insured if the graft is 1mm thick (Fig.616).

As a free gingival graft heals, the original epithelium on the graft is almost completely desquamated, while the subjacent connective tissue is "accepted" (see Revascularization, p. 240). The new epithelialization occurs from the surrounding mucosa (Bernimoulin & Lange 1972). Palatal rugae must not be transplanted, as they would appear in the attached gingiva after complete healing.

Taking a graft using a hand mucotome or scalpel carries with it the danger of penetrating too deeply and severing branches of the palatine artery. Profuse hemorrhage may ensue.

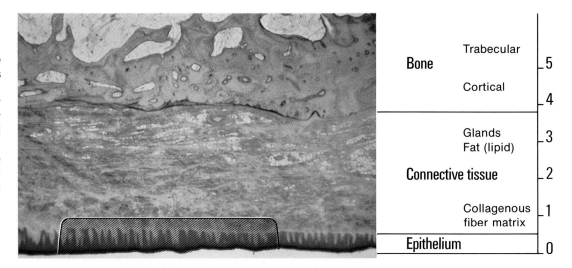

616 Histology of the palate
The soft tissue overlying the palatal bone is about 3–5 mm thick. The ideal graft should be no more than 1 mm thick, so that it contains both epithelium and subepithelial connective tissue. Excessively thick grafts (over 1.5 mm) may contain glandular elements and fatty tissue.

The cross-hatched area at the bottom of the histological section represents a graft that is 6 mm wide and 0.7 mm thick.

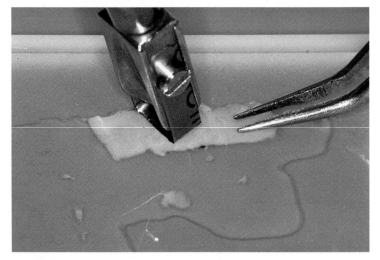

617 Thinning an excessively thick graft
The mucotome, scalpel or surgical scissors can be used to thin a graft that was harvested too deeply. The thinning procedure is performed on a sterile glass slab with sterile saline to prevent dehydration of the tissue.

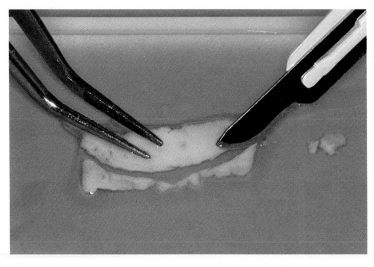

618 Trimming the graft
Grafts harvested with mucotomes are rectangular, and so must be trimmed to fit the recipient bed. This is seldom necessary if the graft is taken from the palate using a scalpel and a template of aluminum foil or wax.

Gingival Extension with Free Gingival Graft (FGG)

Operative procedure

In this 43-year-old female with excellent oral hygiene, *generalized buccal recession* had been diagnosed three years previously. Mild interdental recession was also noted. The patient's brushing method had been horizontal scrubbing, but was changed to modified Stillman three years ago. With this, the progression of recession in the maxilla came to a halt.

However, in the mandible the recession became more severe, especially in the cuspid and bicuspid areas, where attached gingiva is now completely absent. In the following series of photos, the indicated surgical procedure is portrayed.

Presurgical findings:
  HYG 93%   PBI 0.8   TM 0–1
The clinical picture, radiographic findings, recession and width of attached gingiva are presented in the Figures below.

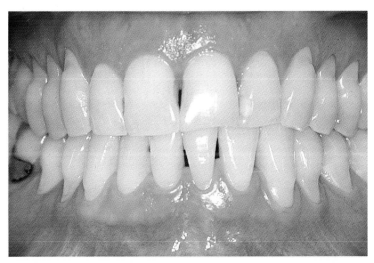

619 Initial clinical view
Areas of recession are visible in maxillary and mandibular cuspid and posterior areas. Teeth with recession also exhibit wedge-shaped defects at the CEJ, probably as a result of improper, traumatic toothbrushing. The areas of recession in the mandible, especially in cuspid and bicuspid regions, are *progressing*. No McCall's festoons are seen.

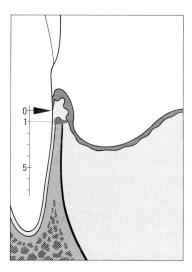
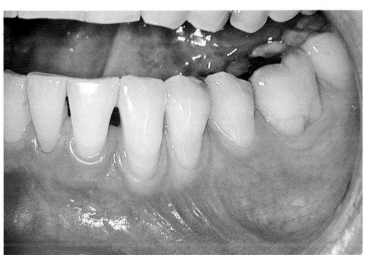

620 Surgical site in lower left segment
There is no attached gingiva present on the buccal aspect of teeth 33, 34 and 35 (area between red and black arrows in the schematic). Tension applied to the vestibular mucosa causes blanching of the gingival margin. A FGG in this area is indicated.

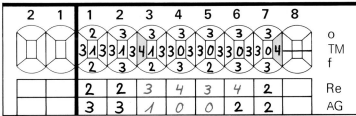

2	1	1	2	3	4	5	6	7	8		
		2	3	3	3	3	3	3		o	
3 1	3 3	3 1	3 4	1 3	0 3	3 0	3 3	0 3	3 0 4	TM	
		2	3	2	3	2	3	3		f	
		2	2	3	4	3	4	2		Re	
		3	3	1	0	0	2	2		AG	

621 Probing depths, tooth mobility (TM), recession (Re), width of attached gingiva (AG) and radiographic findings
From a periodontal standpoint the main problem is the buccal recession. However, the radiographs reveal some horizontal bone loss. Probing depths were normal and tooth mobility was not increasing.

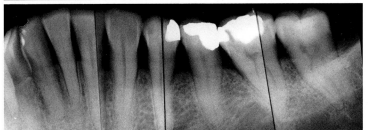

622 Planning the incision

A horizontal incision along the mucogingival line (MGL) is planned. The mesial and distal extents of the incision curve apically toward the vestibule into areas where sufficient attached gingiva is present.

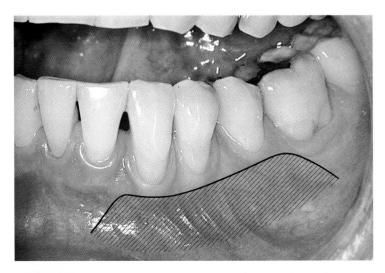

First surgical phase: Extension

623 Horizontal incision

The chairside assistent pulls on the lip to create tension in the vestibular mucosa. Then the no. 15 scalpel is used to make the horizontal incision about 1 mm deep along the mucogingival line, without encroaching upon the periosteum.

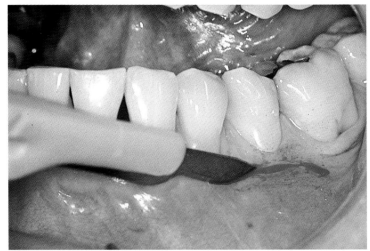
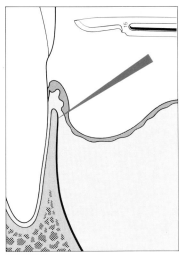

624 Horizontal incision complete

The extent of the incision corresponds to the plan.

Hemorrhage is slight as a result of the terminal anesthetic with vasoconstrictor.

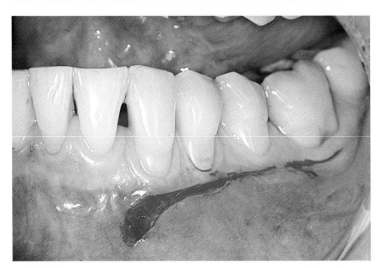

625 Preparation of the recipient site (extension)

Mucosal connective tissue and muscle fibers are sharply dissected away from the periosteum. This procedure is simplified by applying tension to the lip (arrow in schematic). The cutting edge of the scalpel is maintained at an oblique angle to the periosteum.

The recipient bed should consist of periosteum freed of all submucosal tissues so that the graft will be firmly attached in the bed when healing is complete.

Caution: Mental nerve.

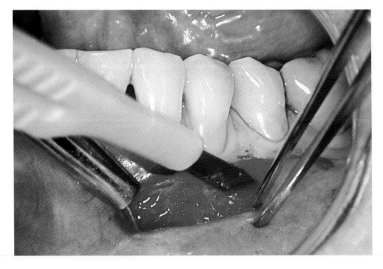
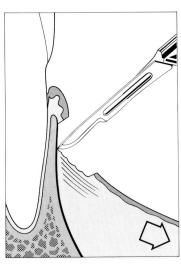

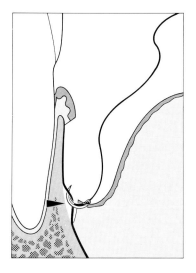

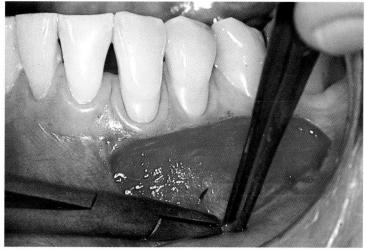

626 Suturing the mucosa apically to the periosteum (optional)
The recipient site, also known as the extension wound, should be wider in its apical extent than the planned graft. The free margin of the vestibular mucosa can be affixed to the periosteum apically using resorbable sutures (see diagram); however, this is *not mandatory*.

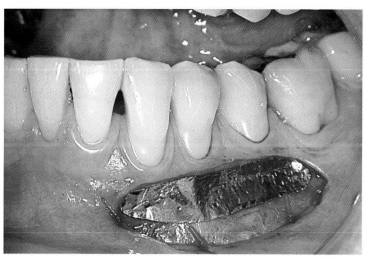

627 Pattern for the free graft
Sterilized aluminum foil is used to make a pattern that precisely fits into the recipient bed. The apical edge of the pattern should be about 2 mm short of the apical border of the bed.

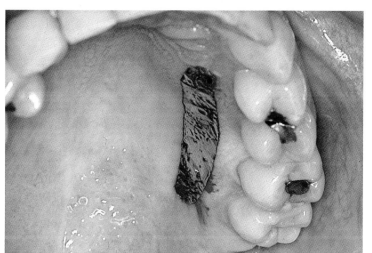

Second surgical phase: Harvesting an individual palatal free graft

628 Aluminum foil pattern on the palate
The foil is placed onto the palate, about 2–3 mm removed from the gingival margin. A scalpel is used to incise around the pattern to a depth of 1 mm.
    For patient comfort, the donor site should be on the same side of the mouth as the recipient site.

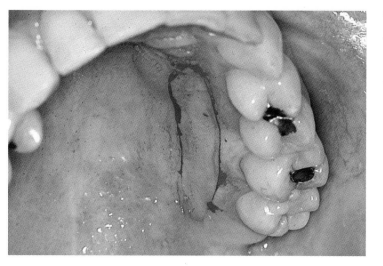

629 Palatal graft outlined by 1 mm incision
The graft must not contain any rugae from the anterior palatal area as these would be transplanted with the graft.

630 Mobilization of the graft margin
A gingivectomy knife is used to undermine and reflect the margins of the graft. A surgical forceps can now be used to lift the tissue.

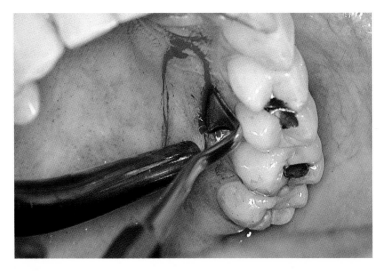

631 Removing the graft
The no. 15 scalpel is used to completely free the graft from the underlying tissue. Visible in the clinical view is yellow fatty tissue on the undersurface of the graft, indicating that it is somewhat too thick.

Right: After removal, the graft is placed on a sterile glass or wooden slab next to the foil pattern. The graft is thinned appropriately and trimmed to correspond exactly to the pattern.

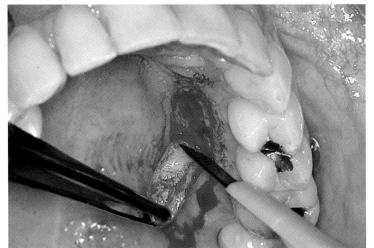
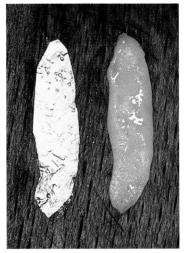

632 Palatal donor site after graft removal
Hemorrhage is generally slight, but if it is persistent, pressure applied over a gauze square, or repeated injection of anesthetic with vasoconstrictor will stop it. In the extremely rare instance of excessive hemorrhage, the severed vessel may have to be ligated with resorbable suture.

A tissue adhesive such as cyanoacrylate may be applied directly to cover the donor site.

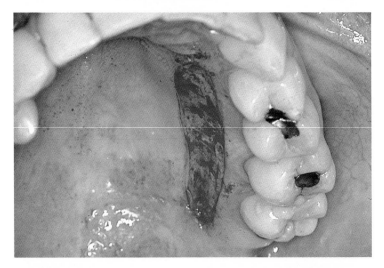

633 Acrylic stent
The donor site may also be covered using a vacuum-formed acrylic stent. This procedure is more complicated than use of tissue adhesive, but is indicated when bleeding is heavy. Furthermore, a stent serves to decrease painful mechanical trauma to the wound by food, tongue and saliva.

The expanse of the stent can be seen on the model. The anterior teeth and the palatal rugae are not covered.

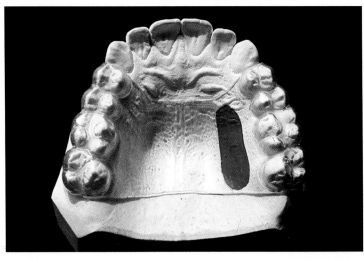

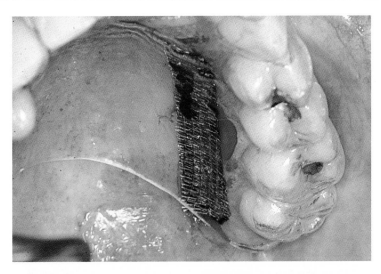

634 Covering the donor site with coagulant-impregnated gauze and an acrylic stent

Most patients wear the stent continuously for only the first few postoperative days, and thereafter only while eating or sleeping.

Re-epithelialization of the palatal wound begins at the wound margins. The rate of regrowth is about 0.5 mm per day. Thus, depending on the expanse of the donor site, complete re-epithelialization can be expected in 10–14 days.

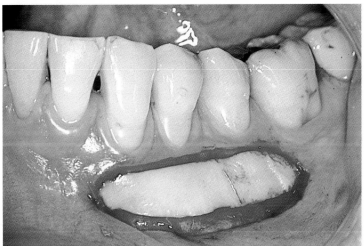

Third operative phase: Graft placement

635 FGG "in bed"

Caution: The graft must be placed with its connective tissue side toward the periosteum.

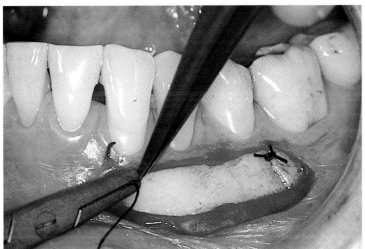
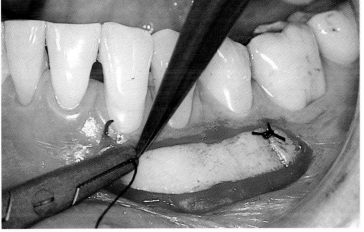

636 Suturing the graft to place

In this case sutures are first placed at the mesial and distal ends of the graft, then one additional suture is placed at each interdental area on the coronal graft margin. Thin, sharply curved atraumatic needle/suture combinations are indicated for this suturing procedure (e.g., 4–0 or 5–0 silk).

Alternative: A FGG may also be placed without sutures. After application of finger pressure to the graft, tissue adhesive is used along the coronal graft margin for fixation.

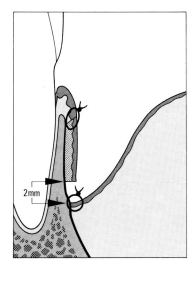
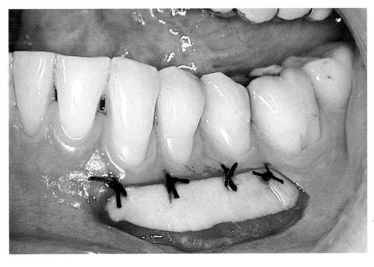

637 End of the surgical phase

The finished graft should be held to place on the periosteum for 2–3 minutes using a moist gauze square under finger pressure. This prevents formation of a thick blood clot beneath the graft, which would tend to lift the graft from the bed. Periodontal dressing is generally not used. The patient is instructed not to brush in the area for 8 days.

Schematic: The FGG is about 2 mm smaller in coronoapical dimension than the extension wound.

2mm

Healing phase

638   3 days after surgery
The surgical site usually looks unappealing several days after the operation. The necrotic superficial cell layers of the graft are desquamating.

Plaque accumulates because of the lack of home care, causing gingivitis in the surgical area.

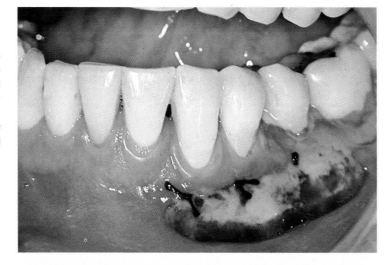

639   8 days postoperatively
The sutures have already been removed. The site is cleansed gently using 3% hydrogen peroxide, and the teeth are cleaned using a rubber cup and toothpaste. The graft appears to be firmly adherent to the bed. The patient may now be permitted to begin home care in the area; gently at first, using a soft toothbrush.

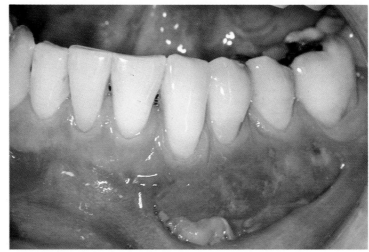

640   1 month postoperatively
The graft is completely healed. It is beginning to exhibit the pale color of heavily keratinized palatal mucosa. Due to shrinkage, the graft is about 20% smaller than when placed, but may be expected to remain this size for years without additional change.

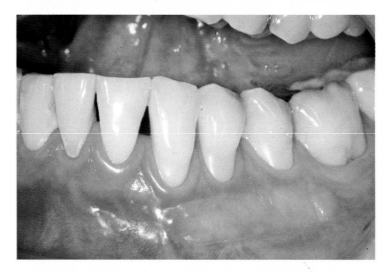

641   4 years postoperatively
The graft remains immobile upon its periosteal base, as does the attached gingiva.

The recession, which was progressing before the operation, has been halted.

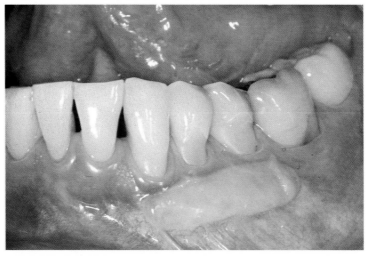

Gingival Extension Using Free Gingival Graft

Summary

The 43-year-old female had employed a gross but intensive horizontal scrub toothbrushing technique for years. Cuspid and bicuspid areas exhibited pronounced, progressiving recession with wedge-shaped defects at the CEJ. The dentition was almost plaque-free and there were no signs of inflammation.

Following a change to the modified Stillman technique and a subsequent 3-year period of observation (compared models), recession in the maxilla came to a halt; however, in the mandible the recession continued.

Mucogingival surgery involving free gingival grafts was performed bilaterally in the mandible, thereby halting the recession. The newly created 5–6 mm of attached gingiva prevented further recession and made it possible for the patient to practice atraumatic home care.

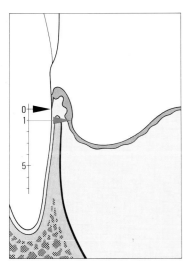
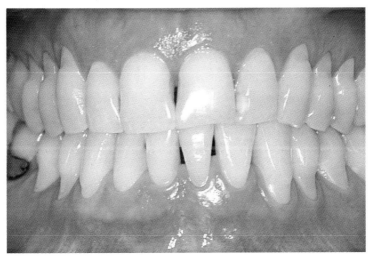

642 Initial findings
Recession in the maxilla remained stable for 3 years after the toothbrushing technique was changed to modified Stillman.

However, recession in the mandible progressed, especially in cuspid and bicuspid areas. Eventually all of the attached gingiva was lost (to the mucogingival line, red arrow).

643 Recession (Re) and width of attached gingiva (AG) in the mandible

		8	7	6	5	4	3	2	1	1	2	3	4	5	6	7	8		
Mand.	Re	X	2	3	3	4	3	2	2	2	2	3	4	3	4	2	X	Re	Mand.
	AG	X	3	1	0	0	2	3	3	3	3	1	0	0	2	2	X	AG	

Before

After

Re and AG 5 years later
Gingival width in the treated areas is 5–6 mm. The progress of recession has been halted. Re values are identical to those before the surgery.

		8	7	6	5	4	3	2	1	1	2	3	4	5	6	7	8		
Mand.	Re	X	2	3	3	4	3	2	2	2	2	3	4	3	4	2	X	Re	Mand.
	AG	X	3	5	5	5	2	3	3	3	3	5	6	6	2	2	X	AG	

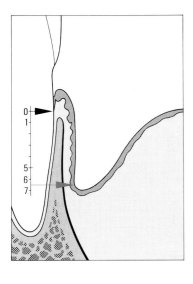
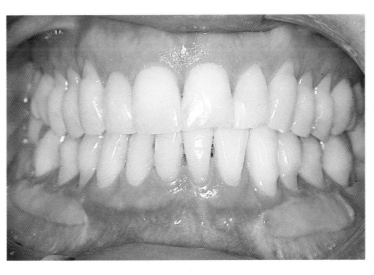

644 5 years postoperatively
The surgical outcome (increased amount of attached gingiva) has halted the recession in the mandible. The rest of the mouth exhibitis no further recession, probably as a result of the change in toothbrushing technique. The recall interval for recession patients is variable, usually every six months or longer.

FGG – Revascularization and Healing

Fluorescence angiography is a technique that can be used to visualize the revascularization and healing in a free gingival graft (Mörmann et al. 1975).

15 seconds after an i.v. injection of sodium fluorescein (20%), the infiltrated capillaries of the periodontal tissues can be photographed under ultraviolet light.

The vascularization of a free gingival graft begins as early as 2 days after surgery. One week later, the healing process is almost complete, but full keratinization of the "new gingiva" requires an additional 1–2 weeks. Only then does the graft take on the typical pale pink appearance of palatal mucosa.

FGG – Fluorescence angiographic examination

645 Immediately after surgery
The entire extension area is devoid of blood circulation (no fluorescence). Nutritive supply to the free graft occurs only by diffusion of tissue fluid from the surrounding recipient bed.

The dashed line demonstrates the margin of the FGG, ca. 6 mm in width.

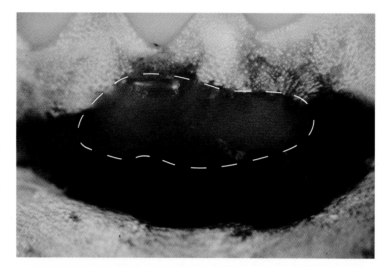

646 2 days postoperatively
Initial vascularization of the free graft is noted, but several areas of ischemia persist (arrows). Extensive areas of the periosteum in the recipient bed apical to the free graft have not yet vascularized, while the entire gingival margin and the apical mucosa exhibit normal blood circulation.

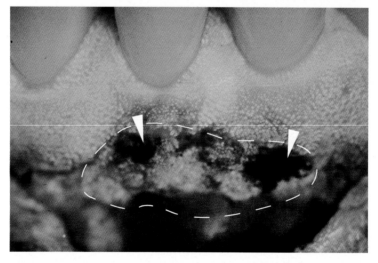

647 7 days postoperatively
The free graft is completely "accepted" and vascularized.

The apical region of the extension wound (not covered by the graft) appears to be closing slowly, with a narrow band (arrows) still completely devoid of vasculature.

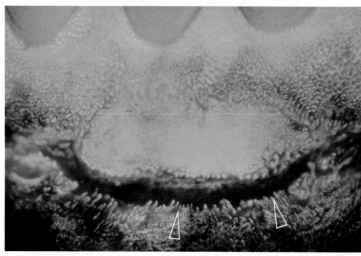

Courtesy of *W. Mörmann*

FGG – Abutment Teeth

Abutment teeth for fixed bridges and removable partial dentures represent areas of particular concern because plaque accumulation is enhanced by crown margins and clasps. Oral hygiene is often difficult. If gingival recession occurs around an abutment tooth, or if the width of attached gingiva is minimal, adequate plaque control may become extremely difficult. The free gingival graft offers one opportunity to resolve at least a portion of the problem.

In the case depicted below, a 30-year-old female was to be treated by means of a fixed bridge seated over an intraosseous implant in the edentulous mandibular molar region using the bicuspid and cuspid (43, 44) as mesial abutments with full cast crowns. No periodontal pockets were present around 43 and 44, but attached gingiva was practically nonexistent, and a FGG procedure was planned.

Findings:

HYG 93%	PBI 0.5
TM 0 at 43; 1 at 44	

The Figures below depict the procedure.

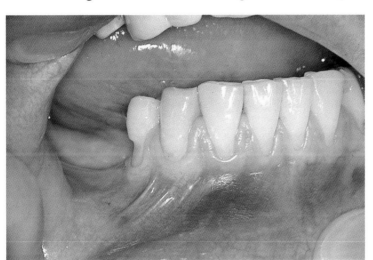

648 Initial clinical appearance
43 and 44 exhibit severe recession. A wedge-shaped defect and lack of attached gingiva are visible on 44. The treatment plan includes 43 and 44 as mesial abutments for a fixed bridge, which will be seated distally on an intraosseous implant.

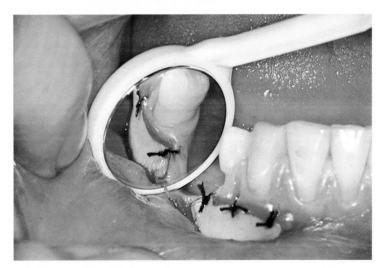

649 Extension operation with FGG
The arcuate free graft was taken as a customized explant from the palate. The graft extended from anterior to 43, around the distal surface of 44, and was sutured to place at its coronal margin. No periodontal dressing was placed.

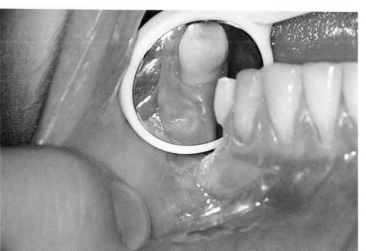

650 2 months postoperatively
The newly created 5 mm band of immobile attached gingiva creates a favorable periodontal condition around the prospective abutments.

When the reconstruction is complete, patient home care will be simple and atraumatic.

FGG over Large Areas – The Mesh Graft

The palate does not provide an unlimited expanse of mucosa for free grafting procedures. The rugae area is not indicated as graft material, and an expansive palatal wound may be uncomfortable for the patient. For these reasons it is advisable to refrain from trying to cover very large defects with a FGG in a single surgical procedure. The mesh graft provides a method whereby a free graft can be "stretched" to cover a larger area. By placing alternating incisions on either edge of the graft, it can be expanded as much as 50%.

In the case depicted, a 35-year-old female presented with progressing areas of recession and Stillman's clefts in the upper left quadrant. The treatment plan included use of a free gingival mesh graft to halt the recession. No periodontal pockets were present after initial therapy.

Findings:

HYG 80%   PBI 0.7   TM 0

Clinical appearance is depicted in the Figure.

651   Recession and Stillman's clefts
This initial clinical view exhibits the progressive recession and Stillman's clefts on teeth 22, 23 and 24. The mucogingival line is clearly visible because the area has been stained with Schiller's iodine solution.

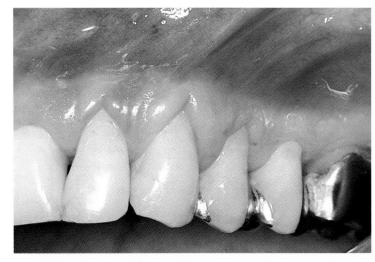

652   Recipient bed for free graft
The bed is over 30 mm long, extending from tooth 22 to 25.

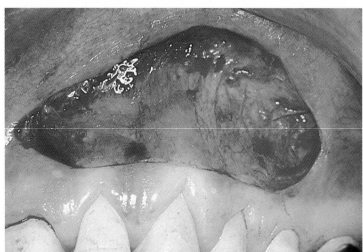

653   Mesh graft before and after expansion
The free graft, harvested from the palate using a mucotome, is 17×7 mm. A scalpel was used to make alternating incisions on each edge of the graft. When tension is applied, the tissue can be expanded to cover the recipient bed, which is 1.5 times longer than the original free graft.

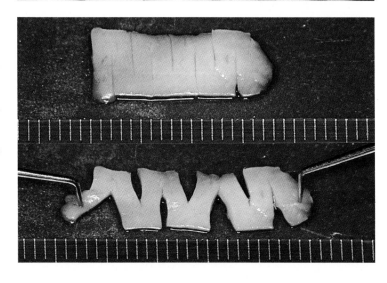

Before

——

After

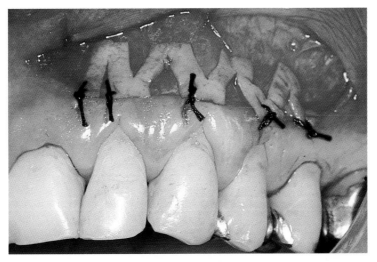

654 Immediate postsurgical view
The graft has been expanded over the recipient bed and sutured at the coronal margin in five locations. Note that the "gaps" in the graft are positioned immediately coronal to the interdental papillae, while grafted tissue is located adjacent to the Stillman's clefts.

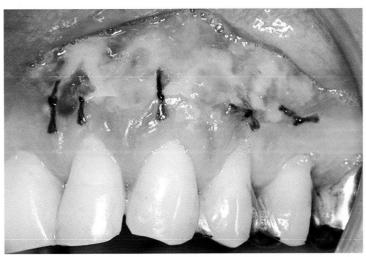

655 7 days postoperatively
The graft has vascularized. The whitish patches represent desquamated epithelial cells from the free graft.
   At this time, the sutures are removed, the tissue is cleansed using hydrogen peroxide (3%) on cotton balls, and a rubber cup with dentifrice is used to clean the tooth surfaces.

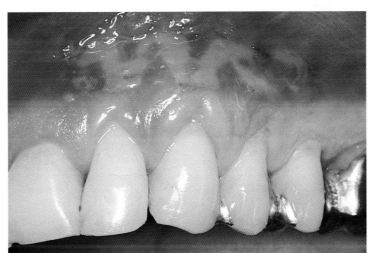

656 28 days postoperatively
After staining with Schiller's iodine solution, the glycogen-free mesh graft is clearly visible (iodine negative). Islands of mucosa (iodine positive) are still present between the graft segments.

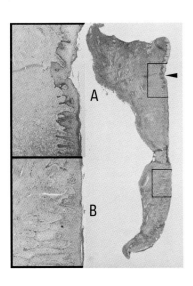
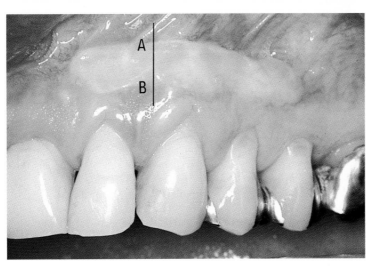

657 2 years postoperatively
The original shape of the clearly visible free graft is not discernible. Keratinized epithelium has filled in the "gaps" in the original mesh graft. A biopsy was taken as indicated by the line A–B in the clinical view.

Left: In this histologic section, the border between mucosa and the transplant is at A. *Keratinized* epithelium from the region between mesh graft segments is shown at B. The mucogingival line is indicated by the arrow.

Frenotomy – Frenectomy

A frenum may exert excessive tension on the gingival margin, resulting in localized recession. To preclude or treat this condition, lip or cheek frenula should be eliminated surgically if they contain fibers that radiate into the marginal gingiva. This can be accomplished by either simply cutting through the frenum (frenotomy) or by excision of the entire fibrous element (frenectomy). These procedures represent the most simple type of mucogingival surgery. Without the use of a FGG, recurrence of 20–50% is the rule, but the remaining band of attached gingiva is usually sufficient. The triangular wound created by frenotomy/frenectomy can be covered with a mini-FGG if desired.

The case depicted below is that of a 17-year-old female with healthy periodontal tissues. The maxillary labial frenum extends to the gingival margin between 11 and 21. A frenectomy is indicated.

Findings:

HYG 95%	PBI 0.4
TM 0	

Clinical apprearance is depicted in the Figure.

658 Labial frenum
The pull exerted by the high frenum attachment has caused the interdental papilla to recede, leaving a space between the central incisors in this young patient (arrows). The area is traumatized each time the patient brushes her teeth.

Schematic: The expanse of the frenum is depicted when the upper lip is reflected. The thin red arrows indicate the planned incisions, which will be performed using scalpel and scirrors.

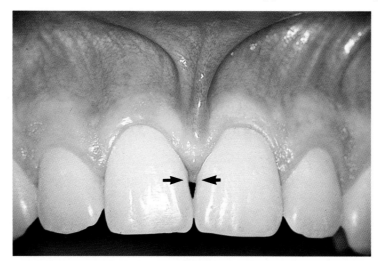 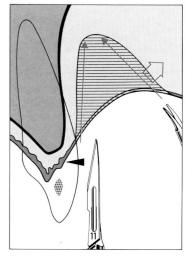

659 Immediate postsurgical view
The Excision of the frenum leaves a rhomboid-shaped wound. A sharp elevator is used to remove muscle and connective tissue fibers from the periosteum of the alveolar process, and the mucosal edges are approximated with sutures.

It was not possible to close the wound completely at its coronal extent due to the immobility of the attached gingiva.

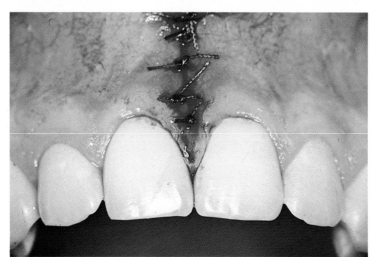

660 2 years postoperatively
Elimination of the frenum pull led to complete regeneration of the interdental papilla (arrows). The interdental space between the central incisors filled completely with connective tissue covered by epithelium.

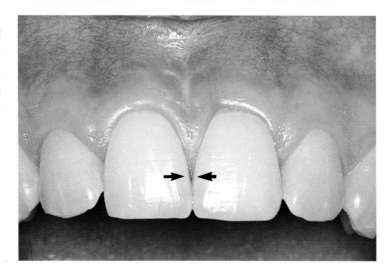 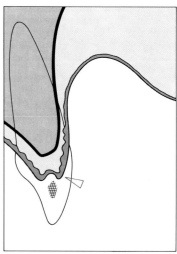

Vestibuloplasty
Modified Edlan-Mejchar Procedure

The submucosal vestibuloplasty described by Edlan-Mejchar (1963) is similar to that used pre-prosthetically in edentulous patients for expansion of the prosthesis bed. A modified Edlan procedure (Schmid & Mörmann 1976) may be an alternative to the free gingival graft (FGG), but is seldom used in periodontal practice today.

Indication

In contrast to the FGG, the Edlan procedure can be used in cases of generalized recession over large arch segments. It can also be employed for treatment of localized recession or for frenum reduction. The esthetic result after the Edlan procedure is better than that after free gingival grafting, because no obvious color discrepancy results.

Contraindication and disadvantages

The Edlan procedure is contraindicated if the treatment plan calls for subsequent coronal repositioning to cover a recession area. In contrast to the FGG, no new keratinized gingiva is created by an Edlan procedure, only attached mucosa, which is not suitable for coronal repositioning.

Principles of the Edlan procedure

The vestibuloplasty begins with a 1–2 mm deep *horizontal incision* through the mucosal epithelium, about 10 mm apical to the mucogingival line. The incision should extend 1–2 teeth beyond the affected area and should terminate bilaterally with a smooth curve upwards toward the mucogingival line (MGL).

A 1–2 mm thick *mucosal flap* is then created by undermining the incision line. The flap consists of epithelium and subepithelial connective tissue. The base of the flap approximates the MGL. The flap is reflected coronally and a scalpel is used to cut through the periosteum horizontally at the base of the flap.

Using an elevator, the periosteum, muscle fibers and residual connective tissue elements are freed from the underlying alveolar bone and reflected 15–20 mm *toward the vestibulum*. It may be necessary in some cases to make lateral releasing incisions to accomplish this. The surface of exposed bone must be large enough to accept the previously prepared mucosal flap. *Be cautious* during the reflection of periosteum in the area of the mental nerve.

The final procedure involves *adaptation of the mucosal flap* to the periosteum-free alveolar bone. Using a moist gauze square, the flap is directed apically and held immobile in place for 3–5 minutes under finger pressure. This helps control hemorrhage, thereby reducing the chance of the flap being dislodged due to a blood clot. Neither sutures nor a periodontal dressing are placed.

If the displaced periosteum shows a tendency to push the mucosal flap coronally as the patient performs lip and cheek muscle movements, the margin of the periosteum in the vestibule may be shortened with scissors or affixed to the mucosa (margin of the horizontal incision).

Edlan Vestibuloplasty

Operative Procedure

Advanced and progressive generalized recession was diagnosed in the mandibular arch of a 26-year-old female. Her home care technique had been changed to the atraumatic modified Stillman method 2 years previously and was reinforced at frequent recalls, but recession continued to progress. The patient still complained of trauma to the gingiva and mucosa during toothbrushing.

At the preoperative examination, several teeth ex-

hibited practically no remaining attached gingiva. A mucogingival surgical procedure was indicated to stabilize the remaining narrow zone of attached gingiva. The Edlan procedure was selected over free gingival grafting because the area requiring treatment extended over eight teeth, from 34 to 44.

Preoperative findings:
  HYG 90%   PBI 0.8   TM 0
The clinical view is depicted in Figure 661.

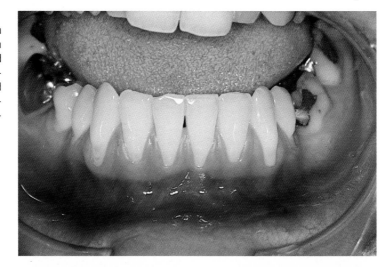

661 Initial clinical view
Advanced, progressive recession in the mandible. Staining with Schiller's iodine solution revealed an area with minimal attached gingiva. The recession was observed only on the facial surfaces. The interdental spaces were still completely filled with gingival tissue.

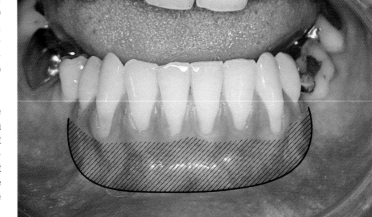
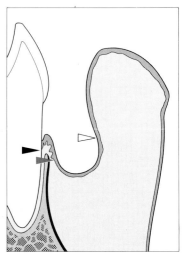

662 Surgical plan – Incision
The horizontal incision (black line) in the mucosa ca. 10 mm apical to the mucogingival line is planned. At its distal extensions, the incision curves back to the mucogingival line, in this case just distal to the first bicuspids.

Schematic: The incision line should be marked on the mucosa with a fine felt-tipped pen without placing tension on the lip (open arrow). The width of the still present attached gingiva is depicted as the distance between the red and the black arrows.

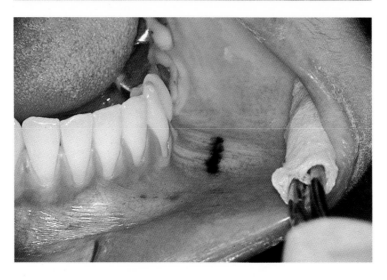
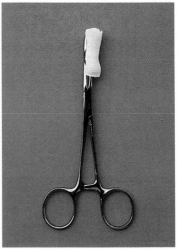

663 Creating tension in the vestibular area
The assistant uses a hemostat with a gauze square to reflect lip and cheek, creating tension in the vestibule. The black mark indicates the distance from the planned horizontal incision to the mucogingival line.

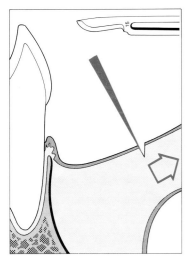

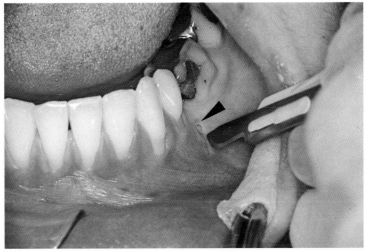

664 Initiating the incision

The first incision begins apical to the mucogingival line just distal to tooth 44 (black arrow in clinical view), curving apically and anteriorly. The incision is 1–2 mm deep and is best performed using the No. 15 scalpel.

The incision severs the epithelium and the superficial connective tissue, without touching the deeper vasculature, nerves and muscle fibers. Nevertheless, this incision usually elicits *profuse hemorrhage.*

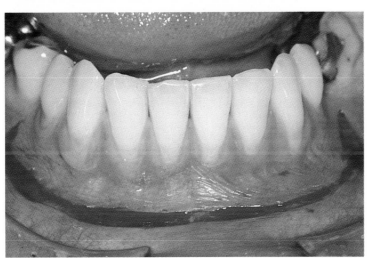

665 Incision completed

The tension created by the photographic cheek / lip retractors causes the wound to open slightly.

The incision is usually covered progressively with gauze squares. Application of light finger pressure will control hemorrhage.

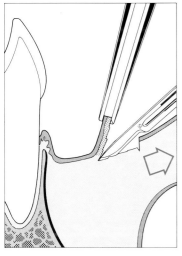

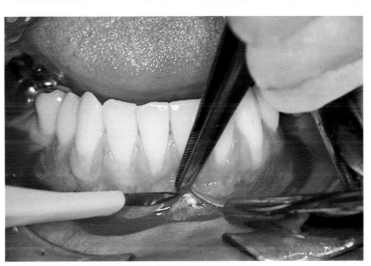

666 Preparing the mucosal flap, beginning at the incision line

The mucosa is grasped with a forceps at the incision line, and the No. 15 scalpel is used to undermine a mucosal flap by sharp dissection, forming a split-thickness flap.

The flap, at least 1 mm thick, consists of epithelium and nutritive subepithelial connective tissue.

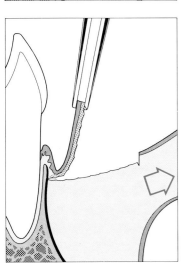

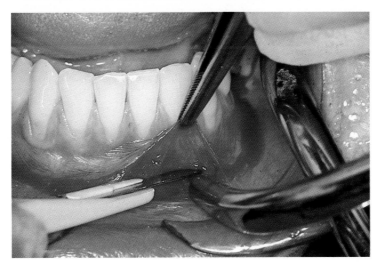

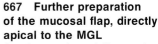

667 Further preparation of the mucosal flap, directly apical to the MGL

Starting at the midline and proceeding in both directions, the delicate tissue flap is gently reflected coronally with a forceps or tissue hook as the submucosal tissues are dissected away with a horizontally held scalpel.

The flap is reflected to the level of the mucogingival line.

668 Problems commonly encountered during flap elevation
There is often considerable hemorrhage at the surgical site, necessitating frequent rinsing, evacuation or application of pressure with a moist gauze to maintain direct vision in the field.

Without direct vision, the danger of grossly perforating the relatively thin flap is great, though tiny perforations are not significant.

An *excessively thin* flap may become necrotic due to inadequate blood supply.

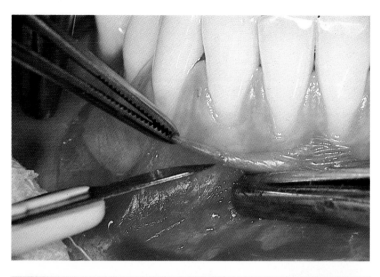

669 Mucosal flap complete
The mucosal flap is reflected coronally using forceps. The mucogingival line represents the base of the flap.

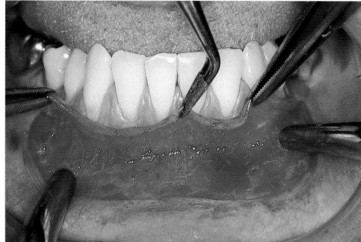

670 Severing the periosteum
The periosteum is severed immediately below the base of the mucosal flap. Frequently several strokes are necessary to cut through the tough periosteum, and the scalpel becomes immediately dull when it contacts the bone.

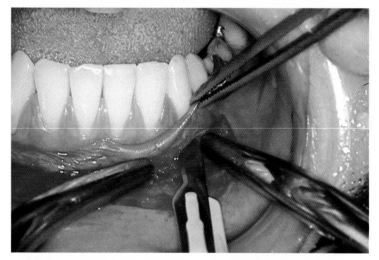
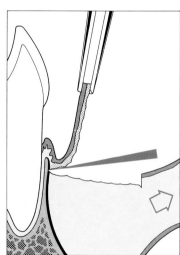

671 Periosteum severed
The periosteum should be incised continuously from right to left. While severing the periosteum the flap may be unintentionally perforated at its base, compromising the nutritive blood supply to the flap. The process of cutting through the periosteum must therefore be performed with extreme care, keeping the mucosal flap elevated at all times.

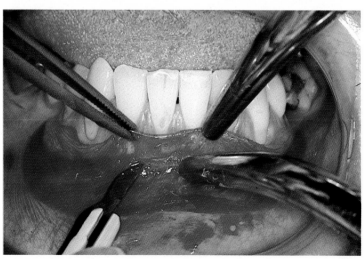

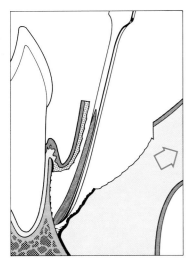

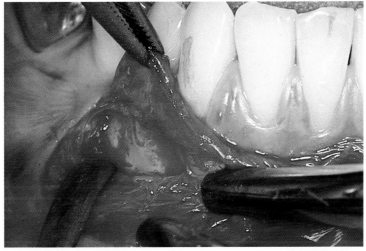

672 Separating the periosteum from bone
A broad elevator is used to apically reflect the periosteum and any adherent submucosal muscle and connective tissue.

Folds of periosteal tissue are thus created. It may be necessary to make vertical releasing incisions so that the periosteum will remain in its apically repositioned location.

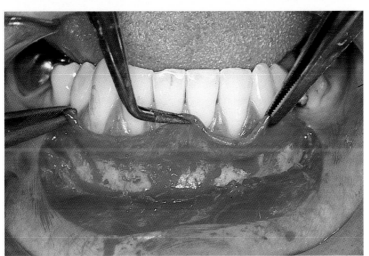

673 Periosteum reflection complete
The periosteum should be reflected apically at least 2 mm beyond the extent of the mucosal flap. This creates a "pocket" between the bone and the periosteum, which the apical end of the mucosal flap eventually occupies.

It may be necessary to shorten the tough periosteum somewhat using a surgical scissors.

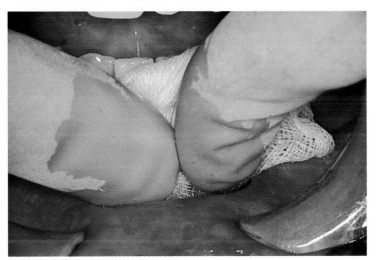

674 Controlling hemorrhage and securing the flap
The mucosal flap is held with pressure onto the osseous surface for 3–5 minutes using a moist gauze square. Bleeding must be stopped completely, to prevent the formation of a large blood clot, which would separate the flap from the bone. Pressure should be carefully applied as excess manipulation can elicit necrosis in the delicate mucosal flap.

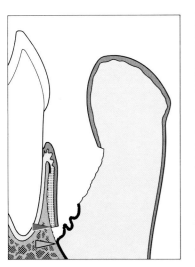

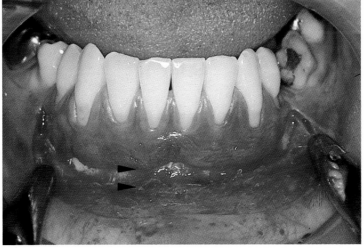

675 Clinical view immediately postsurgically
Neither sutures nor a periodontal dressing are used for fixation of the mucosal flap. The exposed bone (depicted between open and red arrows in the schematic, left) is eventually covered by the mobilized periosteum.

The vestibular wound heals by secondary intention. Home care in the operated area is proscribed for 10 days.

Edlan – Wound Healing, Clinically...

Nourishment for the mucosal flap is severely compromised as a result of the horizontal incision and the undermining flap preparation. As a result, an initial livid discoloration and swelling of the pedunculated flap are clinically evident. This should not concern patient or practitioner as there has never been a reported flap necrosis with proper technique.

Revascularization is initiated from the base of the flap. As blood circulation increases, normal tissue color returns within a week. Wound healing is complete three to four weeks after the procedure and the area apical to the mucosal flap is also completely re-epithelialized at this time. The new firmly attached mucosa maintains its mucosal characteristics forever. It does *not develop into a keratinized gingiva.*

The esthetic result with the Edlan procedure is usually superior to that achieved with free gingival grafting.

Edlan procedure – Wound healing

676 4 days postoperatively
The mucosal flap, with its base at the mucogingival line, has poor blood circulation and exhibits a livid coloration and edema.

The apical extent of the soft tissue wound and the exposed bone are covered with fibrin.

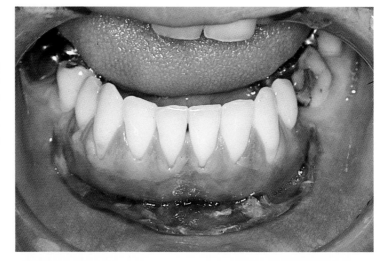

677 10 days postoperatively
Wound healing in the area of the mucosal flap is essentially complete. The reflected periosteum appears as a slowly epithelializing scar. Although the scar is raised at this point in time, after several months it will no longer be palpable.

The patient can now begin gentle home care in the area.

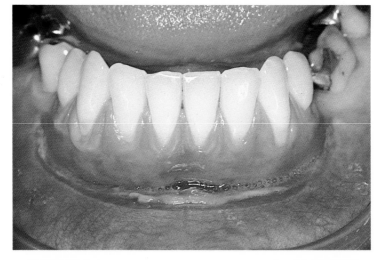

678 2 months postoperatively
The ''Edlan mucosa'' is firmly attached to the underlying bone by means of new periosteum that has formed. The apical margin of the mucosal flap represents the new mucogingival line.

The attached mucosa retains its original character in that it is nonkeratinized. The width of the attached mucosa shrinks by about 50% during the healing phase. From the original 10 mm of reflected flap, 4–6 mm remain.

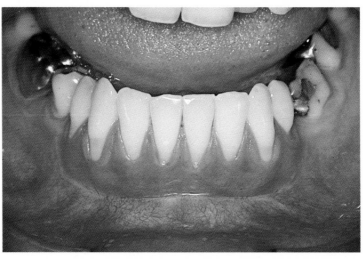

...and as Observed with Fluorescence Angiography

The technique for fluorescence angiography was described in the section on free gingival grafting (p. 240).

Revascularization of the Edlan flap begins immediately after the surgery, starting at the base of the flap. It is therefore important that the flap base not be perforated during surgery. The apical aspect of the flap derives its nutrition initially via diffusion. Revascularization of the entire width of the mucosal flap is complete after only 7 days (Mörmann et al. 1976).

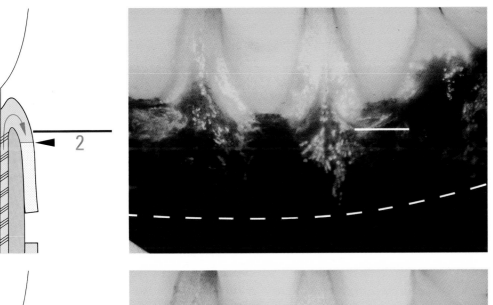

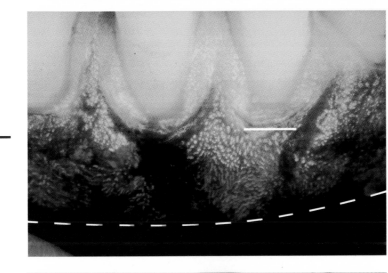

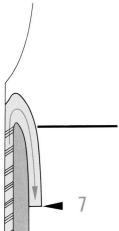

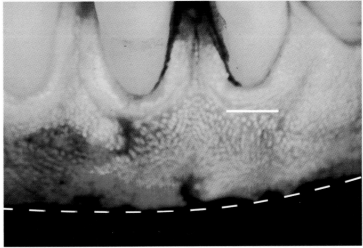

Fluorescence angiographic study of the Edlan procedure

679   2 days postoperatively: Diffusion and initial revascularization
The mucosal flap remains generally ischemic. Early nutrition is via diffusion of tissue fluids.

The vascularization (red arrow in schematic) begins slowly from the mucogingival line (black line in diagram, white line in UV-light view). Areas coronal to the mucogingival line retain their normal circulation.

680   4 days postoperatively: Advancing revascularization
At least 3/4 of the mucosal flap has been revascularized. Several persistent areas of ischemia remain on the facial root surface.

681   7 days postoperatively: Complete blood circulation
The Edlan flap is completely vascularized and firmly attached to the underlying bone via periosteum.

The area apical to the flap margin (dashed line) heals by secondary epithelialization. No blood circulation is evident at this time (dark zone).

Courtesy of *W. Mörmann*

Edlan Procedure

Summary

Despite patient, conservative treatment and revised home care technique, the progress of recession in the anterior, cuspid and bicuspid areas in this 26-year-old female continued. The treatment of choice for increasing the width of attached mucosa was the modified Edlan-Mejchar procedure. It was possible to document the case for a 3-year period postsurgically. During this time, a 5 mm band of attached mucosa remained immobile upon its subjacent periosteum. This widening of the attached mucosa also led to a slight deepening of the vestibule, which made home care easier.

In contrast to a free gingival graft, the Edlan procedure results in a gain of attached mucosa that exhibits no color change, i.e., the esthetic result is superior.

682   Initial clinical view
Advanced, progressive recession in the mandibular anterior, cuspid and bicuspid areas. Minimal attached gingiva remains (between red and black arrows in schematic).

Oral hygiene is difficult; injury during toothbrushing frequently occurs.

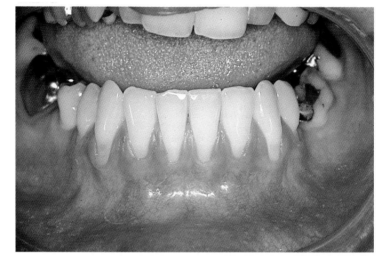 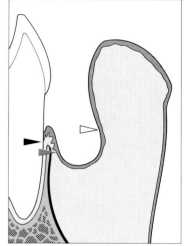

683   Facial recession (Re) and width of attached gingiva (AG)
In the area destined for surgery, the width of attached gingiva is 0–1 mm (red = AG less than 2 mm).

Before

		8	7	6	5	4	3	2	1	1	2	3	4	5	6	7	8		
Mand.	Re	2	2	X	1	3	5	2	3	3	2	4	4	X	X	2	2	Re	Mand.
	AG	2	2	X	3	1	1	1	0	0	1	0	1	X	X	3	2	AG	

After

Re and AG after 3 years
Two years postoperatively, the attached mucosa (''gingiva'') averages 5 mm in width and the recession on the facial aspect has been halted. Recession values are identical to preoperative ones.

		8	7	6	5	4	3	2	1	1	2	3	4	5	6	7	8		
Mand.	Re	2	2	X	1	3	5	2	3	3	2	4	4	X	X	2	2	Re	Mand.
	AG	2	2	X	3	3	5	5	5	5	5	5	4	X	X	3	2	AG	

684   3 years postoperatively
The extent of recession has remained stable since the Edlan operation. The *attached mucosa* achieved by the procedure remains firmly adherent to the underlying periosteum. There is virtually no difference in color between the mucosal flap and the surrounding normal mucosa.

The apical scar tissue is no longer palpable or visible (red arrow in diagram). The incision line (empty arrow in diagram) on the inner surface of the lip and the vestibular mucosa can no longer be distinguished clinically.

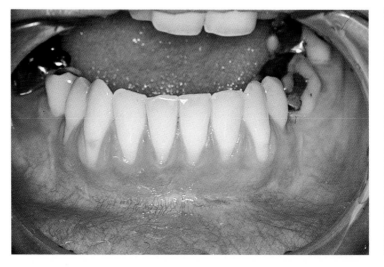 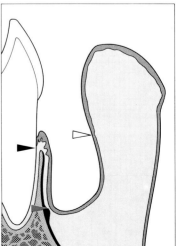

Covering Areas of Recession?

The free gingival graft and the Edlan-Mejchar procedure just described are procedures used to *halt* recession. This is the primary goal of mucogingival surgery.

In contrast, the indications for *covering* a denuded area are limited indeed. They usually relate more to the esthetic aspirations of the patient than to biological necessity.

Indications

– Extremely advanced areas of recession which, despite treatment via free gingival grafting or the Edlan procedure, are still difficult to clean adequately
– Esthetic concerns, especially in the maxilla
– Severe and persistent hypersensitivity of the root surface.

Contraindications

A denuded area that is not becoming larger or which has been successfully treated via free gingival graft or the Edlan procedure does not require coverage. Attempting to cover such an area would have to be viewed as overtreatment or *"l'art pour l'art"* if one of the rare indications listed above were not present.

Treatment options

– Laterally repositioned flap (sliding flap)
– Direct coverage via free gingival graft (FGG)
– Coronal repositioning subsequent to FGG.

1. One of the oldest methods for covering an area of recession is the *sliding flap* (Grupe & Warren 1956). It is only indicated for use in areas of localized recession. The principle of the operation is to elevate and reflect the gingiva and mucosa from a tooth exhibiting *no* recession, and reposition it laterally as a "pedicle graft" onto the adjacent tooth to cover the exposed root surface. This method is plagued by a relatively high rate of recurrence. Furthermore, the donor site, which previously exhibited no recession, may develop recession after the sliding flap procedure.

2. *Direct coverage* of a denuded area with a free gingival graft was described by Sullivan and Atkins (1968 a, b). This procedure can only be successful in cases with clefts of 3 mm or less.

3. *Coronal repositioning* subsequent to free gingival grafting *(FGG),* as described by Bernimoulin (1973) is the method that shows the most promise for covering root surfaces denuded by recession.

   An initial surgical procedure is performed to position a free gingival graft just apical to the area of recession. A waiting period of at least 2–3 months follows. In some cases a "creeping attachment" occurs without any additional surgery, i.e., the gingiva simply grows coronally (see p. 254). If this does not occur, the area can be covered by a second surgical procedure that involves repositioning the grafted tissue coronally.

   Follow-up studies have shown that 50% of all denuded roots treated in this manner remain covered without formation of a periodontal pocket (Bernimoulin et al. 1975). It has not been demonstrated whether the attachment of the gingiva to the root surface occurs via a long epithelial attachment or by means of apposition of new connective tissue.

"Creeping Attachment" after FGG

A 38-year-old female presented with a chief complaint of "worsening denudation" of the cervical area of tooth 34. This tooth had been restored with a full cast crown four years previously during the course of the construction of a fixed bridge. The etiology of recession could not be immediately ascertained, although one could suspect that tension from the movable mucosa played a part as there was practically no attached gingiva present. In addition, oral hygiene was rendered difficult by the high buccal frenum attachment.

A free gingival graft halted the progress of recession. At the same time, the patient's home care regimen was modified to the vertical-rotatory method (modified Stillman). As a result, not only was the recession halted, the gingival margin spontaneously migrated coronally, a process known as "creeping attachment."

This type of creeping attachment after FGG is not the norm and can only be expected in favorable cases (Matter 1980; Dorfman et al. 1982).

685 Initial clinical situation
2 mm of gingival recession are observed on the buccal aspect of the crowned abutment tooth 34. The crown margin is clearly supragingival.

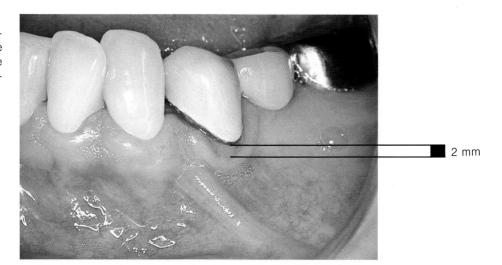

2 mm

686 1 month after free gingival grafting
The clinically visible exposed root surface is now only 1 mm wide.
A spontaneous coronal migration of the stabilized attached gingiva has occurred. The sulcus on the buccal surface of 34 is not deepened.

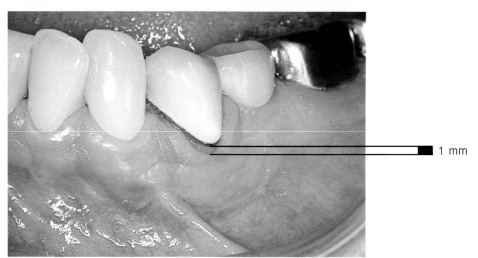

1 mm

687 2 years after free gingival grafting
The recession on tooth 34 has almost completely disappeared. Less than 0.5 mm of root surface is exposed on the facial surface.

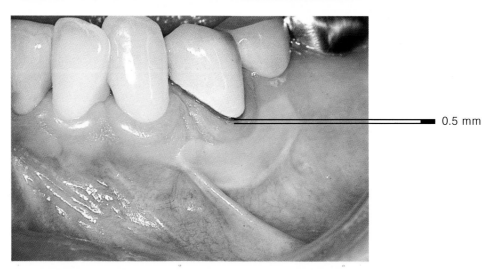

0.5 mm

Coronal Repositioning after FGG

Operative procedure for the 2-stage operation

This 26-year-old female complained of a pronounced, secondarily inflamed and esthetically disturbing area of recession on the facial aspect of tooth 41. The recession extended into the movable oral mucosa.

Home care was above average, but in the area of 41 oral hygiene was difficult. In the area of exposed root surface there was plaque, calculus and a resultant mild chronic gingivitis. Lip movement caused direct tension on the gingival margin at 41 (pumping effect?).

Although it was possible to *halt* the progress of recession by means of a FGG, the patient also wished to have the existing defect *covered*.

Findings after FGG:

HYG 88%	PBI 0.8
TM 0 except tooth 41 (TM = 1)	

No periodontal pockets were present. The Figures below depict clinical and radiographic findings.

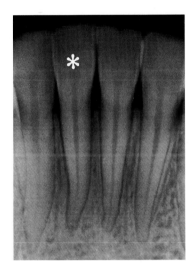 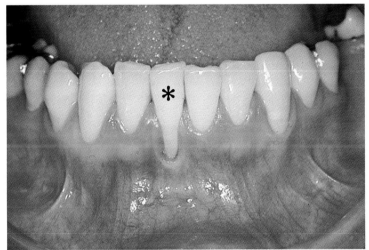

688 Initial clinical view
The entire mandible exhibits mild facial recession of 1–3 mm.

Pronounced 6 mm recession is clinically obvious on the facial surface of 41 (∗), extending to the movable oral mucosa and manifesting marginal inflammation. No periodontal pocketing was detected.

The radiograph does not reveal the facial dehiscence on tooth 41.

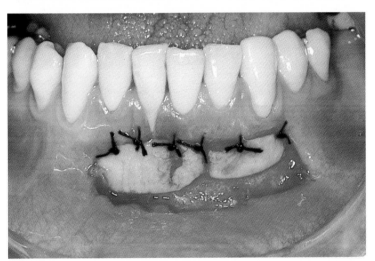

First procedure: FGG

689 Free gingival graft
Two small free gingival grafts have been sutured to place in the anterior area between 42 an 33. This would be expected to halt the recession.

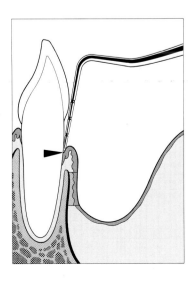 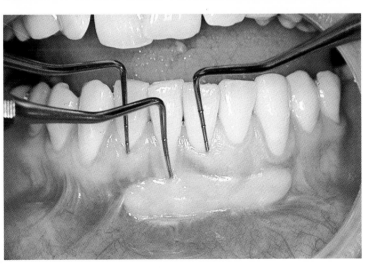

690 2 months after FGG
The clinical situation is one of freedom from inflammation and pockets, including the labial surface of 41 (arrow in diagram at base of sulcus).

It would be reasonable to wait 1–2 years for the possibility of creeping attachment. However, the patient demanded an immediate covering of the defect, which she found esthetically disfiguring.

Second surgical procedure: Coronal repositioning

691 Surgical plan – Incisions

1. *Marginal:* An arcuate incision is planned for the facial surface of 41. The "new papillae" are outlined by this initial incision.
2. *Vertical:* The horizontal incision is carried vertically over teeth 42 and 31.
3. *Gingivectomy:* Only the epithelium of the papillae coronal to the horizontal incision is excised to prepare a recipient bed (see Fig. 693 R).

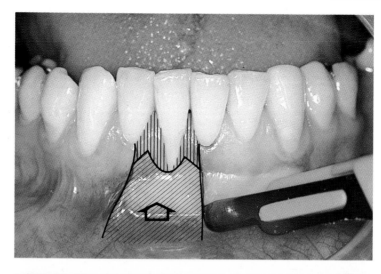

692 Incisions 1 + 2
– Horizontal incision: A scalloped incision outlines the shape of the future gingival margin.
– Vertical incisions bilaterally.

The schematic depicts the recession, the sulcus (arrow), the free gingival graft and the horizontal internal bevel incision at the cervix of the tooth.

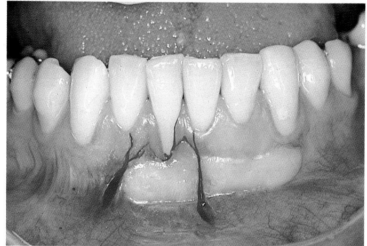
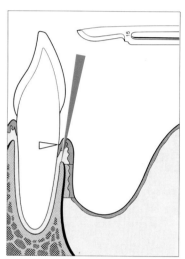

693 Creating a flap – Gingivectomy of the "old" papillae

After reflection of a mucoperiosteal flap, the facial epithelium of the adjacent papilla is excised almost vertically using a gingivectomy knife. This provides a connective tissue bed for the flap that will be repositioned coronally.

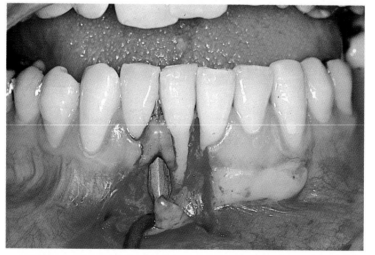
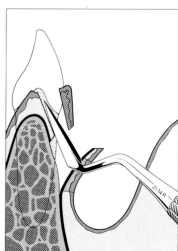

694 Root planing
After reflection of the soft tissue flap, it became clear that the facial dehiscence was more pronounced than the gingival recession.

Only the root surface exposed by the gingival recession is thoroughly cleaned and planed. Root surface exposed by flap reflection should not be treated, as the tissue can reattach to pre-existing healthy fibers.

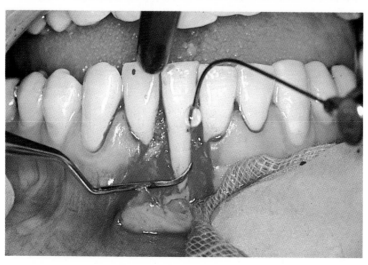

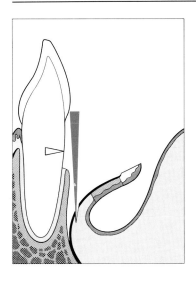

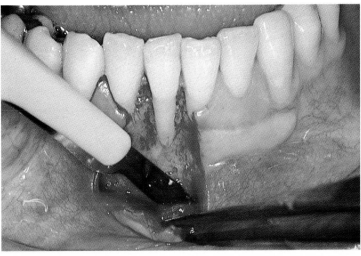

695 Severing the periosteum

At the base of the flap, in the area of the movable oral mucosa, the resilient periosteum is incised completely along the entire extent of the flap, using a No. 15 scalpel. This permits coronal repositioning of the flap without tension.

This incision must be made with care to avoid severing the supraperiosteal blood vessels or the flap itself.

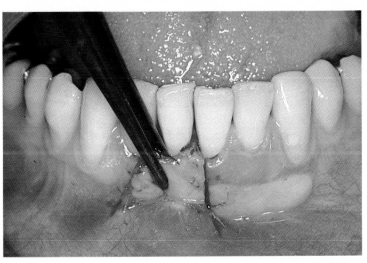

696 Coronal repositioning

The flap has been completely mobilized and can be positioned coronally without tension.

If tension exists, e. g., because the periosteal incision was incomplete, the flap may become necrotic and the recession will recur.

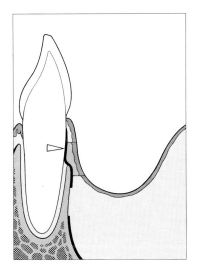

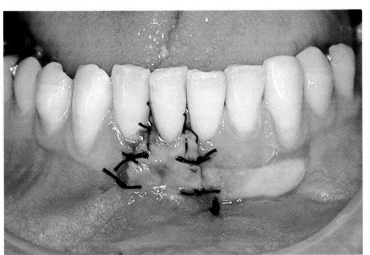

697 Immediately after surgery

The incisions described above have led to the creation of a new gingival margin and new papillae. After coronal repositioning of the flap, the new papillae lie directly upon the highly vascular recipient beds prepared by the gingivectomy procedure. The flap is held firmly in its new location by interrupted sutures.

The schematic shows the effect of severing the periosteum.

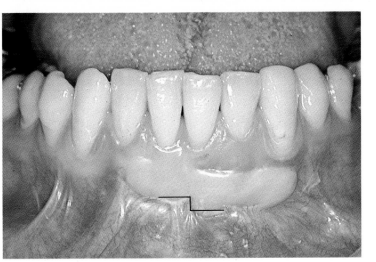

698 6 months after coronal repositioning

The denuded area on 41 is completely covered, and *no* pocket can be probed on the facial aspect. The step-like indentation in the free graft (line) demonstrates the degree of coronal displacement of the attached gingiva.

Coronal Repositioning after FGG

Summary

A localized area of recession was noted, extending into the mobile oral mucosa. Home care in the area was difficult and the gingival margin was inflamed. A free gingival graft was placed to halt the progress of recession. Nine weeks after graft placement, a second surgical procedure involving coronal repositioning of the grafted tissue was performed at the patient's request in an attempt to cover the root surface of 41. Four years later, no recurrence of the recession had occurred.

This degree of success is not always achieved by coronal flap repositioning. Recurrent recession of about 50% may be expected (Bernimoulin et al. 1975).

The labial plate of bone will not regenerate. Attachment of the gingiva to the root surface is probably via a long junctional epithelium.

699 Initial clinical view
The mandible exhibits mild generalized recession, while the labial root surface of tooth 41 is exposed by the pronounced 6 mm recession that extends beyond the mucogingival line. No attached gingiva remains in this region, nor is there any periodontal pocket (arrow in diagram depicts the base of the sulcus).

Plaque accumulation and the resultant inflammation are obvious in the area of deep recession. The rest of the dentition is well maintained by home care.

Before

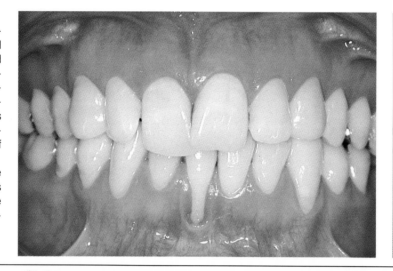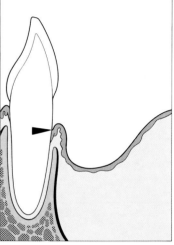

After

700 Four years after surgery
The 6 mm defect on tooth 41 that was covered by coronal flap repositioning (vertical red arrow in diagram) remains free of recurrence, and there is no periodontal pocket on the labial surface. The zone of attached gingiva in the area is 5 mm wide.

Recession on other teeth in the mandible has not become more pronounced.

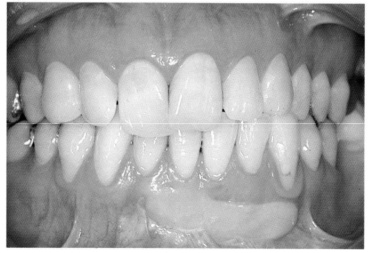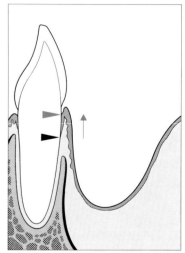

Periodontics – Endodontics

The relationship of the periodontium to the endodontium (pulp contents) is indeed an intimate one. These two anatomic entities are quite literally connected to each other at the apical foramen and via lateral canals. Thus, pulpal pathology may directly effect the periodontal tissues. On the other hand, advanced periodontitis or severe recession may occasion pulpal necrosis by way of the apex, lateral canals or the furcation.

In their comprehensive textbook, Guldener and Langeland (1982) proposed a *classification* of the reciprocal relationships between the periodontium and the endodontium:

Class I: Primarily endodontic problems
Class II: Primarily periodontal problems
Class III: Combined endodontic and periodontal problems.

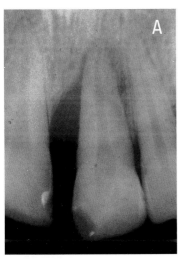 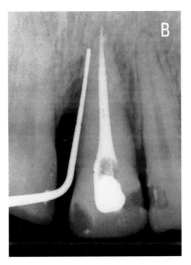 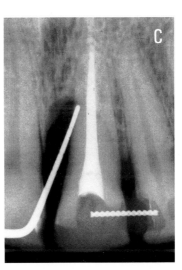

701 Endo / perio lesion, Class II b

A. The localized 11 mm periodontal pocket on the mesiopalatal aspect of tooth 21 has led to a retrograde pulpitis.

B. Following endodontic treatment, root planing in the area is performed after reflecting a flap. The tooth is "temporarily" splinted to the adjacent tooth.

C. 12 years later, new bone formation is observed on the radiograph. The "temporary" splint has now been in situ for 11 years.

Class I – Primarily endodontic problems

A *necrotic pulp* can elicit an acute or chronic lesion in the apical periodontal region. Endodontic treatment is generally sufficient to alleviate the periodontal problem if there is no concurrent periodontitis.

Class II – Primarily periodontal problems

a) If hemisectioning of a tooth is necessary for periodontal reasons, or if root planing for a deep pocket approaches the apical foramen, it may be necessary to devitalize the tooth.

b) *Pulpal necrosis* may result from a periodontal infection that approaches the apex of the tooth. Combined endodontic-periodontal treatment may be indicated (see Fig. 701).

Class III – Combined endo / perio problems

An apical lesion resulting from a necrotic pulp may develop simultaneously with a deep periodontal lesion. If the two expanding pathologic processes approach each other and fuse, the result is an inflammatory lesion extending from the gingival margin to the apex of the tooth.

Periodontal Healing
Reattachment – New Attachment

In recent years, the dental profession has moved away from the more radical treatment modalities (pocket elimination) in cases of periodontitis. The primary goals of therapy today are elimination of the etiology, and enhancement of healing in diseased tissues.

Numerous research studies performed during the last several years have provided answers to questions concerning whether or to what extent healing is possible in the form of reattachment or regeneration (cf. Schroeder 1983). The most basic classification of healing possibilities is:

1. Epithelial reattachment
2. Epithelial regeneration (new attachment)

---

3. Connective tissue reattachment
4. Connective tissue regeneration (new attachment).

702 Periodontal pocket (infrabony)

Original gingival margin

A. Before treatment
The blue horizontal lines represent the original location of
– Gingival margin
– Base of the pocket
– Intact periodontium.

The inflammatory infiltrate (INF) extends apically beyond the last vestiges of the intact junctional epithelium, to the bony crest.

Original base of the pocket

Level of intact periodontal ligament

B. Pocket therapy
Healing (red arrows, right) ensues subsequent to root planing and curettage:
– Rapidly from the epithelium
– Somewhat slower from the gingival connective tissue
– Very slowly from the bone
– Extremely slowly in terms of new cementum.

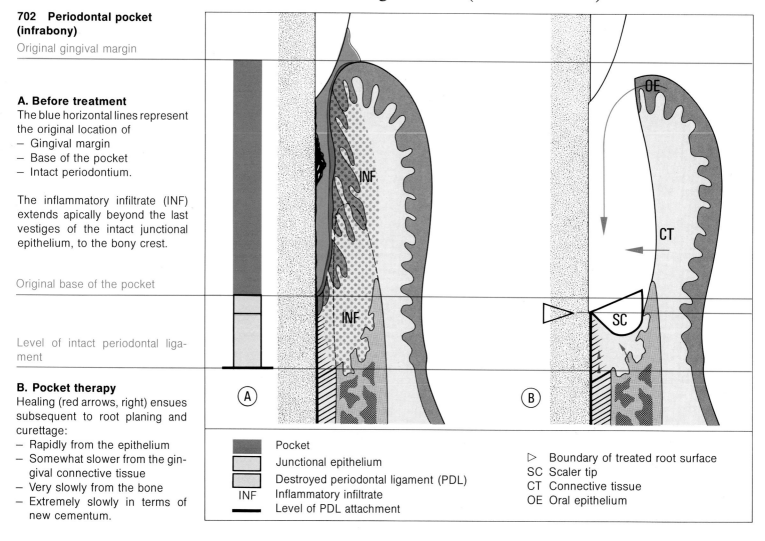

Pocket
Junctional epithelium
Destroyed periodontal ligament (PDL)
INF Inflammatory infiltrate
Level of PDL attachment

▷ Boundary of treated root surface
SC Scaler tip
CT Connective tissue
OE Oral epithelium

Epithelium

1. *Reattachment of diseased epithelium is impossible.* During periodontal therapy, all pocket epithelium is removed (curettage).

2. *Epithelial regeneration* ("new attachment," de novo formation) occurs after many types of periodontal treatment. The new epithelium is generated from the surrounding oral epithelium. Daughter cells resulting from mitotic activity quickly cover the connective tissue wound surface and develop into a new long junctional epithelium with a basal lamina and hemidesmosomes along the root surface (Listgarten 1976a, b). The new epithelium generally covers the entire length of the treated pocket; this may explain why some investigators have observed new epithelial tissue *apical* to new bone that has formed (Caton & Nyman 1980; Stahl et al. 1982, 1983; Magnusson et al. 1983).

Connective tissue

3. *Connective tissue reattachment* may be expected only in the most apical regions (infiltrated but *not infected*) subjacent to the junctional epithelium, where no mechanical treatment (root planing) has been per-

formed. It is in these areas that remnants of periodontal ligament fibers and intact root cementum remain (see 3 in Figs. C & D, below; Listgarten & Rosenberg 1979; Nyman et al. 1982).

4. *Connective tissue regeneration* (new attachment): Formation of new cementum with insertion of newly generated connective tissue fiber bundles may be expected only in the deeper areas of the treated periodontal pocket, if at all (see 3B in Fig. D).
Connective tissue accumulating postsurgically parallel to the root surface but not inserting into new cementum probably derives from gingival fibroblasts and not from periodontal ligament cells (see 3A in Fig. D, below; Caton et al. 1980).
Whether or not acid conditioning of the root surface can enhance true connective tissue attachment remains under study (Ririe et al. 1980; Cole 1981; Polson & Proye 1983; Stahl et al. 1983).

Alveolar bone

Radiographically detectable formation of new bone and reduction of clinical probing depth are possible, but this is not proof of true periodontal regeneration (Listgarten 1980).

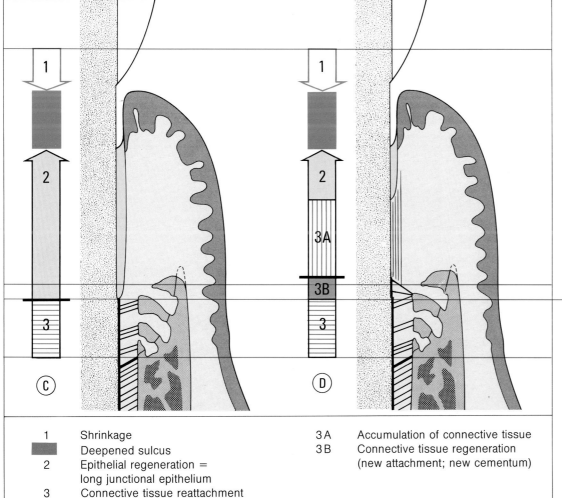

703 Types of healing
Healing can occur by generation of a new junctional epithelium (2), by connective tissue accumulation (3A), connective tissue regeneration (*new attachment,* 3B), and connective tissue *reattachment* (3).

C. Long junctional epithelium
During the healing process the tissues shrink (1), cells of the oral epithelium grow out, contact the tooth surface and develop into a new junctional epithelium (2). This new JE continues apically until the first connective tissue fibers embedded in cementum are encountered (3).

Boundary of treated root surface

D. Connective tissue accumulation, periodontal regeneration
In coronal areas, healing occurs as described under C. Apical to the new junctional epithelium (2), collagen fibers accumulate parallel to the root surface (3A). Only seldom does *new* cementum form with insertion of collagen fiber bundles (3B). In the most apical region of the treated area, reattachment of residual fibers may occur (3).

1	Shrinkage	3A	Accumulation of connective tissue
	Deepened sulcus	3B	Connective tissue regeneration
2	Epithelial regeneration =		(new attachment; new cementum)
	long junctional epithelium		
3	Connective tissue reattachment		

Negative Results of Treatment

Periodontal therapy such as root planing, curettage, and surgical procedures may be accompanied by unpleasant side effects, some of which are unavoidable. Among these are:

- Hypersensitivity of exposed root surfaces
- Poor esthetics (maxillary anterior area)
- Phonetic difficulties.

The patient must be warned of these possible consequences before initiation of periodontal therapy.

Sensitive teeth may be treated by means of desensitizing solutions and dentifrices. In refractory cases, the dentist may attempt electrosurgical fulguration, or place cervical restorations, or – in extreme situations – the teeth can be devitalized (pulp extirpation). Problems of *esthetics* and *phonetics* may be successfully treated by fabrication of a customized gingival mask ("party gums"). Full cast crowns may alleviate the situation in some cases; however, the latter procedure may only exacerbate the poor esthetics, as crown margins may be exposed supragingivally.

Successful periodontal therapy

704 Exposure of the CEJ and coronal root surface ("long teeth")
This 32-year-old female exhibited periodontal recession prior to the surgical procedure, and esthetics became worse still after periodontal surgery. After treatment, the chief complaints were poor esthetics and phonetic difficulties.

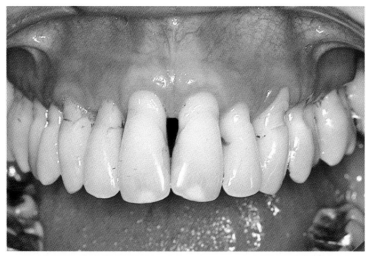

705 Gingival mask
A customized impression tray is used to obtain a precise model of the anterior maxillary segment, including the attached gingiva to the mucogingival line. The gingival mask is fabricated on the model, finished to a knife edge just short of the mucogingival line. Retention is achieved by extension of the acrylic into interdental areas.

Denture base acrylic in various shades and textures can be used to blend the gingival mask perfectly with the patient's own tissues.

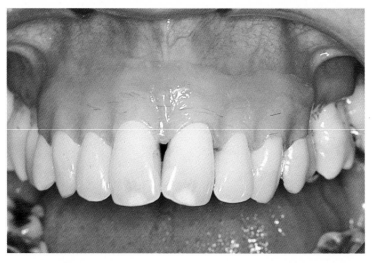

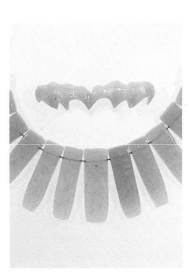

706 Improved esthetics with the gingival mask in situ
The gingival mask may provide a significant esthetic improvement, especially for patients with a high smile line, who expose maxillary anterior teeth and gingiva when speaking or laughing.
  A prerequisite for this kind of therapy is excellent home care.

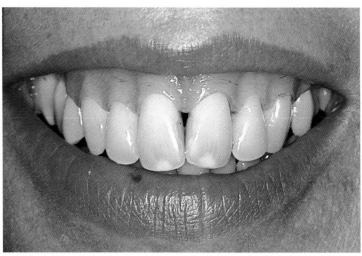

Medicaments

Medicaments are frequently used before, during and after periodontal therapy. The specific mechanisms of action, side effects, indications and contraindications as well as possible interactions of such medicaments must be understood by the dentist. The spectrum of activity of such medicaments permits their classification into four groups:

1. Gingivitis/periodontitis treatment (topical, systemic)
2. Wound treatment (analgesic, anti-inflammatory)
3. Antibiotic coverage
4. Physician-prescribed medicines for various systemic disorders.

1. Medicaments for Treatment of Gingivitis and Periodontitis

There exist today no medicaments or vaccines that are effective over the long term for prevention or treatment of gingivitis and periodontitis. One may differentiate between medicaments for topical application and those for systemic administration to support local (mechanical) therapy (see Table, pp. 264–265).

Most of the agents available to the dentist may be regarded as *"causal therapy"* directed generally against the microorganisms of supra- and subgingival plaque and their accumulation on tooth and mucosal surfaces, or targeted toward specific pathogenic flora.

The *symptoms* of disease, such as acute inflammation, are approached primarily with topical agents.

In periodontics medicaments are used:

- For treatment of acute conditions
- For pre-treatment and post-treatment in conjunction with the mechanical therapy
- For support of mechanical treatment of juvenile periodontitis (LJP) and rapidly progressive periodontitis (RPP)
- For treatment of symptoms that develop after periodontal therapy, e.g., hypersensitive teeth.

Therapy for acute conditions

Acute infections, especially Gingivoperiodontitis ulcerosa (ANUG), may be treated in the initial stages by means of *topically* applied ointments containing *antibiotics* and *corticosteroids,* sometimes mixed with an adhesive salve such as Orabase. Disinfectant and cleansing rinses may also be employed (see Table, p. 264).

Medicinal treatments before and after local (mechanical) periodontitis therapy

In cases of simple gingivitis and slowly progressive adult periodontitis (AP), local mechanical therapy is generally the only treatment required.

Topically applied rinsing solutions that inhibit plaque (*chlorhexidine, hexetidine, H_2O_2*) may be prescribed as adjunctive therapy for short-term use. These rinses are indicated before and after hemorrhage-inducing procedures (curettage, flap surgery) to reduce the quantitative microbial counts in the oral cavity. Such rinsing solutions are not intended for long-term use over months or years.

Systemic administration of antibiotics is *not* indicated for treatment of adult periodontitis (AP), except in patients with a history of focal infection.

(text continued on p. 266)

Medicament (Concentration)	Effect Indication (Ind.)	Side effects Contraindication (Contr.)
Chlorhexidine (CHX)	inhibits plaque formation	reversible staining of teeth and tongue influences taste sensation desquamation of mucosa and disturbance of wound healing with excessive CHX concentration

Medicament (Concentration)	Effect Indication (Ind.)	Side effects Contraindication (Contr.)
– **CHX digluconate** mouthwash (p. 119), 0.1–0.2% Products: – **Corsodyl** 0.2% *(ICI)* – **Chlorhexamed** 0.1% *(Blend-a-med)* – **Plak-Out** concentrate *(Hawe)*	*Ind.:* adjunct to mechanical plaque control before and after periodontal surgery initial therapy for ANUG	*Contr.:* exposed bone long-term use
– **CHX dihydrochloride** powder (p. 120) Product: – pure substance, 100% *(ICI)*	*Ind.:* use under periodontal dressing	*Contr.:* exposed bone

Medicament (Concentration)	Effect Indication (Ind.)	Side effects Contraindication (Contr.)
Hexetidine	plaque inhibition (less effective than CHX, but research shows it to be extremely effective when used in combination with ZnF_2)	slight, reversible staining mild influence on taste sensitivity
Product: – **Hextril** *(Warner-Chilcott)* 0.1% rinsing solution	*Ind.:* instead of CHX (e.g., in USA where CHX not available!)	*Contr.:* –

Medicament (Concentration)	Effect Indication (Ind.)	Side effects Contraindication (Contr.)
Hydrogen peroxide (H_2O_2) *Products:* – 3–10% solution for topical application – 0.3–0.5% rinsing solution	cleansing and disinfection some plaque inhibition	tissue damage with long-term use? "emphysema" if applied under pressure (syringe)
	Ind.: wound clean-up perio pocket rinsing initial therapy for ANUG	*Contr.:* –
Sodium perborate in a combined preparation Products: – **Amosan** *(Cooper),* – **Kavosan** *(Cooper)* sodium perborate, sodium bitartrate, menthol, powder for making rinsing solution	analgesic	tissue damage with long-term use?
	Ind.: for home use by patient initial therapy for ANUG	*Contr.:* –
Sodium bicarbonate concentrate ($NaHCO_3$) Product: – paste made from powder, H_2O_2 and water	some disinfectant and plaque inhibitory action possibly bactericidal (hypotonic)	none known
	Ind.: "Keyes technique" (1978) as a dentifrice in gingivitis and periodontitis	*Contr.:* effectiveness?

Medicament (Concentration)	Effect Indication (Ind.)	Side effects Contraindication (Contr.)
Tetracycline (ointment)	antibacterial bacteriostatic	hypersensitivity reaction
Products: – **Achromycin ophthalmic ointment** *(Lederle)* (1% tetracycline-HCl) – **Aureomycin ointment** *(Lederle)* (chlortetracycline-HCl, 1% or 3%)	*Ind.:* acute pocket exacerbation under periodontal dressing in combination with an adherent salve (e.g., Oratran, Orabase) to cover apthae or infected ulcerations	*Contr.:* ANUG lesions (necrosis, gram-negative anaerobes!)

Medicament (Concentration)	Effect Indication (Ind.)	Side effects Contraindication (Contr.)
Corticosteroids in combination with antibiotics (ointments) (formula: prednisone)	anti-inflammatory analgesic (antibacterial)	none known
Products: – **Terracortril** with tetracycline-HCl *(Pfizer)* – **Locacorten** with neomycin *(Ciba)* – **Dontisolon** with neomycin *(Hoechst); and others*	*Ind.:* initial therapy for ANUG acute, painful lesions of gingiva and mucosa	*Contr.:* acute infections (inflammation) that do not heal within a few days (mycotic, luetic, tuberculous or viral lesions)

Periodontitis Therapy – Medicaments for Systemic Adjunctive Treatment

Side effects Contraindications (Contr.)	Effect Indication (Ind.)	Medicament (Dosage: Number × tablets × days)
sensitivity to light hypersensitivity reactions	effective against *gram-positive* and *-negative* organisms, incl. Actinobacillus actinomycetemcomitans (Aa)! (broad spectrum antibiotic) bacteriostatic	**Tetracycline** (tablets, capsules)
Contr.: severe liver or kidney disfunction (acidosis) *relative Contr.:* children to age 8 pregnancy	*Ind.:* adjunct to local mechanical treatment in *juvenile periodontitis* **(LJP)**	Products: – **Hostacyclin 500** *(Hoechst,* 500 mg tetracycline-HCl) 2 x 1 x 8 to 2 x 1 x 14 – **Ledermycin** *(Lederle,* 300 mg demethylchlortetracycline) 2 x 1 x 8 to 2 x 1 x 14 – **Vibramycin** *(Pfizer,* 100 mg doxycyclin) 2 x 1 x 8 to 2 x 1 x 14
gastrointestinal disturbance including nausea, vomiting, diarrhea allergy (rare) *Contr.:* none known	effective against *gram-positive* (and *-negative*) organisms bactericidal *Ind.:* adjunctive to local mechanical therapy in *rapidly progressive periodontitis* **(RPP)** and possibly during *active, suppurating phases of adult periodontitis* **(AP)**	**Spiramycine** (tablets) Product: – **Rovamycine 500** *(Specia,* 500 mg spiramycine) 3 x 1 x 8 to 4 x 1 x 10
digestive disturbance nausea reversible leukopenia	especially effective against *gram-negative anaerobes* such as Bacteroides, Fusobacteria, Spirochetes and Protozoa bactericidal	**Metronidazole** (tablets) Product: – **Flagyl** *(Specia,* 250 mg metronidazole) 3 x 1 x 8 to 4 x 1 x 14
Contr.: CNS disorders blood dyscrasias 1st trimester of pregnancy (alcohol intolerance) *interaction with hydantoin!*	*Ind.:* adjunctive to local mechanical therapy in rapidly progressive periodontitis **(RPP)** and possibly in ulcerative periodontitis **(ANUG)** (in combination with *penicillin* (p. 266), for protection against osteomyelitis etc.)	**Ornidazole** (tablets) Product: – **Tiberal** *(Roche,* 500 mg ornidazole) 2 x 1 x 8 to 2 x 1 x 14
nausea, vomiting disgestive disturbances diarrhea allergic reaction (rare)	effective against *gram-positive* and *-negative aerobes* such as Staphylococci and Streptococci, and against *gram-negative anaerobes* such as Bacteroides, Spirochetes etc. bactericidal	**Combined preparations:** **Antibiotic & chemotherapeutic** (tablets) Product: – **Rodogyl** *(Specia,* 250 mg spiramycine plus 125 mg metronidazole) 4 x 1 x 8 to 6 x 1 x 10
Contr.: neurologic disorders hematopoietic disturbances *(alcohol intolerance)*	*Ind.:* adjunctive to mechanical therapy in *progressive* **(RPP)** and *juvenile* **(LJP)** periodontitis (also indicated for presurgical antibiotic coverage)	

Treatment of juvenile and rapidly progressive periodontitis

Systemic therapy for these relatively rare periodontal diseases is possible because research has clarified the nature of the bacterial infection. Today, aggressive LJP and RPP lesions are treated by local therapy but also systemically with *tetracycline* (LJP) and *metronidazole* or *ornidazole* (RPP). Administration of these drugs is generally over an 8–14 day course, simultaneous with initial therapy. A second course of drug therapy may be instituted during the surgical procedures or several months later, for example at the first recall. *Caution:* Side effects, contraindications (see Table, p. 265).

Treatment of problems resulting from therapy

One unpleasant consequence of local therapy for periodontitis is sensitivity of exposed root surfaces.

There are numerous commercial products for treatment of this condition; most are protein-denaturing astringents. Dentifrices are also available containing strontium chloride (Sensodyne) or formalin (Emoform). However, it is often months or years before the condition can be controlled to the patient's satisfaction.

If hypersensitivity is severe, superficial fulguration may be attempted, or the tooth can be devitalized and treated endodontically.

2. Prevention of Pain and Swelling – Wound Treatment

The surgical procedure most often employed is the conservative modified Widman procedure, which is relatively atraumatic and requires neither preoperative nor postoperative systemic medications.

If surgery is more complex, a pain medication may be required, such as *paracetamol* (Seymour 1983) or Tylenol no. 3.

For prevention of postoperative edema, medicaments from the *antiphlogistic* and *antirheumatic* categories may be administered immediately prior to surgery and for several days thereafter. Examples include *Motrin 400, Ponstan 500, Voltaren 50* etc.

A periodontal dressing or cyanoacrylate tissue adhesive may be indicated (see Periodontal Surgery, p. 162).

3. Antibiotic Coverage

Bacteremia is a universal consequence of any dental procedure that results in hemorrhage. Such a transient bacteremia is usually of no consequence for a healthy patient, but some patients with specific systemic disorders require premedication. Every patient who has ever had *endocarditis* or *acute polyarthritis* must be covered, as must patients who have undergone *allogenic organ transplant, joint replacement, heart valve replacement* etc. The American Heart Association recommends penicillin p.o. as first drug of choice. If this is not

tolerated, *erythromycin* is substituted, also p.o. The third possibility is *Vancomycin* administered intramuscularly.

Because Bacteroides species (RPP) and Actinobacillus actinomycetemcomitans (LJP) may play a role in endocarditis, several recent publications have advocated a combination of penicillin derivatives and metronidazole (for treatment of RPP) or tetracycline (for LJP) to ensure adequate antibiotic coverage of patients at risk (Mühlemann 1983; Slots et al. 1983).

4. Systemic Medications

Many patients requiring periodontal surgery will already be taking one or more drugs. Drugs of particular concern include anticoagulants, antihypertensives, digitalis, hormones, phenytoin, psychotrophics, immunosuppressants (cortisone, azathioprine, cyclosporine-A) and cystostatics.

Periodontitis therapy for the patient with a systemic disorder may have to include some compromises. In some cases, the only recourse is to provide exclusively palliative treatment. If the patient can be treated normally, the course of periodontal therapy should be performed in coordination with the patient's physician.

Maintenance Therapy – Recall

The long-term success of periodontal therapy depends less upon the manner in which the case was treated than on how well the cases is "maintained" in subsequent recall. Many clinical investigators have demonstrated clearly that different treatment methods for periodontitis all lead to essentially the same good result if the postoperative recall interval does not exceed 3 months (Rosling et al. 1976b; Nyman et al. 1977; Knowles et al. 1979; Ramfjord et al. 1982). Research by Axelsson and Lindhe (1981a) showed dramatically the effects of preventive measures performed during recall (Fig. 709). The study revealed that regular and short-interval (2–3 months) prophylaxis by the dental hygienist leads to *freedom from caries and attachment loss*. This 6-year study casts some serious doubts about "classical" reparative dentistry.

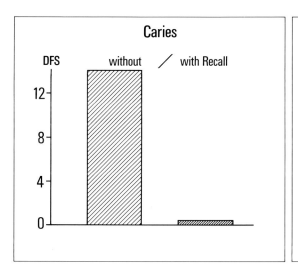

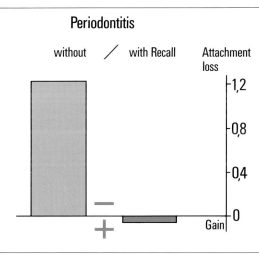

709 Caries and attachment loss with and without recall (Axelsson study)
Patients who received neither home care motivation nor dental prophylaxis at "one visit to the dentist per year" exhibited 14 new carious lesions and progressive attachment loss over a 6-year period.

Similar patients who received professional dental prophylaxis every 2–3 months developed essentially no new carious lesions and actually exhibited a slight attachment gain.

The primary goals of maintenance therapy are:

– Prevention of new infections
  (gingivitis, periodontitis)
– Prevention of re-infection of inactive residual pockets (periodontitis)
– Prevention of dental caries
– Maintenance of optimal chewing function.

These goals can be achieved through:

– Re-examination and re-evaluation
– Re-motivation of the patient
– Re-instruction in home care procedures
– Professional plaque and calculus removal, especially in those areas exhibiting signs of renewed disease activity (bleeding on probing).

Recall Organization – Recall Effect

The introduction of a recall system into the dental practice demands a special organization that can only be accomplished with auxiliary personnel, especially the dental hygienist.

A conventional or a computerized system for timely recall of each patient is a must. However, each practitioner must realize that the perfect recall interval will not be possible for all patients. Some patients will not accept the recommended recall schedule, preferring to make their own appointments at an interval of their own choosing. One factor that may play a role in such choice is proximity of the patient to the dental office. A factor of concern to the dentist is that with a growing number of recall patients there will be less and less time for accepting new patients and performing initial therapy.

With initiation of a comprehensive recall system, the practice gradually makes a transition from *reparative dentistry to preventive dental medicine*. Such a transition is a laudable goal, but it is achieved by too few preventive-minded practitioners.

Both private and governmental medical/dental insurance programs must come to accept that preventive measures are more meaningful and, in the long run, more cost effective than reparative dentistry.

It is eminently wiser for a third party payor to cover the cost of prevention than to repeatedly pay out large sums for treatment of disease that could have been prevented. Indeed, it may be prudent and justifiable for preventive services to take precedence over restorative measures.

A recall interval may vary between 2–12 months depending on severity of the case, degree of motivation and manual dexterity of the patient, as well as the capacity of the dental practice team.

The challenge presented by a regular recall system and a preventive approach to dentistry is not yet accepted in all western countries. Even some university dental schools include preventive dentistry only peripherally in the curriculum, and periodontology is not an individual department in some European schools as yet. The capacity for training dental auxiliary personnel such as dental hygienists is completely lacking in some universities, and too small in others.

Certain clinical data must be gathered at every recall appointment, before professional prophylaxis is performed and before any required follow-up therapy. Other kinds of data need to be re-evaluated at longer intervals.

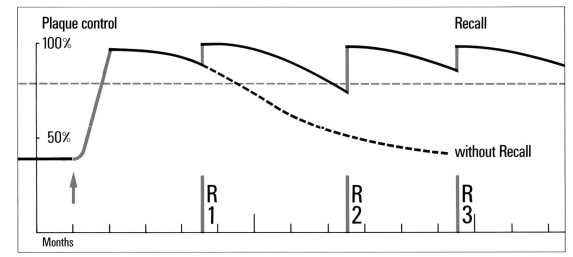

710 Recall effect
Initial therapy (blue line) enhanced by surgical intervention (red line) leads to healthy periodontal tissues if plaque control is optimal. If the patient is left on his own, the original suboptimal condition will be quickly achieved (dashed black line).

With regular re-motivation and professional prophylaxis at recall appointments (R 1, R 2, R 3 etc.), the successes achieved by initial therapy and/or surgery can be maintained for years.

Data gathering

- *At each recall appointment* (e.g., every 3–4 months):
  - Gingival condition (PBI, bleeding on probing)
  - Plaque accumulation (HYG, disclosing agent).
- *In addition, every 6–12 months:*
  - Probing depths
  - Activity of residual pockets (exudate, pus; possible microbiologic evaluation)
  - Occlusion, reconstructions, caries.
- *In addition, every 2–4 years:*
  - Complete radiographic survey, vitality testing.

Procedures

Depending on the findings at data gathering, the following procedures may be necessary:
- *At every recall appointment:*
  - Re-motivation of the patient
  - Repeated OH instruction, and correction of brushing and interdental cleaning procedures
  - Plaque and calculus removal.
- *At longer intervals:*
  - Treatment of recurrence (root planing, curettage, flap procedure)
  - Restorative work as necessary.

Recall – Auxiliary Personnel

Highly qualified auxiliary personnel such as the dental hygienist and certified dental assistants actually *replace* the dentist at chairside in many procedures such as data gathering, prophylaxis, and maintenance therapy.

A fulltime dental hygienist can care for the needs of over 500 periodontal recall patients per year, calculated at 1 hour per visit and 3–4 visits per year. Such care is, of course, performed under the supervision and control of the dentist. The evaluation and supplementation of data gathered by the dental hygienist, as well as checking work performed by the DH, remains the domain of the dentist or periodontist.

In addition to the duties in patient care, the dental hygienist can also take care of the organization of the recall system. In "emergency" situations, the DH can also perform all the functions of a dental assistant.

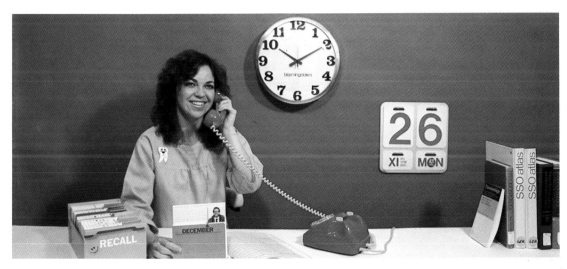

711 Patient recall
The recall interval for periodontitis patients will vary individually from 2–12 months, depending on the diagnosis, the patient's degree of motivation and manual dexterity, as well as the extent of original attachment loss. In general, a 3-4 month recall interval is satisfactory for maintenance of results achieved by initial therapy and surgery.

The recall interval is determined in the dental office; only seldom can it be left to the patient's discretion.

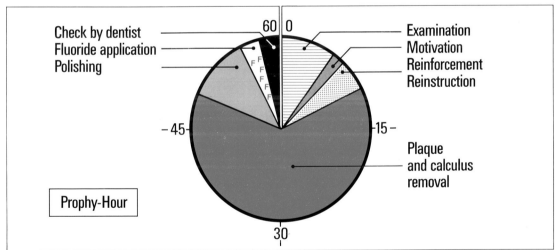

712 The "Prophy Hour"
The standard length of a recall appointment is one hour. This diagram depicts the work to be accomplished by the dentist (black) and the dental hygienist (blue) during the hour, and the time required by each task.

For removal of plaque and calculus, about 40 minutes are allocated. If the patient is fully dentulous, that means less than 2 minutes per tooth! Generally, teeth with symptoms of active periontal disease (bleeding) require more time (scaling).

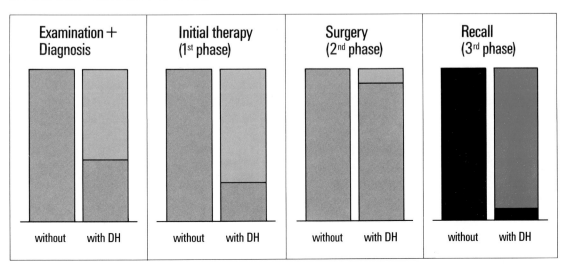

713 Relief of the dentist (black) by the hygienist (blue)
The hygienist is responsible for about 90% of the recall hour. Also, more than half of the time required for information gathering and initial therapy can be assumed by the hygienist. Even during the surgical treatment phase the DH can assume some of the tasks, e.g., debridement, wound cleansing and dressing removal.

Successful periodontal therapy

- Elimination of inflammation (gingival bleeding)
- Elimination of pocket activity
- Reduction of pocket depths
- Attachment loss halted
- Tooth mobility stabilized or reduced.

Failure of periodontal therapy

- Persistent bleeding
- Persistent pocket activity
- Increasing pocket depths
- Advancing attachment loss
- Increasing tooth mobility.

Most failures in the treatment of periodontitis can be explained. The most common causes of failure include: Incorrect local and systemic medical history, incorrect diagnosis and prognosis, incorrect treatment plan, inadequately performed therapy, *insufficient patient cooperation, and lack of maintenance.*

714 Rapidly progressive periodontitis (RPP) with advanced destruction
When this patient presented, she had never been instructed in oral hygiene methods. This 38-year-old woman just wanted a check-up; she had no complaints!

Clinical evaluation revealed pockets to 8 mm, some of which exhibited signs of activity. HYG = 0; PBI = 3.8.

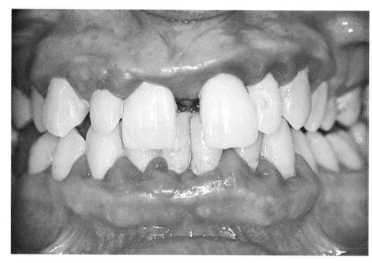
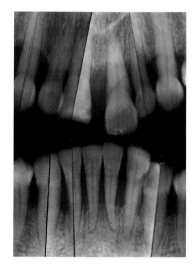

715 After initial therapy
The clinical picture is significantly improved after thorough scaling, root planing and soft tissue curettage. The patient's cooperation in home care was inadequate from the beginning. Because of this, no surgical procedures were performed. Shortly after initial therapy, plaque and calculus accumulations occurred in the mandibular anterior area. The patient refused to go on regular maintenance recall.

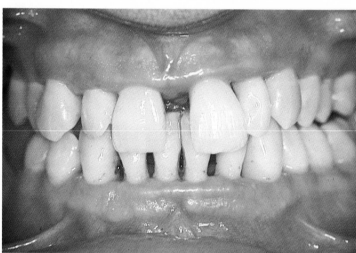

716 5 years later, without recall
The patient presented again after teeth 22, 23, 32 and 42 had exfoliated spontaneously. The dentist elected not to begin periodontal treatment again.

The new treatment plan included a complete denture in the maxilla and a partial denture in the mandible, maintaining the four bicuspids as abutments.

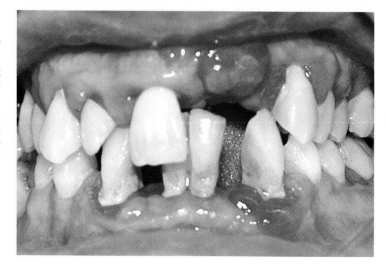
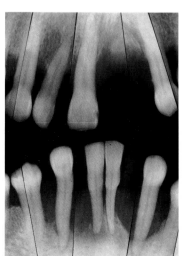

Function – Occlusal Therapy

The masticatory system is composed of the jaws, the temporomandibular joints, the muscles of mastication, the nervous system, the teeth with their occlusal complex, and the periodontal tissues. The various parts of the system are physiologically and morphologically synchronized when function is normal, but if any disturbance, alteration or disease in any *one* of the component parts of the masticatory system occurs, one or more of the other components may also be affected. On the other hand, within the limits of physiological tolerance the masticatory system has the capacity to deviate from the norm and adapt to or compensate for disturbance(s). This chapter will present:

- Causes and types of functional disturbances
- Functional analyses
- Consequences of functional disturbances, occlusal periodontal trauma
- Boundaries of mandibular movement
- Treatment of functional disturbances by selective grinding and bite guards.

Causes and Types of Functional Disturbances

General causes

– *Psychic stress* that may lead to neuromuscular tension in the masticatory muscles.

Oral causes

– *Premature occlusal contacts* in retruded centric, also known as centric relation (CR), and/or in maximal intercuspation, also known as habitual closure or centric occlusion (CO).
– *Interferences* during lateral excursion of the mandible, both on the working side and on the balancing side, as well as during protrusive movement.
– *Loss of vertical dimension* resulting from lost teeth or severe occlusal attrition. This can lead to premature contacts, lateral interferences, or to increased neuromuscular tone.

Parafunction, bruxism

– In occlusal parafunction, *unphysiologic loading time* combined with *elevated loading pressure* have a traumatic effect on the periodontium. In clenchers (usually daytime) and bruxers (usually at night), the teeth and the periodontium are unphysiologically loaded for longer periods of time than by normal swallowing and chewing.

Other types of functional disturbances

– Loading of teeth in an *unphysiologic direction,* for example when a tooth has drifted or tipped
– *Hypofunction,* as observed in unilateral chewers
– *Afunction,* when antagonists are missing.

The various types of functional disturbances may also occur in combination.

Functional Analysis

The cause and type of functional disturbance are determined *in the patient's mouth* by performing a functional analysis. The following examinations should be performed on every patient with periodontitis, as well as on patients complaining of TMJ discomfort and neuromuscular disturbances:
– Examination for signs of occlusal abrasion (parafunction)
– Consideration of tooth mobility in relation to bone loss and occlusal trauma
– Determination of premature contacts in centric relation (CR) and centric occlusion (CO)

– Determination of lateral interferences
– Neuromuscular findings (pressure sensitivity at muscle attachment areas)
– TMJ evaluation.

In difficult cases, bite registration and *evaluation of mounted study models* may enhance the clinical findings.

Thorough descriptions of various functional analyses are available in the dental literature (Ramfjord & Ash 1981, 1983; Bauer & Gutowski 1975).

Consequences of Functional Disturbances

Functional disturbances, especially bruxism, can result in a wide range of symptoms that may manifest in damage to one or several components of the functional system:
– *Occlusal surface* (excessive attrition)
– *Neuromuscular system* (neuralgiform pain, muscle spasm, muscle pain)

– *TMJ* (discopathies, abnormal joint mobility, asymmetric mandibular movements resulting from "interferences" in the joint, popping, friction, pain and swelling
– *Periodontium* (increased tooth mobility, *occlusal trauma*). For the periodontist, occlusal trauma may be of special importance.

Occlusal Periodontal Trauma

The significance of *occlusal trauma* in the initiation of periodontitis was a source of controversy for decades. Today, we know from experimental studies that abnormal occlusal forces can elicit neither gingivitis nor periodontitis. However, the progression of an already present (active) periodontitis may be accelerated (Svanberg & Lindhe 1974; Polson et al. 1976 a, b; Lindhe & Ericsson 1982).

Definition: Occlusal trauma is defined as "a microscopic alteration of the structures adjoining the periodontal ligament that manifests clinically as a (reversible) elevation of tooth mobility" (Mühlemann et al. 1956; Mühlemann & Herzog 1961).

The histologic changes include circulatory disturbances, edema and hyalinization of periodontal ligament fibers, mild inflammatory infiltrate, and nuclear pyknosis of osteoblasts, cementoblasts and fibroblasts (Svanberg & Lindhe 1974). The periodontal ligament space *adapts* by becoming wider, and assumes an hour-glass shape.

There are *no* histologic changes in the supracrestal (gingival) collagen fibers nor in the junctional epithelium.

The histologic alterations in the periodontium are completely *reversible* if the cause of the trauma is eliminated. Tooth mobility also returns to normal when the etiology is removed.

Adaptation to unphysiologic loading:
If occlusal trauma persists over a long period of time, the tissues of the periodontium may *adapt* to the insult, even without any treatment. The periodontal ligament space remains widened, but its histological structure is normal in appearance. Tooth mobility remains *elevated, but does not increase.*

Progressive tooth mobility from unphysiologic loading:
If abnormal occlusal forces are heavy and *persistent,* tooth mobility may continue to increase. Therapeutic elimination of the cause of the trauma may be possible by selective occlusal grinding, inserting a bite guard, splinting of teeth (stabilization), or reconstruction (e.g., bridgework).

Idealized Mandibular Border Movements

Man's two temporomandibular joints permit three-dimensional mandibular movements. The *boundaries* of these movements, recorded by an incisal reference point between the two mandibular central incisors, are represented by the so-called Posselt figure (Posselt 1952). These border movements are usually diagrammed in their ideal form (Figs. 717–719). However, large individual differences exist, especially in the occlusal relationships when mandibular teeth come into contact with and intercuspate with their maxillary antagonists

(Figs. 724–726). Mandibular border movements may also be altered or limited by dental, skeletal or TMJ anomalies, but functional disturbances (muscle spasm) are most commonly involved.

Minimum physiologic opening of the mandible is generally accepted as 40 mm (2 fingers wide), while protrusive and lateral movements are 5 mm. Many patients, however, exhibit excursive movements that are considerably larger than these means.

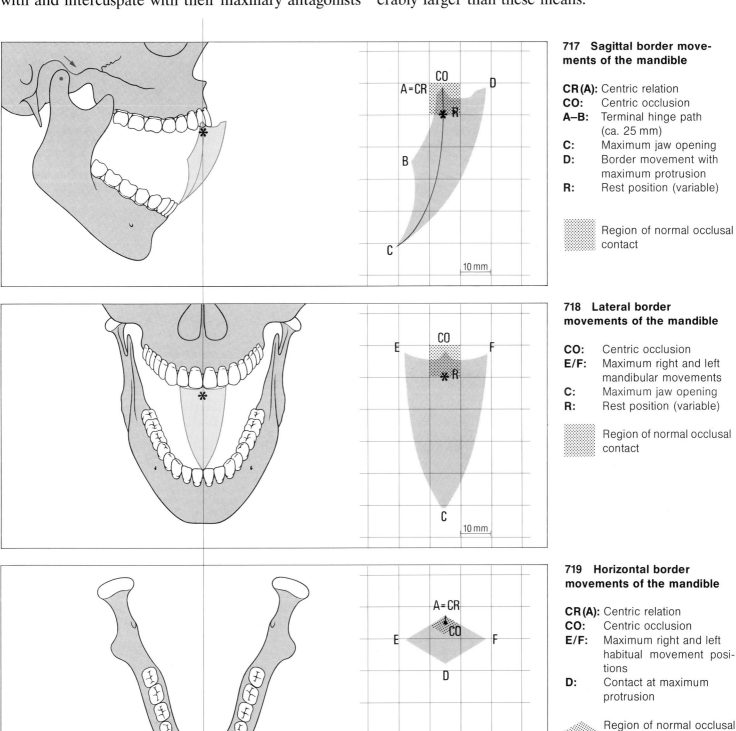

717   Sagittal border movements of the mandible

CR(A): Centric relation
CO: Centric occlusion
A–B: Terminal hinge path (ca. 25 mm)
C: Maximum jaw opening
D: Border movement with maximum protrusion
R: Rest position (variable)

Region of normal occlusal contact

718   Lateral border movements of the mandible

CO: Centric occlusion
E/F: Maximum right and left mandibular movements
C: Maximum jaw opening
R: Rest position (variable)

Region of normal occlusal contact

719   Horizontal border movements of the mandible

CR(A): Centric relation
CO: Centric occlusion
E/F: Maximum right and left habitual movement positions
D: Contact at maximum protrusion

Region of normal occlusal contact

With increasing jaw opening the possibility for lateral excursions is progressively limited.

Function and functional disturbances are influenced by occlusion, mandibular movements and interarch relationship.

Joss & Graf (1979) and Graf (1981) registered mandibular movements at tooth contact in normal, healthy, symptom-free subjects using three-dimensional computerized plots. The critical area between centric relation (CR) and maximum intercuspation (CO) was recorded, as well as the movement of the mandible at initial protrusive and lateral excursions.

Large physiologic variation was detected between *normal bite,* above average *overbite* and abraded dentition, probably as a result of occlusal guidance during mandibular movements.

Significant differences were also detected among test subjects in terms of the distance between CR and CO. A more or less pronounced distance between CR and CO was the rule. This appears to be normal physiologic variation, and should be kept in mind during selective grinding in the natural dentition when attempting to attain a "long centric" or "freedom in centric."

720   Normal bite (model)
Points of light between the central incisors of maxilla and mandible are the reference marks for the 3-dimensional computer plot of mandibular movements at tooth contact. Two Selspot TV cameras (left and right) record the movements of the red (mandibular) point of light. The green light is the stationary reference point (maxilla).

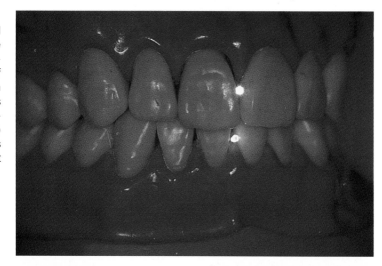

721   Overbite
This patient exhibited a true overbite, slight Class II interarch relationship, and pronounced cuspid guidance. The patient was symptom-free.

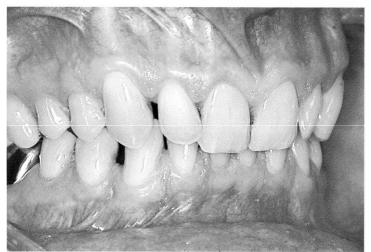

722   Abraded dentition
This patient exhibited severe attrition, but was symptom-free despite parafunctions. Depicted is a protrusive-lateral movement, demonstrating the patient's bruxing position.

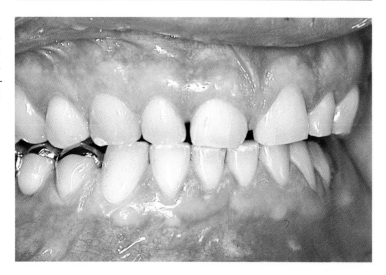

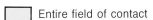
Entire field of contact

● CR: Centric relation

○ CO: Centric occlusion

CR: Position at centric relation

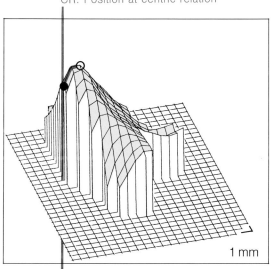

1 mm

1 mm

1 mm

723 Idealized representation of the horizontal field of movement of the mandible
Mandibular movements performed with no tooth contact provide a tracing that is identical to a *gothic arch* tracing as seen in prosthetics. The only limitations to mandibular movements are the boundaries provided by the anatomical structures of the TMJ.

Color code of the fields of contact (Figs. 724–726)
☐ Entire field of contact
▨ Incisor contacts
▨ Cuspid contacts
▨ Bicuspid contacts

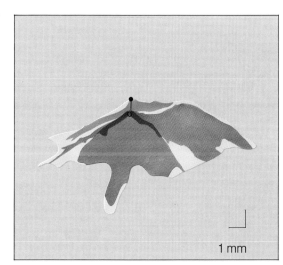

1 mm

1 mm

724 Normal bite – Computer plot and composite
The mandibular movement tracing with tooth contact depicts a physiologic distance (1 mm, red) between CR and CO. The mandibular movement is guided by incisors and cuspids in maximum intercuspation, and by bicuspids in the most retruded position.

Plot: Elevation 30°; angle 75°.

725 Overbite – Computer plot and composite
Only a short guidance path (0.8 mm, red) exists between CR and CO. The mandible is guided by incisors and cuspids around the narrow intercuspation region.

Plot: Elevation 30°; angle 75°.

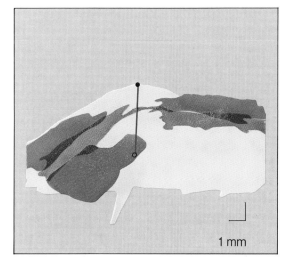

1 mm

726 Abraded dentition – Computer plot and composite
Excessively expansive *"long centric"* (3 mm, red). Movements to the right occur with incisor, cuspid and bicuspid guidance; to the left, guidance is primarily on bicuspids (helicoid abrasion).

Plot: Elevation 30°; angle 75°.

All three variations depicted in Figures 724–726 are within physiologic limits and require no therapeutic corrections.

Courtesy of *H. Graf*

Goals of Occlusal Adjustment

Even though occlusal trauma does not cause periodontitis, it can weaken periodontal health. Therefore, occlusal trauma should be eliminated in the course of therapy for periodontitis, especially if tooth mobility is becoming progressively more severe (Ramfjord & Ash 1979, 1983; Ash & Ramfjord 1982). The method of treatment is occlusal adjustment via selective grinding. There are simple rules for the removal of premature contacts in centric relation, for harmonizing the lateral occlusion ("BULL" rule, Fig. 742), and for elimination of balancing side contacts.

Selective occlusal grinding has additional effects in addition to elimination of occlusal trauma:
– Prevention or elimination of parafunctions
– Creation of symmetrical left / right chewing function
– Stabilization of the occlusal plane
– Adjustment of occlusion *after* orthodontic treatment
– Adjustment of occlusion *before* prosthetic replacement.

No effort should be made to attain the "ideal" occlusion!

727 Contact of antagonists in intercuspation (CO)
With maximum closure there exist habitual contacts of the buccal cusps of mandibular teeth in the fossae of the maxillary teeth, or of the maxillary palatal cusps in the mandibular fossae. In an ideal, non-abraded dentition, these contacts may be 2- or 3-point in nature, i.e., the cusps of maxillary teeth occlude at more than one point (example on second molar).

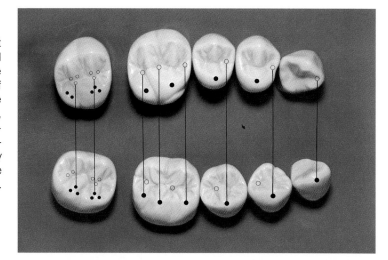 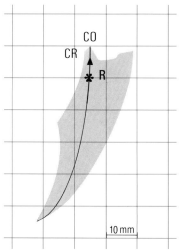

728 "Tapping test" for determination of tooth-tooth contacts in centric relation (CR)
The patient's mandible is moved by the dentist along the joint-guided hinge axis without pressure, until first contact between maxillary and mandibular teeth occurs.

With this technique, the head of the *condyle* achieves its zenith in the fossa (right).

Caution: Application of presure can force the condyle dorsally and inferiorly, into an unphysiologic, unstable position.

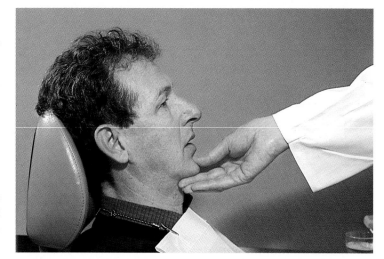 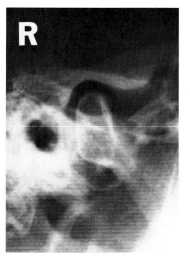

729 Slide from premature contact in CR into intercuspation (CO)
When the mandible is manipulated by the dentist along its hinge axis, the movement may be stopped by one or more premature contacts. If the patient then bites into full intercuspation, the mandible shifts (usually in an anterior direction, and many times anterior-lateral). The shift is noted on the diagram (right) by the red arrow.

Such premature contacts should be eliminated.

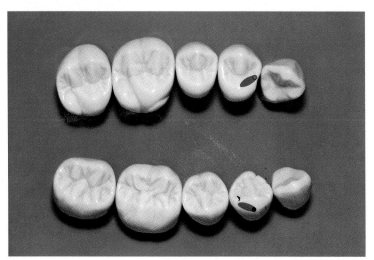 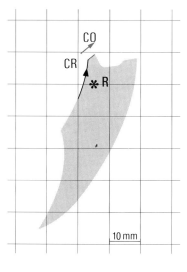

Practical Occlusal Adjustment – Premature Contacts

Premature contacts in centric relation are detected using the "tapping test" (Fig. 728). If the test reveals that at least three pairs of opposing teeth on each side of the arch make contact at the same instant, and if an interference-free slide in centric of no more than 1 mm occurs, *no* corrective occlusal adjustment is indicated.

If only one or two pairs of teeth makes contact initially, and/or if the subsequent slide to centric is greater than 1 mm or has a lateral component, selective grinding is indicated.

An experienced dentist can perform selective grinding immediately. Only in difficult cases or with complex, expansive rehabilitation is it necessary to first mount the case in an articulator to study the precise interarch relationship.

The goal of selective grinding is the creation of *freedom in centric* (Ramfjord & Ash 1983), i.e., free horizontal guidance of the cusps between CR and CO.

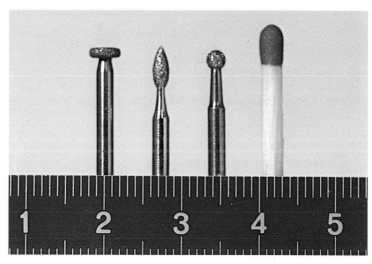

730   Instrumentarium for selective grinding
Selective grinding is performed using fine wheel, flame and ball-shaped diamonds.
    The occlusal surfaces of the teeth are dried thoroughly, then the premature contacts are marked with ribbons of various colors.

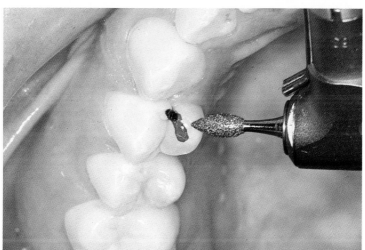

731   Premature contact in CR, with slide (red) into CO (black)
The red marking is shaped into a gentle depression using a flame-shaped diamond, without encroaching upon the palatal cusp tip or the contact point in CO (black dot).

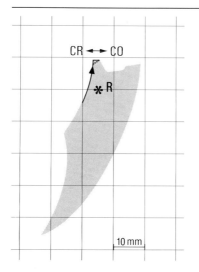

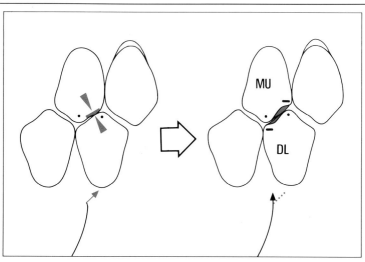

732   Premature contact on cuspal inclines
This results in a forward/sagittal mandibular shift. The mesial cusp incline is recontoured on the maxillary tooth (MU) and the distal cusp incline in the mandible (DL). It is necessary to repeatedly check the selective grinding by re-marking with color ribbon. If secondary prematurities develop on other antagonist pairs, they should also be eliminated.

A *long centric* is created between CO and CR, i.e., a horizontally located sagittal guide path not more than 1 mm in extent.

733 Premature contact on buccal cusp inclines
Teeth 15 and 45 exhibit premature contact (red) in centric on the buccal cusp inclines. This causes a lateral shift of the mandible, and must be eliminated because at maximum intercuspation the TMJ position is asymmetric (see situation 1, Fig. 734).

Right: Mandibular shift (red arrow) in the frontal segment of the Posselt figure.

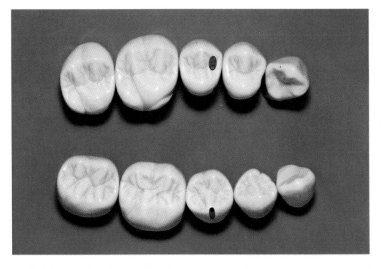
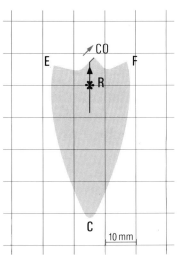

734 Buccal-lingual inclines – Possible premature contacts (right) between:

1. Inner aspect of maxillary facial and outer aspect of mandibular facial cusp;
2. Inner aspect of maxillary palatal and inner aspect of mandibular facial cusp;
3. Outer aspect of palatal and inner aspect of mandibular lingual cusp.

Situation 1:
Widen the maxillary fossa facially. It may be necessary to reduce the facial surface of the mand. tooth.

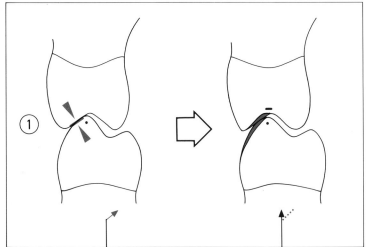
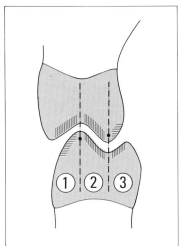

735 Situation 2:
The premature contact is eliminated through minimal widening and lateral shifting of the fossae of both teeth. Neither *cusp tip* is altered in any way.

It is wise to keep in mind that the contacting surfaces often represent balancing side interferences (p. 281).

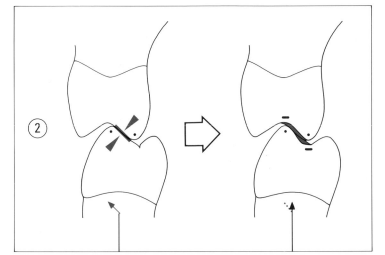

736 Situation 3:
The fossa of the mandibular tooth is widened somewhat to accomodate the cusp of the maxillary tooth. The outer aspect of the palatal cusp may also be lightly reduced at the point where it contacts the fossa of its antagonist.

Right: By eliminating the prematurities (Situations 1–3), a *wide centric* is created (see Posselt figure).

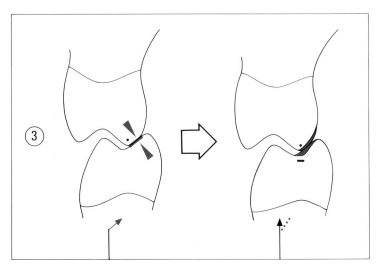
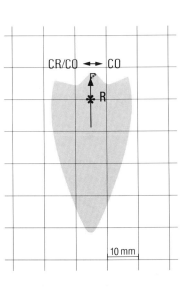

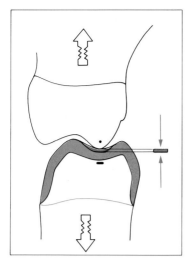

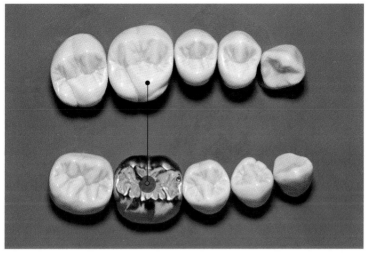

737 Premature contact between cusp and fossa
This type of prematurity is often detected after seating a crown or a bridge, and may occur in CR or in CO. The two involved teeth are depressed into their sockets each time the jaws close, often resulting in increased axial tooth mobility.

The procedure for eliminating this situation involves *deepening the fossa* by occlusal grinding. The corresponding cusp may be reduced if it also represents a balancing side interference.

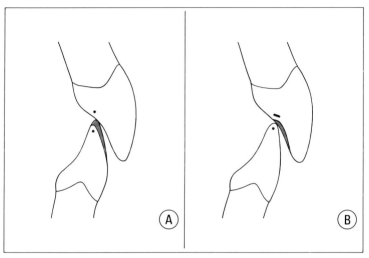

738 Anterior prematurity
Naturally occurring prematurities in the anterior segment are rare, but may be detected after a crown or bridge is seated.

The contacts during mandibular protrusive movement should be checked before any selective grinding is performed. If the effected teeth are found to exert an interference during protrusive, then selective grinding is performed on the mandibular tooth (A).

If there is no interference during protrusive movement, the palatal surface of the maxillary tooth (B) is reduced.

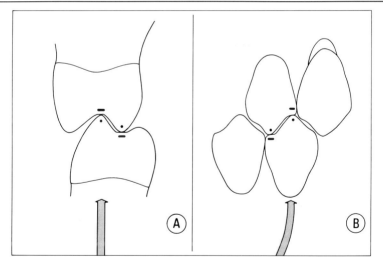

739 Selective grinding of "centric" completed
The patient can now assume a multipoint occlusion in both CR and CO without any interference or slide. A mesiodistal *long centric* has been created (B) that permits a degree of mandibular movement against the maxillary teeth.

Similarly (A), a *wide centric* has been created that permits ca. 0.5 mm of free mandibular movement buccolingually.

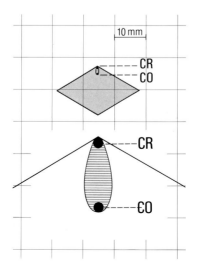

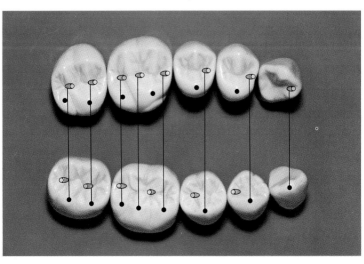

740 "Freedom in centric"
There exists between CR and CO a teardrop-shaped field measuring about 1 × 0.5 mm within which free movement of the mandible, i.e., of the cusps within their respective fossae *(freedom in centric)* is possible. These areas are depicted on the occlusal surfaces of opposing teeth in this Figure, with lines connecting the cusp tips to their CR positions in fossae.

Left: This horizontal section through the Posselt figure depicts the approximate size of this zone of free movement.

Working Side

The goals of selective grinding in the posterior segments of the dental arch are the creation of interference-free, harmonic movements in intercuspation and the elimination of broad guidance surfaces that are the sites of parafunctions (clenching, brusixm). Physiologic, non-traumatic posterior segment guidance on the working side is left unchanged; this situation may be characterized by anterior cuspid guidance or group function.

Interferences are removed by selective reduction and flattening of the interfering, excessively steep cusp inclines ("BULL" rule, Fig. 742). The goal is to achieve cuspid guidance during lateral mandibular movements if possible.

The posterior segment guidance pathways that are created by selective occlusal grinding should be contact *lines,* not broad contact surfaces, for example, the line contact of the buccal cusp inclines in the maxilla. Expansive contact areas between antagonists may provide the stimulus for renewed parafunction.

741 Interference – Dysharmonious lateral movement

The most commonly encountered interferences on the working side (see green pathway, right) are found on bicuspids. The involved surfaces are usually the buccal cusp in the mandible and the inner aspect of the buccal cusp in the maxilla (e.g., between 14 and 44 as depicted here).

Such interferences are encountered less often between the palatal maxillary cusp and the inner aspect of the mandibular lingual cusp.

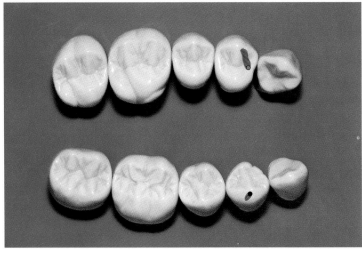
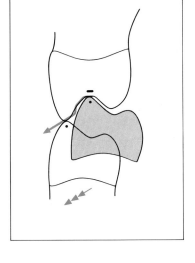

742 Selective grinding of interference on the working side – "BULL" rule

The contacts in centric must *not* be eliminated ("long centric") during the selective grinding procedure. Above all, the cusp tips (black dots) must not be touched.

This can be accomplished by performing selective grinding in the maxilla to eliminate an interference on the buccal aspect, and by grinding in the mandible to eliminate an interference in the lingual aspect (*the BULL rule:* **B**uccal **U**pper, **L**ingual **L**ower).

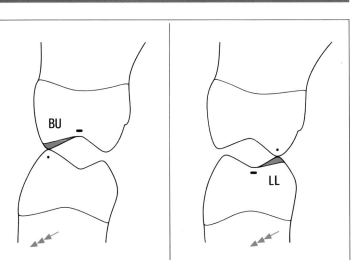
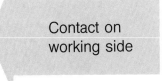

Contact on working side

743 Harmony in the posterior segment after selective grinding

The goal in elimination of an interference on the working side is to integrate *cuspid guidance* into posterior segment guidance.

Group function, e.g., guidance involving incisors, cuspids and bicupids is acceptable in the fully dentulous situation, but is not a goal to be sought aggressively.

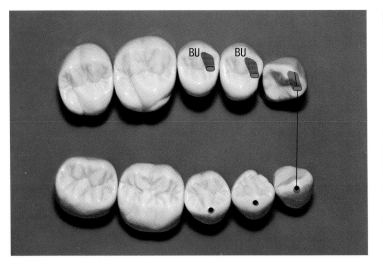
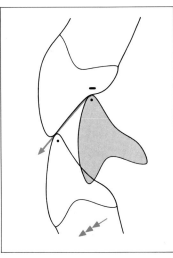

Balancing Side

In the natural dentition, balancing side contacts are neither necessary nor desirable. *Balancing side interferences* can actually be injurious insofar as they may elicit parafunctions, particularly clenching. The effected teeth are usually the second molars and, if present, the third molars, which may become hypermobile or undergo periodontal damage as they must bear the clenching forces.

Balancing side interferences should be *eliminated* by means of selective grinding of the balance pathway. However, centric contacts and guidance contacts on the working side must be maintained. The centric contacts will determine whether the balance pathway to be eliminated by grinding is on the inner aspect of the palatal cusp or on the inner aspect of the mandibular buccal cusps. If both upper and lower cusps are involved simultaneously in the balancing side interference, it will be necessary to relieve the situation with maintenance of at least one cusp-fossa contact in centric.

Heavy balancing side interference on a third molar may be an indication for extraction of this tooth.

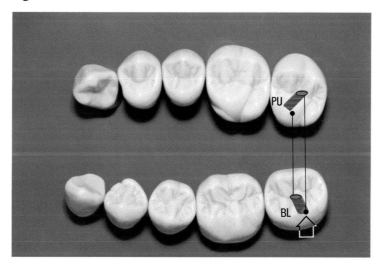

744   Balancing side interference in posterior segment
A balancing side interference (red marking) exists during lateral mandibular movement to the right, between the inner aspect of the buccal cusp of the lower second molar and the inner aspect of the palatal cusp of the upper second molar.

Centric contacts exist on the palatal cusp in the maxilla and on the buccal cusp in the mandible; the latter should preferentially be maintained (arrow).

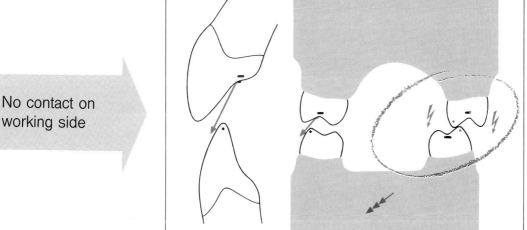

No contact on working side

745   Balancing side interference in the left molar area during mandibular excursion to the right
The excessively steep cusp inclines on the balance side (circled red) prevent any tooth contact on the working side (green). Even the cuspid region is devoid of guiding contact (see long green arrow).

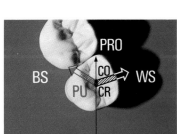
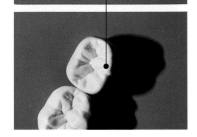
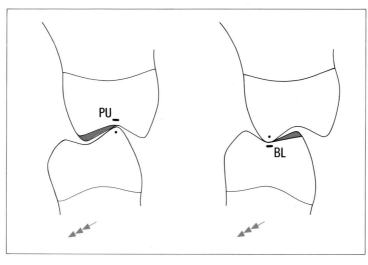

746   Elimination of balancing interference – "PUBL" rule
Centric contacts (CR/CO) must also be maintained when performing selective grinding on the balancing side.

If centric contact is between the mandibular buccal cusp and the maxillary fossa, the upper palatal balance pathway (PU) should be eliminated (left, red arrow).

If centric contact consists of the upper palatal cusp in the lower fossa, the balancing side interference is removed by grinding the inner aspect of the lower buccal cusp (BL).

Protrusive Movement – Interferences

If interferences occur on anterior teeth during protrusive movements, they must be eliminated. Any interferences in the posterior segments should also be eliminated via selective occlusal grinding, analogous to mesiodistal elimination of balancing side interferences as described above. In patients with anterior open bite, no corrective efforts should be made (e.g., by excessive grinding on posterior teeth).

Reduction of Wear Facets

Pronounced wear facets are frequently observed in patients with parafunctions, and can be eliminated according to the *Jankelson* (1960) principles (see also Occlusal adjustment, situation 1, Fig. 733, and situation 3, Fig. 734, p. 278).

747   Selective grinding in protrusive movements
Centric contacts on the anterior teeth should occur only in CO (not in CR). Occasionally the teeth make contact only when a slight mandibular protrusive movement is made from CO. These contacts (black dots) must be maintained when selective grinding is performed during protrusive movement:
A: Grinding the palatal surface in the maxilla.
B: Grinding the maxillary palatal and mandibular lingual surfaces.
C: Grinding the buccal surface of the mandibular anterior teeth.

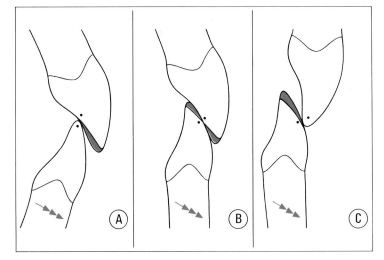

748   Elimination of balancing contact during protrusive movement
Molars that are tipped or that lack antagonists (circled in red) may make it impossible to achieve contact in the anterior area during mandibular protrusion (green arrows).
  Extraction of such molars will certainly eliminate the interference, but selective grinding can achieve the same goal. The grinding is similar to that employed for eliminating a balancing side interference in the posterior area, but in a mesiodistal plane.

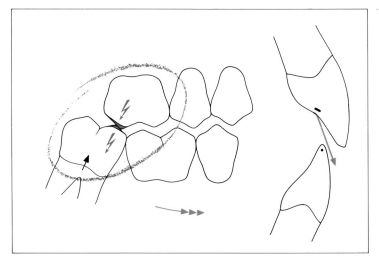

749   Reshaping wear facets
Parafunctional habits can result in expansive attrition in the area of the maxillary buccal cusps and mandibular oral cusps (wear facets). The buccolingual field of occlusion is expanded (A: blue bar – *widening* of occlusal field).
  By selective occlusal grinding of the external surfaces of the cusps (Jankelson), the wide facets can be reduced to point contacts with the newly created cusp tips (arrows); the field of occlusion is thereby reduced (B: *narrowing*, coronoplasty).

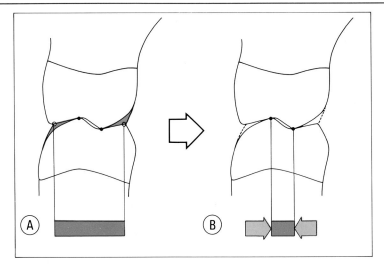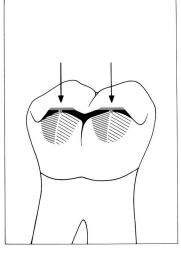

Occlusal Bite Guard – The Michigan Splint

When parafunctional habits (e.g., bruxism) result in occlusal periodontal trauma (increased tooth mobility), the dentition should undergo selective occlusal grinding and facets should be eliminated.

However, selective grinding is often impossible due to masticatory musculature spasms. Reciprocal functional relationships exist among occlusion, periodontium, TMJ, musculature and central nervous system (CNS). The CNS may also be influenced by psychic components (Fröhlich 1966). Psychic stress situations are relieved through elevated activity of the masticatory musculature (clenching, bruxing). In such situations, if occlusal dysharmonies are also present a "vicious circle" is created, which can best be broken through use of a bite guard, e.g., the Michigan splint (Geering 1978; Ramfjord & Ash 1983). The result is that the occlusion is taken out of the "circle" and the masticatory musculature relaxes (Graf 1969). If the psychic component is not too great, selective occlusal grinding can be accomplished in the mouth after only a few weeks.

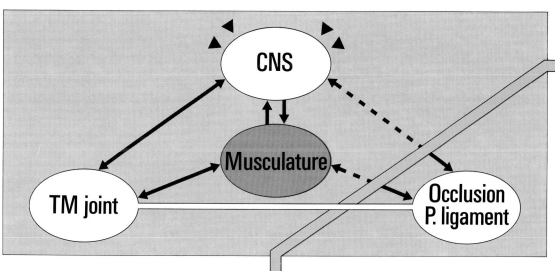

750 Reciprocal influences of the masticatory musculature

Interruption by splint

The tone of the masticatory musculature (red) is a product of influences from the central nervous system, the occlusion and the TMJ.

The *feedback mechanisms can be interrupted* quite simply through use of a bite guard (blue bar).

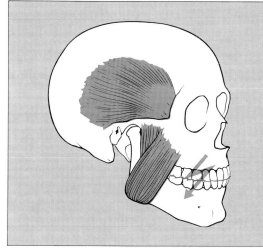
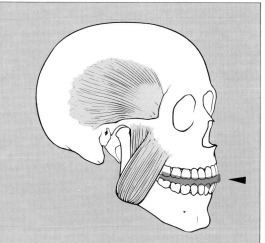

751 Spasm (left) and normal tone (right)

Elevated activity of the masticatory musculature (masseter, temporalis) is an etiologic factor for occlusal trauma.

Insertion of an occlusal bite guard (blue) can elicit an immediate and dramatic reduction of this hyperactivity. The heavy, destructive forces exerted upon the periodontium by clenching or bruxing are reduced to more physiologic levels. Also, the forces are evenly distributed over the entire dental arch by the bite guard.

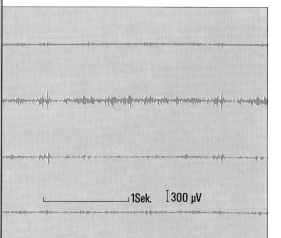

M. temporalis dexter

M. masseter dexter

M. masseter sinister

M. temporalis sinister

1Sek. ⌶300 µV

752 Electromyography before and after insertion of a bite guard

The electromyograms *before* (red) and *after* (blue) insertion of a bite guard reveal the quieting of the masticatory muscles' previous hyperactive states.
EMG courtesy of *H. Graf*

If the patient's level of psychic stress is very high, however, clenching and bruxism on the bite guard itself may ensue. The possibilities for alleviating this situation include oral physiotherapy or the administration of tranquilizers to calm the CNS component.

753 Michigan splint in the articulator
Fabrication of the bite guard (depicted here is a Michigan splint) out of clear acrylic is performed only after registration of the occlusal relationships in an adjustable articulator. This usually means that only slight alterations will have to be made on the bite guard at the time of insertion. The thickness of the occlusal surface of the bite guard should be minimized to avoid opening the bite excessively. The Michigan splint is almost always seated in the maxilla.

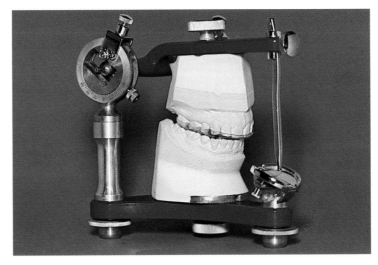

754 Characteristics of the Michigan splint
The buccal cusps of mandibular molars and bicuspids, as well as cuspids and incisors, occlude onto the smooth acrylic surface (left).

Right: In the *cuspid region (A)* a "cuspid rise" is built into the splint. This provides the only guidance for the mandible during lateral and protrusive excursions. The principle of "freedom in centric" is thus also applied during fabrication of a bite guard (splint centric).

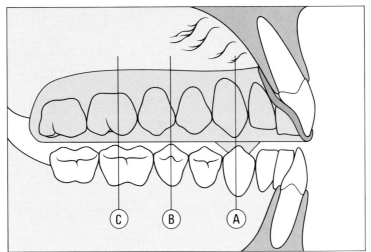
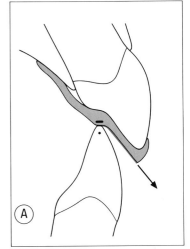

755 Michigan splint
Occlusal contacts of the mandibular buccal cusp tips are marked in red, cuspid guidance pathways for protrusive and lateral excursions in green.

Right: Transverse section through the *bicuspids (B)* shows that the splint surface incorporates a depression in the fossa area to accept the steep cusp of the mandibular bicuspid. This precludes excessive bite elevation, but occlusal contact is lost immediately with lateral mandibular movement (arrows).

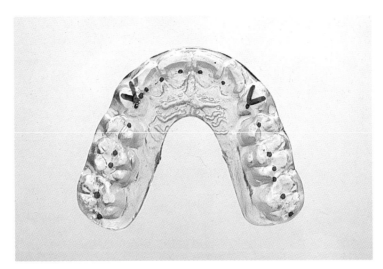
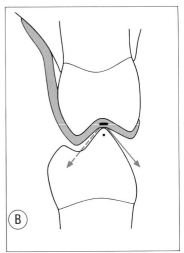

756 Cuspid rise
Cuspid rise (black arrow) incorporated into the Michigan splint opens the occlusion during lateral excursions.

Right: Section through the *molar region (C)* shows that the acrylic is flat since cusp inclines are not as steep and the bite therefore is not opened excessively. Molar contact is lost immediately due to the cuspid rise (working and balancing side excursions, blue arrows).

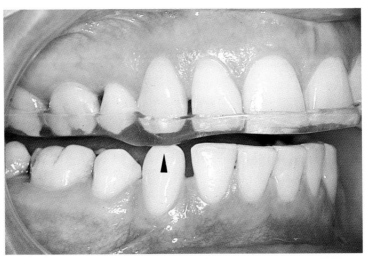
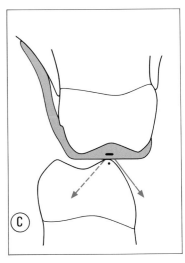

Orthodontics

A casual relationship between dental malocclusion and periodontitis is difficult to document (Ainamo 1972; Geiger et al. 1973, 1974; Stahl 1975; Ingerval et al. 1977; Buckley 1972, 1981; Hug 1983). However, dental crowding may make plaque removal difficult, and this favors the progression of inflammatory disease in the periodontal supporting tissues.

One must differentiate between malocclusion that has existed since complete eruption of the permanent dentition and tooth drifting that occurs over a period of time, perhaps as a consequence of periodontitis. The latter may be due, at least in part, to the periodontal disease process itself, and includes tipping, rotation, extrusion and especially protrusion of the maxillary anterior teeth. Realignment of teeth that have drifted in a dentition manifesting periodontitis can usually be accomplished by means of simple orthodontic movement.

The factors involved in the development of dental malocclusion following loss of periodontal support are not always obvious. Possible causes include oral parafunctions such as tongue thrust or lip biting, occupation-related peculiarities such as holding nails or pins between the teeth, and tipping of adjacent teeth into an extraction site resulting in occlusal imbalances. It has also been speculated that the granulation tissue present in deep periodontal pockets may exert a force that causes drifting, or that the intact fiber structure on the side of a tooth opposite a deep pocket may exert a *pull* that results in tipping or drifting of a tooth.

Orthodontic treatment of a periodontally compromised dentition should never be started until the initial therapy phase is completed and the infection has been brought under control. The rationale for various treatment options should be considered: Is the proposed tooth movement for functional or esthetic reasons? Could the patient's problem be solved by other means, for example by recontouring teeth (odontoplasty) to correct functional, morphologic or esthetic problems? Is a prosthetic solution feasible?

If the final decision is to go ahead with orthodontic treatment, an array of possible methods including simple wire ligatures, removable plates and fixed appliances is available. The choice will depend in large measure on the diagnosis, the goals of therapy and the difficulty of the tooth movement desired.

Another factor in selection of treatment modality is the concerns of the patient, especially the adult patient, who is often not prepared or willing to submit to long-term orthodontic therapy with fixed appliances. Thus, compromises often have to be made. In a dentition that has been ravaged by periodontal disease, orthodontic treatment represents a particular trauma for the remaining supporting structures. It has been amply demonstrated that orthodontic treatment results in temporarily increased tooth mobility, which is greatly accelerated by occlusal trauma. For this reason, if the destruction in the periodontium is severe, major orthodontic treatment may be contraindicated.

Space Closure in the Maxillary Anterior Segment

Following completion of periodontal therapy for moderate periodontitis (AP), the 40-year-old female depicted below requested that the space between 21 and 22 be closed orthodontically for esthetic reasons. The diastema had developed over the previous several years. Gingival shrinkage following the periodontal treatment further enlarged the interdental area, making the esthetic problem greater.

Space closure was accomplished in 2 months by means of a *removable appliance* with a *labial bow* and finger spring on 21. The entire anterior segment was retracted and tooth 21 was moved distally.

After such treatment, retention is required. This can be accomplished using a *cast metal splint* (Wolf & Rateitschak 1965), a composite resin splint, or a lingual bonded retainer.

Tipping movement of a single tooth can be performed by the general practitioner or by the periodontist. An orthodontist is not necessary for this simple tooth movement.

757 Before treatment – After completion of periodontal therapy
Protrusion of the anterior segment. An unesthetic diastema has developed between 21 and 22. The brown staining is due to chlorhexidine rinse, which was prescribed for plaque inhibition postsurgically.

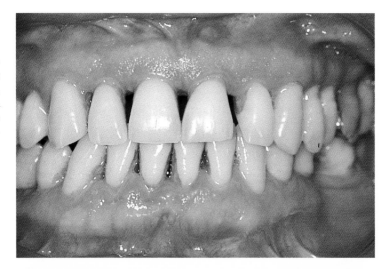
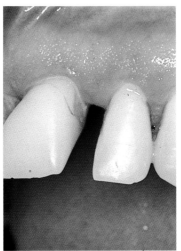

758 Removable appliance
An acrylic palatal plate with a labial bow for correction of the anterior protrusion and a finger spring for distal movement of 21.

Right: In order to avoid elongation (supereruption) of the anterior teeth or apical movement of the arch wire, the practitioner may elect to place small "bumps" of acid-etched composite resin (blue) on the facial surfaces of some teeth above the arch wire.

One force vector of the appliance is thereby directed in an apical direction, tending to intrude the tooth (red arrow).

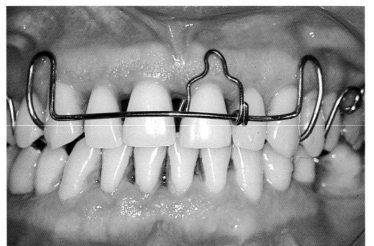
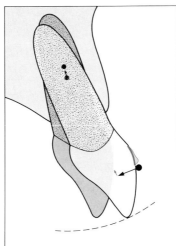

759 Retention after completion of orthodontic treatment – 2 possibilities
Cast metal splint (left): A chromecobalt splint can be worn at night. It is anchored on the bicuspids by means of flexible clasps that grasp the tooth crown.

Composite splint (right): An alternative to a removable retainer is the use of acid-etch resin for semipermanent splinting of groups of teeth (here: 21, 22, 23). This also enhances esthetics by decreasing the size of the interdental spaces.

Courtesy of *P. Stöckli*

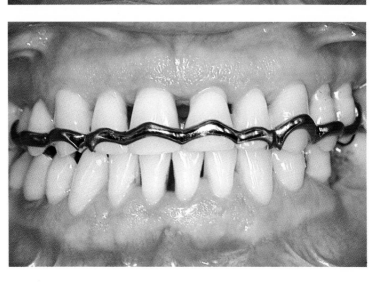
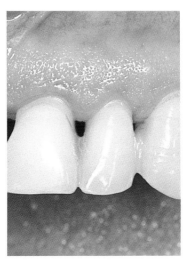

Treatment for Protrusion

This 41-year-old female suffered from generalized periodontitis of moderate severity. Some drifting of the anterior teeth had occurred, and maxillary anterior protrusion had become noticeably more severe in the last several years. The patient requested periodontal therapy, but also desired esthetic improvement.

Orthodontic treatment would be indicated in a patient of this age solely on the basis of her functional problems, which included overbite, overjet and anterior protrusion in both maxilla and mandible. The goals of the orthodontic treatment, following completion of ini-

tial periodontal therapy, were 1) bite opening and 2) retraction of the anterior segments. The treatment was accomplished using fixed appliances in both arches, a transpalatal arch to expand the maxilla, and posterior *high pull headgear* with bite-opening torque. Following orthodontic treatment, restorative procedures should be performed to stabilize the occlusion. Also, the "initial therapy" phase of periodontal treatment is *repeated*, to eliminate inflammation resulting from compromised oral hygiene during the 8-month orthodontic phase.

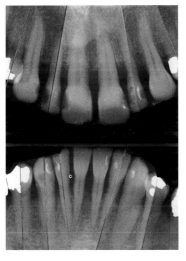
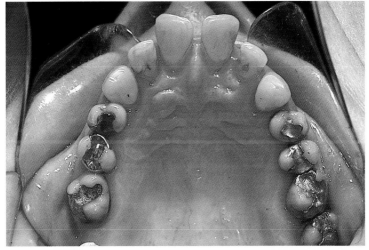

760 Initial clinical view
The patient presented with moderate periodontitis, as well as protrusion and rotation of the anterior teeth. The problem was probably enhanced by the patient's lip-biting habit. Erythema of the palate was caused by a removable orthodontic "plate" worn by the patient for some time but without success.

The radiograph reveals horizontal bone loss and diastemata in both anterior segments, which may have been caused by a tongue thrust habit.

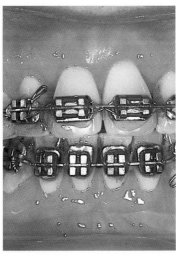
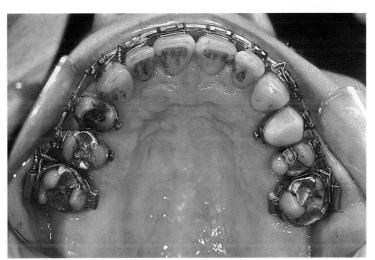

761 Fixed orthodontic appliance
Brackets were affixed by means of acid-etch resin; the treatment involved edgewise technique and headgear. Both maxilla and mandible were fully banded.
These clinical views were taken immediately before removal of the appliances at the termination of active treatment.

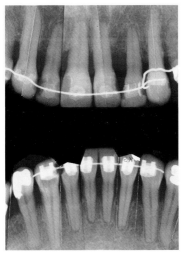
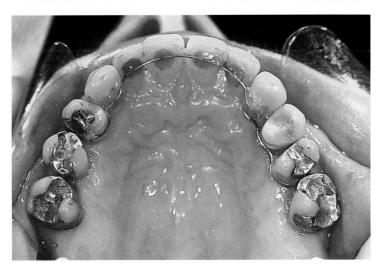

762 Retention
Acid-etched resin was used with a palatal archwire for retention in the maxillary anterior segment; its esthetic value is obvious.
Retention in the mandible was by means of an archwire in the labial brackets, which were left in place after active treatment.
At this time, definitive restorative work and follow-up periodontal therapy can begin. A short recall interval is indicated because of the problems of plaque retention by and around the fixed retention elements.

Courtesy of *P. Stöckli*

Uprighting the Mandibular Second Molar

It is not necessary to prosthetically close every space in the dental arch. If the occlusion is stable and there is adequate periodontal support, no drifting of teeth should occur.

Tipping of a second molar into a first molar extraction site is a common occurrence, and is accelerated in a dentition manifesting periodontal destruction. The mesial surface of the tipped molar becomes an excellent area for plaque accumulation, which promotes the development of a still deeper periodontal pocket on this surface. This was the situation presented by the 48-year-old female with adult periodontitis (AP), whose case is depicted below.

Tooth 38 was extracted during initial therapy, for endodontic reasons. Both lower second molars were uprighted during a 7-month period before seating fixed 3-unit bridges bilaterally.

The tooth movement was accomplished with a removable appliance incorporating a bite plane extending distally to the bicuspid area, a labial bow, and uprighting springs mesial to both second molars.

763 Initial panoramic radiograph – Mesially tipped second mandibular molars
Following extraction of the first molars years ago, the second molars had tipped severely into the spaces. Periodontal pockets had formed on the mesial surfaces of the second molars (plaque retention, difficult home care). The development of mesial pockets may have been accelerated by the change in occlusion that occurred with the initial tipping of the molars, resulting in nonphysiologic forces on the molars and further tipping.

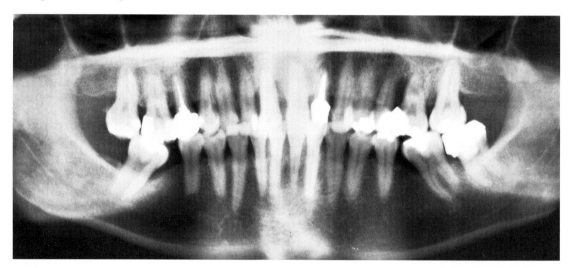

764 Removable appliance – Lateral views
Mandibular appliance was fabricated from clear acrylic and incorporated an anterior bite plane, labial bow with adjustment loops and uprighting springs for the molars.

Opening the bite was necessary to eliminate occlusal interferences on the molars during uprighting.

Although less precise and clumsier than a fixed appliance, the removable appliance is often preferred by adult patients.

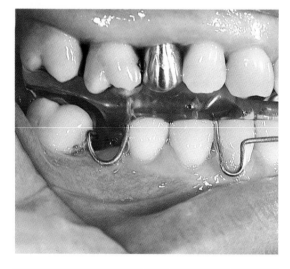
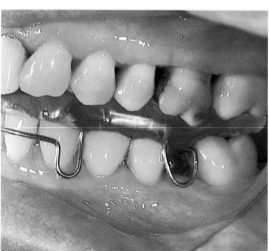

765 Radiograph after completion of orthodontic and prosthetic treatment
Tooth 38 was extracted and the two lower second molars were uprighted.

The 3-unit bridges were prepared and seated soon after completion of orthodontic therapy, serving as retainers for the uprighted molars. The pontics of the bridges permit adequate access for oral hygiene on the mesial surfaces of the second molars.

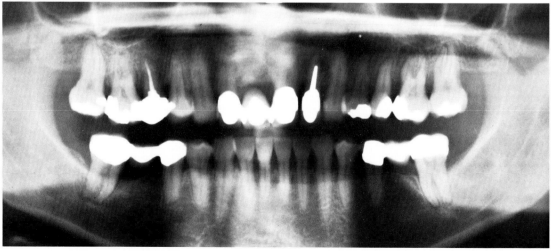

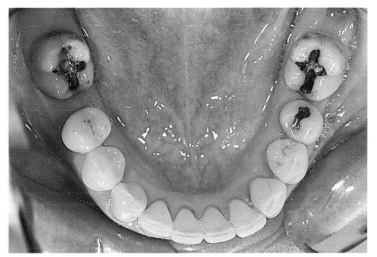

766 Initial view
The second molars (47; 37) are severely tipped mesially.

The tipping has narrowed the extraction site, making adequate oral hygiene difficult and promoting plaque retention (gingivitis, periodontitis).

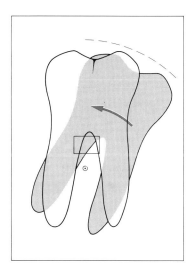

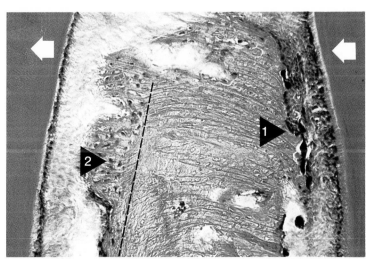

767 Bone resorption and deposition during orthodontic treatment – Histology
White arrows indicate direction of uprighting. In the pressure zone (1), one notes osteoclastic bone resorption, while in the tension zone (2) bone apposition is observed (van Gieson, × 25).
Courtesy of *N. P. Lang*

Diagram: The center of rotation during uprighting of a 2-rooted molar is located between the roots, near the bifurcation.

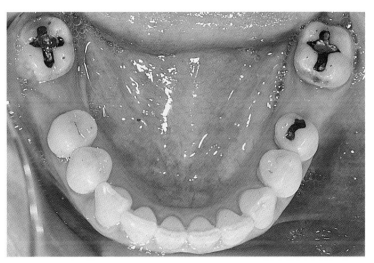

768 Molar uprighting complete
Definitive prosthetic work should begin immediately, to maintain the space created. Note that the buccal surface of 47 is fractured off (not due to the orthodontic treatment!).

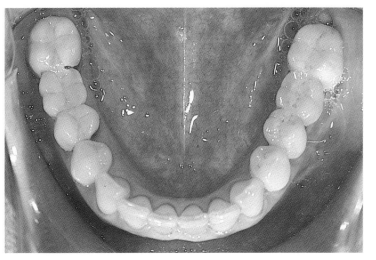

769 Space closure – Retention
Fixed bridgework maintains the uprighted molars, affords replacement of the missing teeth, and provides a pleasing esthetic result.

The interdental spaces and the area beneath the pontics are contoured to permit and facilitate home care by the patient, who can use interdental brushes in these areas.

Courtesy of *P. Stöckli*

Treatment of the Malpositioned Cuspid

Before orthodontic therapy, this 14-year-old female had to be treated for severe gingivitis and incipient juvenile periodontitis (LJP, see p. 72).

Because the patient's home care continued to be less than optimum during the course of initial therapy, a removable appliance was selected for the orthodontic treatment. Fixed appliances require a high level of patient cooperation and motivation for plaque control around brackets and wires. A removable appliance can be easily cleaned at the sink, and the oral cavity is easier to keep clean as well.

Financial considerations may also be a factor in the selection of fixed or removable orthodontic appliances.

**770 Initial view –
Malpositioned cuspid**
The maxillary right cuspid was severely malpositioned. The use of a plaque disclosing agent revealed the very poor oral hygiene. The cuspid and the palatally displaced left lateral incisor created especially difficult plaque-retentive areas. The result was extremely severe gingivitis with pseudopockets in this region of the maxillary arch.

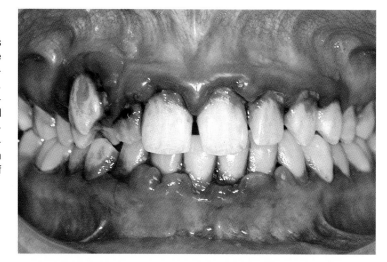
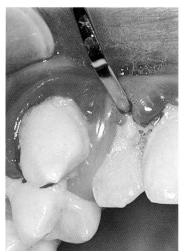

771 Removable orthodontic appliance
Subsequent to periodontal initial therapy, a palatal plate with a labial arch wire was fabricated. The appliance incorporated a finger spring on 11 and a modified adjustment loop for vertical and lingual forces on the cuspid (13).

Extraction of the first bicuspid (14) was necessary to create space for the malpositioned cuspid. The orthodontic treatment lasted about one year.

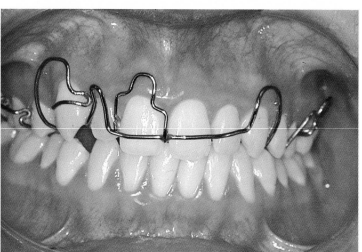

772 Final result 3 years after initiation of therapy
The orthodontic result is acceptable. The patient (now 17 years old) performs home care effectively using the Bass technique and dental floss. Use of a disclosing agent reveals plaque in only a few locations. Bringing the maxillary right cuspid into line makes maintaining oral hygiene in the area easier.

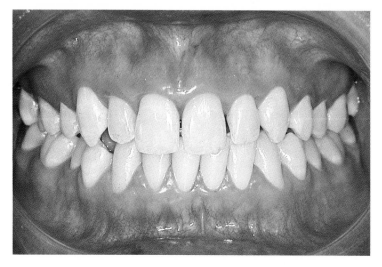
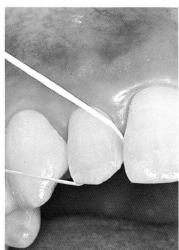

Splinting – Stabilization

The significance and the value of splinting mobile teeth as a periodontal therapeutic technique are questionable. In order to clarify whether there are any indications for splinting, one must first consider the causes of tooth mobility:

  - *Quantitative* loss of supporting structure due to periodontitis
  - *Qualitative* alterations of supporting structures due to trauma from occlusion
  - Short-term trauma to the periodontium due to treatment of periodontitis
  - Combinations of the above.

Mobile teeth whose degree of mobility is not increasing *do not* generally require splinting. Teeth with increased mobility traced to occlusal trauma should be treated by occlusal adjustment, not by splinting (Vollmer & Rateitschak 1975). While it is true that mobile teeth can be immobilized by splinting, and that this may provide some comfort for the patient, is does not lead to any long-term biologic stabilization of the teeth (Galler et al. 1979; Rateitschak 1980).

Depicted below is a classification of splinting possibilities:

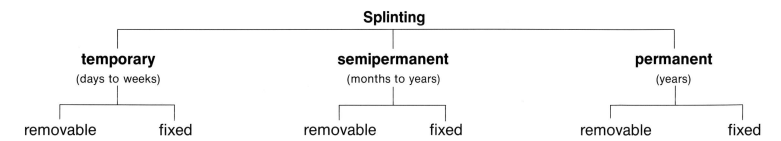

Indications for the various types of splinting

Temporary or semipermanent splinting is indicated for severely mobile teeth before or during periodontal therapy. Such splinting can reduce treatment trauma.

Semipermanent or permanent splinting may be used to stabilize highly mobile teeth that impair the patient's chewing. Orthodontic retention may also be viewed as a type of semipermanent/permanent splinting.

Permanent splinting is employed during complex oral rehabilitation where abutments are highly mobile or where a few abutments must support the entire prosthesis, particularly when such abutment teeth have minimal periodontal support, but have been successfully treated periodontally. If such teeth are not splinted, the danger of progressively increasing tooth mobility exists (Nyman & Lindhe 1979).

Temporary Splinting

The simple wire ligature (Fig. 773) may serve as a *fixed* splint for a few days to several weeks. Wire ligatures are seldom used today, primarily because of the esthetic considerations. A more commonly used fixed temporary splint is the acid-etch composite resin splint without tooth preparation (Fig. 774). Such a splint can be applied quickly and easily with the rubber dam in place; however, it is a temporary measure because adhesion of the resin to tooth structure is not very strong without the additional mechanical retention provided by a cavity preparation, grooves etc. Fracture of the splint is common if more than 3–4 teeth are included in a single splinted unit.

A *removable* temporary splint may be fabricated of clear acrylic pulled under vacuum over a study model (Fig. 775). Such splints are often indicated for temporary stabilization of individual teeth for short periods of time. This type of splint was formerly used as a "bite guard" in the treatment of oral parafunctions, but with very little success.

773 Wire splint
Soft steel wire (0.4 mm dia.) is wrapped around the facial and oral surfaces of the teeth to be splinted, and the ligature is tightened by twisting the ends.

Stabilization of individual teeth is accomplished by application of interdental ligatures. Acid-etch resin "stops" may be applied to the labial surface of each tooth (cf. Fig. 758) to prevent the wire from slipping apically.

A wire splint affords no protection against the forces of occlusion.

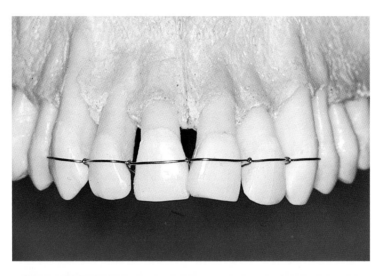

774 Composite resin splint, no tooth preparation
After thoroughly cleaning the teeth, the interproximal surfaces are acid-etched (red in diagram) and resin (blue) is applied. The apical area of the interdental space must be left open to maintain good hygiene.

Right: Above, incisal view of resin splint in place; below, scanning EM view of an acid-etched enamel surface.

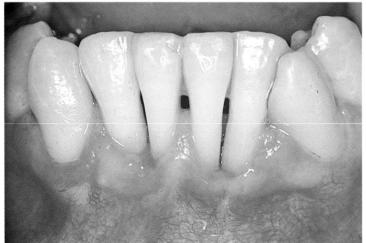
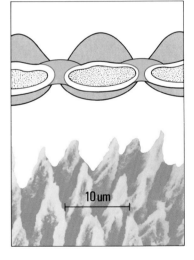

10 um

775 Vacuum formed removable acrylic splint
This splint can be used for short-term retention or stabilization of teeth. The margin of the splint should extend just beyond the height of contour of each tooth (arrows in schematic) on both labial and lingual surfaces, to provide secure retention.

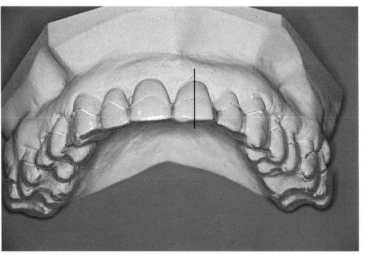
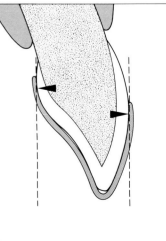

Semipermanent Splinting – Anterior Area

The most commonly used *fixed* semipermanent splint in the anterior area is the acid-etch composite resin splint applied after tooth preparation. It may serve for several months or even years. Often it is possible to remove old anterior restorations and utilize the cavity preparations in the splint. The technique of application is identical to placement of a composite resin restoration using the acid-etch pretreatment.

In the mandibular anterior area, the intracoronal resin splint incorporating polyester fibers has proved useful (Grau & Lutz 1982). Light-polymerized resin is generally used for this type of splint because of its long working time.

Removable semipermanent splints may be fabricated as cast chrome-cobalt alloy frameworks incorporating finger clasps for retention. This type of splint generally is indicated only for wear at night, as a retention appliance after orthodontic treatment or after surgical procedures (see Fig. 759).

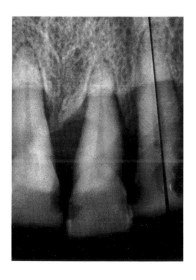
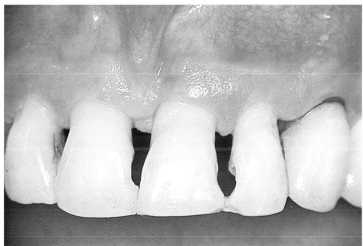
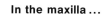

In the maxilla ...

776 Composite resin splint with tooth preparation
This 38-year-old female was adamant in her wish that the almost hopelessly involved maxillary anterior teeth be maintained.

Following initial therapy, the highly mobile teeth 11, 21 and 22 were stabilized by removing the old Class III resins and using the cavity preparations for retention of acid-etch resin splint. The splint remained in place until the definitive prognosis for the entire dentition could be determined.

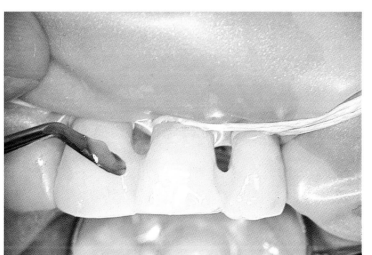

777 Splint application with rubber dam
After etching the cavity margins with phosphoric acid, the cavity preparations and the coronal portion of the interdental spaces were filled with light-cured composite resin, then polished.

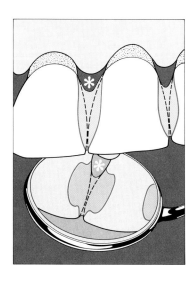
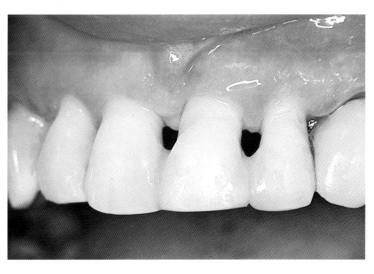

778 3 years later
The interdental spaces were left open beneath the contact areas (∗), which permitted good interdental hygiene using toothpicks and interdental brushes.

Schematic: Red = acid etched areas. Blue = composite resin. The resin is retained by both the acid-etching and by the undercuts of the cavity preparation.

... and in the mandible

779 Disturbing tooth mobility
This 25-year-old female presented with ulcerative gingivoperiodontitis (ANUG) in an interval stage. The radiograph revealed moderate to severe bone loss in the mandibular anterior area.

Teeth 41, 31 and 32 were highly mobile and non-functional. An *intracoronal,* fiber-reinforced semipermanent splint was indicated, to remain in place at least until the treatment planning, definitive prognosis and active therapy could be completed.

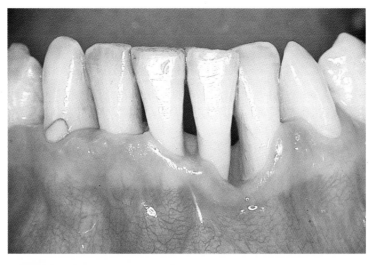

**780 Intracoronal splinting
– Preparation of grooves**
Using a small round diamond, grooves are cut in enamel/dentin ca. 0.7–1.0 mm deep at the level of the interdental contact areas completely around each tooth. The edges of the grooves are rounded off, and a base is placed to protect the pulp wherever the groove extends into dentin.

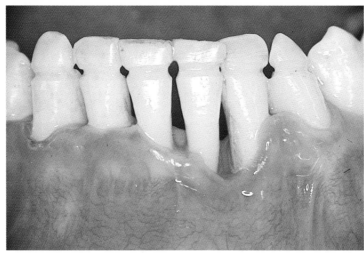

**781 Acid etching –
Application of polyester ligatures**
Two splints, each incorporating three teeth, are to be made. The tear-resistant Kevlar ligature is first coated with resin monomer (right), then applied to the teeth as repeated figure "8s" and tied off.

The work is performed with the rubber dam in place (note floss at the cervical area of each tooth to hold the dam in place) to insure a dry field.

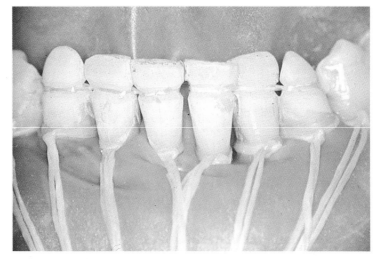

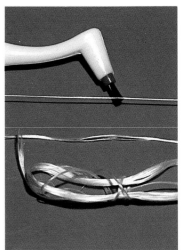

782 Intracoronal splints
The etched and smoothed margins of the grooves (red in schematic) are painted with monomer before filling with light-cured resin (blue).

After smoothing and polishing, the intracoronal resin splint is almost invisible clinically.

The incorporated fibers greatly reduce the danger of resin fracture.

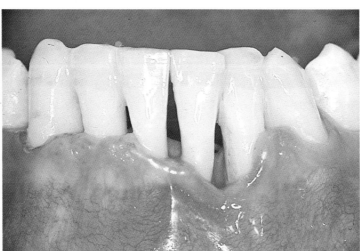

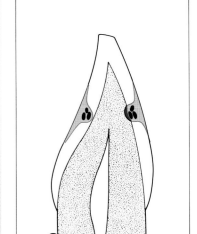

Semipermanent Splinting – Posterior Area

The most common indication for semipermanent splinting in the posterior areas is for interim stabilization of highly mobile teeth subjected to heavy occlusal forces. Such splinting may be necessary before, during or after periodontal therapy, when the long-term prognosis for the mobile teeth has not yet been established.

This sort of "handicraft" temporary splint is inexpensive and easy to fabricate. A popular method involves use of composite resin reinforced with stiff steel wire.

Since composite resin is highly susceptible to abrasion, the dentist may elect to incorporate amalgam or ceramic centric "stops" in the occlusal surface of the splint (Lutz & Leuthard 1978; Lutz et al. 1980).

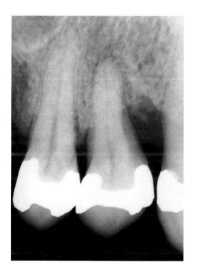
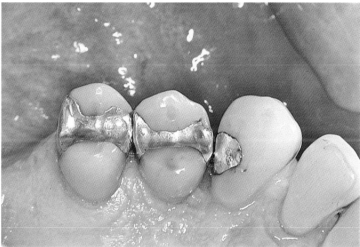

Case 1

783   After initial therapy
A splint is indicated for stabilization of the highly mobile tooth 14 in the interim before definitive planning for the prosthetic reconstruction. The radiograph reveals pronounced bone loss, accounting for the mobility.

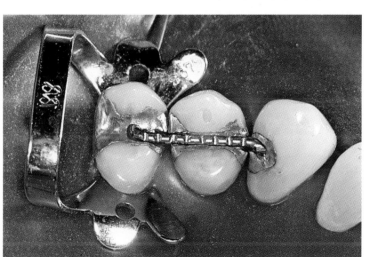

784   Occlusal groove and wire placement
A groove is cut into the occlusal amalgams in teeth 13, 14 and 15, with retentive undercuts. A stiff stainless steel wire (ca. 1 mm dia.) is adapted into the groove for reinforcement.

The grooves are then filled with self-curing acrylic resin, which is subsequently smoothed and polished.

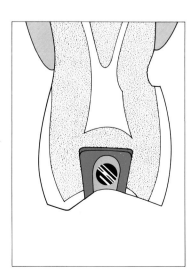
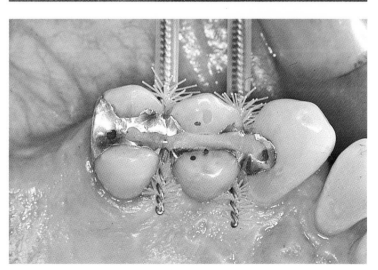

785   Semipermanent splint
It is imperative that the interdental space beneath the splint be left open for cleaning. Here, for example, interdental brushes can be conveniently used.

Schematic: The heavy wire reinforcement (black) is completely surrounded by the composite resin (light blue) and by old amalgam (blue).

Case 2

786   Emergency: Apical abscess with palatal fistula
Virtually hopeless situation for teeth 16 and 17 in a 35-year-old female who is completely dentulous.

The treatment plan involved extraction of 17, with a heroic effort to save the highly mobile 16 by means of endodontic treatment and subsequent resection of the palatal root.

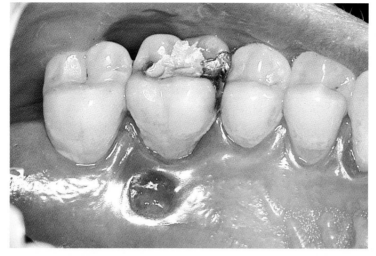
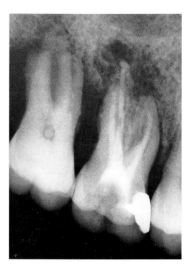

787   Preparation
Following completion of the root canal therapy, the old amalgam restorations were removed from 16, 15 and 14, and a cavity liner was placed in vital teeth 15 and 14.

Cavity margins were acid-etched, and a 1 mm thick stainless steel double-twist wire was adapted. Monomer was then applied to the cavity margins and the entire 3-tooth segment was filled with resin. The wooden wedges insure that the interdental spaces will remain open for hygiene.

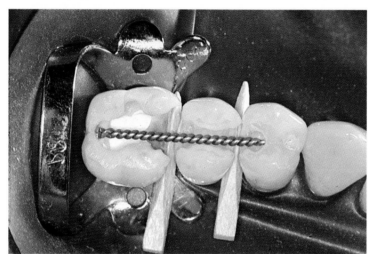

788   Splint complete
The occlusion must be checked and adjusted appropriately.

Diagram: If centric contacts from opposing teeth fall onto the resin splint, and the splint is destined for long-term use, the dentist may elect to put *amalgam "stops"* in the occlusal surface at the contact areas (black arrow).

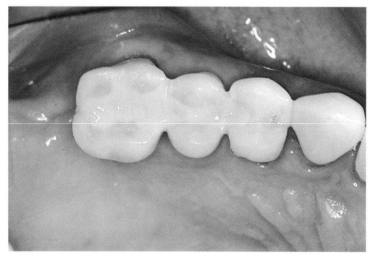
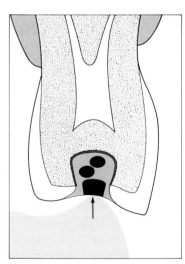

789   Amalgam stops
All of the major occlusal contacts (red marks) of mandibular cusp tips with the splinted unit are either on enamel or on the amalgam stops.

Radiograph: Visible are the remaining buccal roots and the amalgam used in the pulp chamber before resection of the palatal root, one year after treatment.

The definitive treatment planning can now be undertaken.

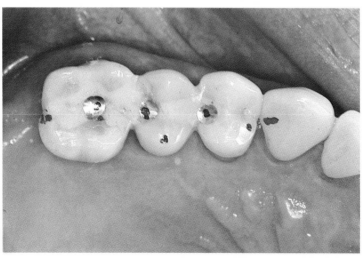
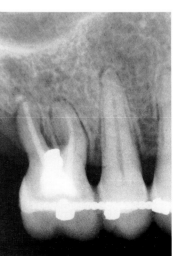

Reconstruction – Prosthodontics

Definitive prosthetic treatment may only begin several months after completion of periodontal therapy, when healing and consolidation have occurred. By this time, the patient's level of motivation is known. The prognosis for each individual abutment tooth can be stated with relative certainty.

The primary goal is to re-establish effective *chewing function.* This does not demand that the patient have 28 teeth, i.e., not every lost tooth must be prosthetically replaced.

Prosthetic planning may be influenced by requirements for maintenance or improvement of *esthetics.*

The *splinting* that is effected by fixed bridgework does not, in and of itself, have any therapeutic advantage. For this reason, splinting *per se* is not included in a prosthetic treatment plan unless there are specific reasons to do so, such as increased tooth mobility that disturbs the patient, or mobility that exhibits increasing severity due to occlusal trauma that is difficult to eliminate.

The insertion of a prosthetic replacement must not be associated with trauma to the gingiva or periodontium. Most important in this regard is that the bridge or denture 1) not promote plaque retention and 2) permit the patient to practice optimum oral hygiene. Consideration must be given to the *characteristics* of different types of prostheses (temporary and definitive):

— *Fixed bridgework*
   Crown margins supragingival; crown contour; interdental
   and sub-pontic areas accessible for hygiene; functional, atraumatic occlusion.

— *Removable prostheses using telescope crowns or precision attachments*
   Telescope crown margins supragingival; attachments accessible for hygiene;
   occlusion functional but atraumatic; major and minor
   connectors should not create plaque-retentive nitches.

— *Cast framework partial dentures*
   Clasps (hold abutments bodily; occlusal rests; no continuous splinting);
   interdental areas accessible for hygiene; major and minor connectors should not
   create plaque-retentive areas; functional but atraumatic occlusion.

Any fixed or removable *temporary* or *definitive* replacement must be planned and executed with regard for its possible effects on periodontal supporting structures. This is particularly important in the periodontitis patient, who often wears some type of temporary appliance throughout the entire treatment and healing phases of therapy.

Fixed Provisional Restoration

Temporary replacements for lost teeth must be "friendly" to the periodontium. This is especially true when the temporary is to be inserted immediately after extraction of hopeless teeth and periodontal surgery. Whenever possible, a fixed temporary should be chosen over a removable one.

A general rule is that extracted teeth should be replaced immediately and that prepared teeth should receive temporary coverage that provides full chewing function.

Usually this type of *immediate temporary* is replaced during the course of healing by a more precise *long-term temporary,* which should resemble the planned definitive replacement as much as possible in terms of tooth position, contour, occlusion and shape of interdental areas.

790   After initial therapy
First appointment: Abutment teeth 13, 11 and 23 are grossly prepared for full coverage restorations, an impression is taken, and individual temporary crowns are seated.

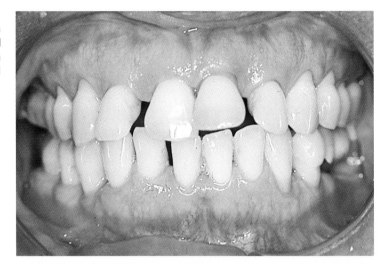

791   Immediately after surgery
Second appointment: Extraction of 12; 21 & 22, pocket elimination around abutment teeth and frenectomy.

Insertion of a heat-cured acrylic temporary bridge prepared in the lab by removing teeth 12; 21, 22 from the study model to simulate the extractions.

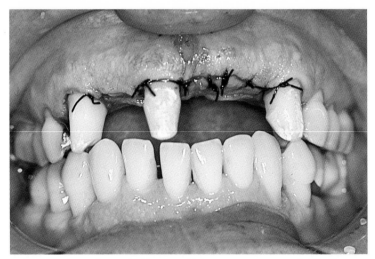

792   Long-term temporary bridge
The acrylic bridge that had been fabricated in the laboratory is adjusted and seated. All crown margins are clearly supragingival (see schematic).

Definitive tooth preparation and construction and seating of the final bridgework can begin only after complete healing of the periodontal surgical areas and the extraction wounds; this is generally a matter of months. The definitive anterior bridge will be of porcelain-fused-to-metal.

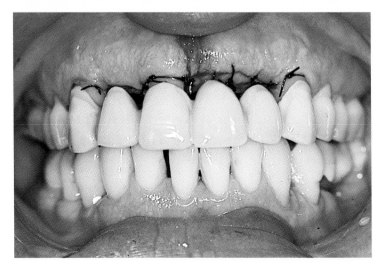
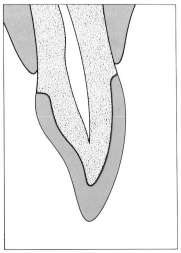

Removable Provisional Appliance

A removable temporary is indicated when the definitive prosthetic treatment is to be a cast framework partial denture or one incorporating telescope crowns, or if only a few abutment teeth remain for anchorage.

The requirements of a definitive removable partial denture should also be fulfilled by the temporary denture: Clasps must hold the abutment tooth bodily, occlusal rests (dental/periodontal support) must prevent apical depression of saddles, the marginal gingiva must not be traumatized by clasps or the denture base.

In order to have an "immediate temporary" ready for insertion after extractions and periodontal surgery, the teeth destined for extraction can be removed from the model in the laboratory and the temporary constructed in advance. A temporary denture made in this way often requires considerable adaptation and adjustment upon insertion, because the postoperative conditions are seldom exactly like those "estimated" in the lab. In many cases it is necessary to reline the denture immediately for good tissue adaptation (e.g., with soft reline material or periodontal dressing).

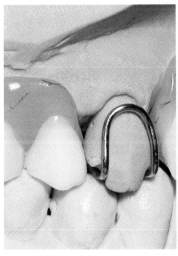
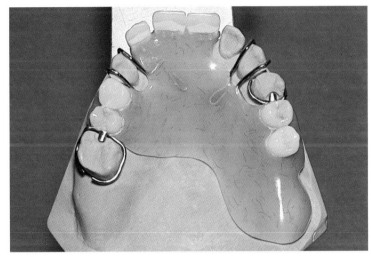

793 Removable maxillary temporary denture on the model
The retentive elements grasp the abutment teeth bodily (left). The cuspids' incisal edges were reduced mesially and distally to provide space for the clasp arms. This was permissible because the treatment plan calls for both cuspids to receive full cast telescope crowns. The ledges created on the cuspids provide dental support for the denture.

Neither the denture base nor the clasps must be permitted to impinge on the marginal gingiva.

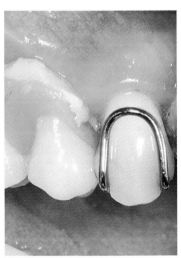
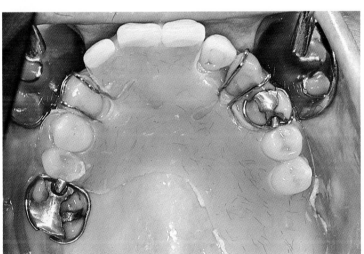

794 Temporary denture after relining
Immediately following the periodontal surgery, which included extractions and flap procedures, the temporary denture is adapted in the mouth and relined using a soft material

The soft reliner also serves as a wound dressing.

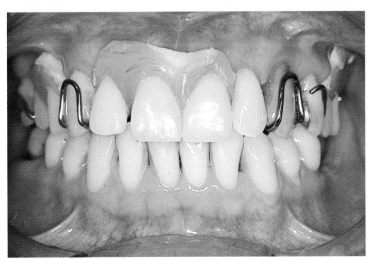

795 Frontal view of relined upper temporary denture
The cuspid clasps are optimum in terms of function, but minimal in terms of esthetics.

Fixed Prosthetics – Crowns, Bridges, Attachments

To protect the periodontal tissues, the following requirements should be met by all crowns, pontics, and crowns with attachments for removable partial dentures:
- *The margins* must be located supragingivally. (The only exception is for esthetics in the anterior area.)
- *The crown* (contour) must not be bulbous in any dimension. Undercontouring is preferable to overcontouring, in terms of plaque retention.
- *A pontic* or *cantilevered unit* should contact the alveolar ridge only at a point or along a line, not an area contact.

- *Interdental areas* must be left open, through-and-through, to permit oral hygiene by means of interdental brushes, perio-aid etc. (compromise in maxillary anterior segment: Phonetics and esthetics).
- *The occlusion* must be free of interferences (see Function/Functional Therapy, p. 271). Occlusal surfaces of replacement teeth should be consistent with the occlusal form of the remaining natural dentition.

796 Crowns – Bridges
For reasons of esthetics, the crown margins of abutment teeth 13, 11 and 23 are located slightly below the gingival margin, but the interdental areas remain open. The tooth preparation at the margin was a shoulder with a beveled edge.

The gingiva remains free of inflammation; there is no bleeding on probing, but stippling is absent and the surface appears "glassy" and friable.

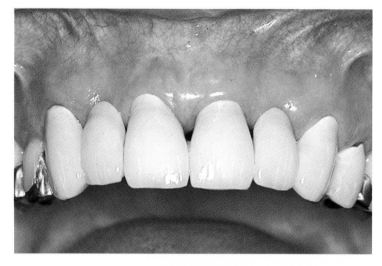
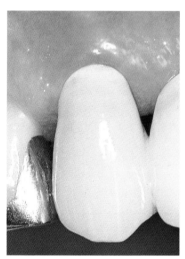

797 Pontic
In the posterior area, interdental areas remain wide open, permitting hygiene by means of interdental brushes. Any contact of the pontic with the alveolar ridge should be along a single line (indicated by the black line); pontics must not encroach on the MGL.

Schematic: The area under the pontic is easily cleaned using Superfloss.

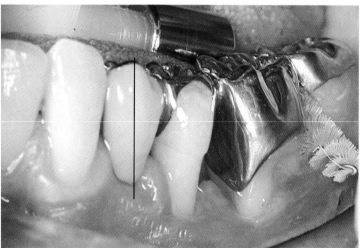
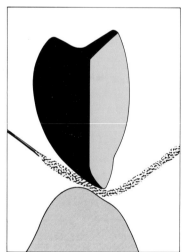

798 Precision attachments
Custom milled precision attachments in the lingual aspects of the porcelain-fused-to-metal crowns on 44 and 43 receive their counterparts from a removable free-end saddle partial denture without clasps.

Margins of the crowns are supragingival and accessible for cleaning. The interdental areas are also accessible, allowing optimal hygiene.

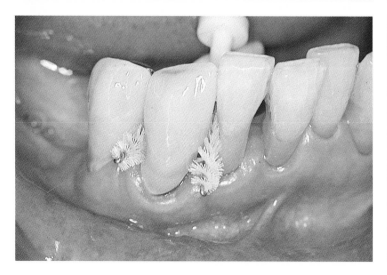
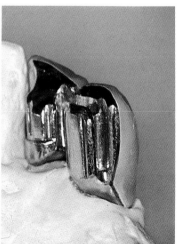

Removable Prosthetics – Construction of Telescopes

Periodontally, the "friendliest" removable partial denture is that based on telescoping crowns, because virtually perfect oral hygiene is enhanced around the single, unsplinted abutment teeth.

A telescope construction can be made to resemble a *removable bridge* or a *partial denture* (Figs. 800 & 801). The decision to use one or the other form will depend on the number and distribution of remaining teeth, as well as esthetic considerations. Problems often arise in anterior and cuspid areas, where abutment teeth must

be severely reduced during tooth preparation in order to preclude having the final restorations be overcontoured.

The margin of the telescope crown should be located *supragingivally*. The denture base and any connectors (e.g., palatal strap, Fig. 801) must not encroach upon gingival margin tissues. The occlusion must be functional, non-interfering and consistent with the patient's mandibular movements.

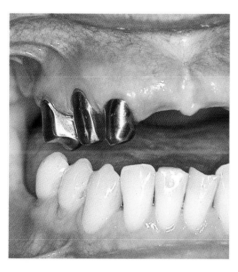
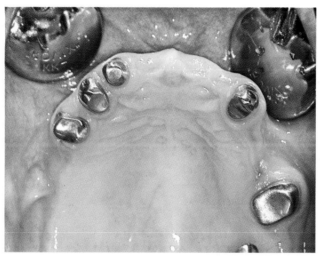

799 Primary anchors for a telescoping construction
Maxillary teeth 14, 13, 12; 23 and 26 received telescope caps 6 months after completion of periodontal therapy (see same case, pp. 68 & 204). All crown margins are located just supragingivally.

The prosthesis that seats onto the primary anchors may be either a removable bridge (A) or a removable partial denture (B). In the 45-year-old female patient depicted here, both types were fabricated and evaluated.

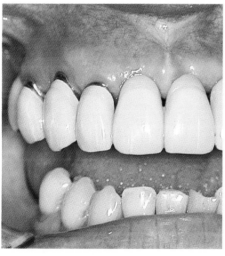
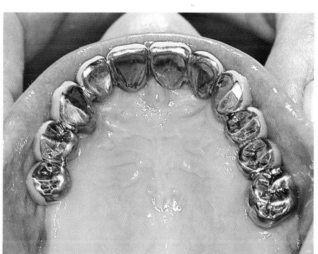

800 A – Telescoping bridge (removable)
The gingiva must not receive any irritation from the bridgework. The patient found the central incisors esthetically objectionable (too long).

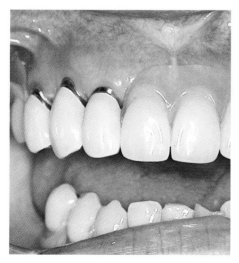
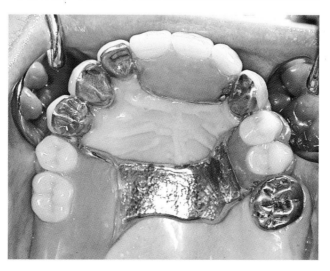

801 B – Telescope partial denture
Using this construction technique, it was possible to improve the esthetics in the anterior region. Neither the saddle nor the palatal strap may encroach on the gingival margin.

When the partial denture is removed, perfect oral hygiene is easy to achieve on the five lone-standing abutments.

The opinion of this patient (not the dentist!) was that the partial denture variation was superior to the removable bridgework (esthetics, stability).

Removable Prosthetics – Cast Framework Partial Denture

The partial denture with a cast framework (usually of chrome-cobalt alloy) is less "friendly" to the periodontal tissues than either fixed bridgework or a telescoping unit. Nevertheless, *socioeconomic circumstances* frequently demand its use.

Bergmann et al. (1983) demonstrated that the useful life of a cast framework partial denture can approach 10 years in a patient with treated periodontitis who performs adequate home care.

Prerequisites for a long and complication-free partial denture lifespan include maintaining proper occlusal relationships (selective grinding), taking perfect impressions using customized trays, maintaining the interdental areas of remaining teeth open for hygiene, and keeping the patient on a regular recall schedule. In addition, the partial denture should be rigid, should have clasps that hold abutment teeth bodily, and should be tooth-born (i.e., through use of occlusal rests). The major connector (palatal strap or lingual bar) should be strong yet not obtrusive.

802 Initial view
All four maxillary anterior teeth are hopelessly involved periodontally (see radiograph). All other teeth can be treated periodontally and retained.

The entire dentition exhibited extremely heavy deposits of plaque and calculus both supra- and subgingivally.

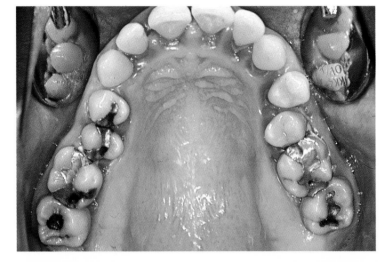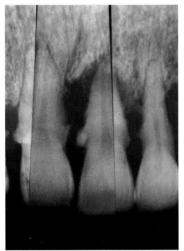

803 After periodontal therapy
The patient was completely informed of the alternatives available for replacement of the anterior teeth, including prognoses for remaining teeth and expected costs. He elected the cast framework partial denture rather than a fixed anterior bridge.

Before taking the final impression, all old restorations were smoothed and polished. The teeth were recontoured according to the requirements of a removable cast framework partial denture (occlusal rests, parallelism, space for minor connectors, retention).

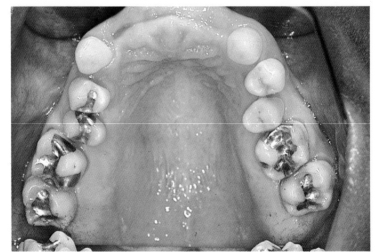

804 Cast framework partial denture
The gingival margins of all remaining teeth are not encroached upon by the major connector or the clasps. The unit does not add new plaque-retentive areas. Clasps and clasp tips are located far from the gingival margin (right).

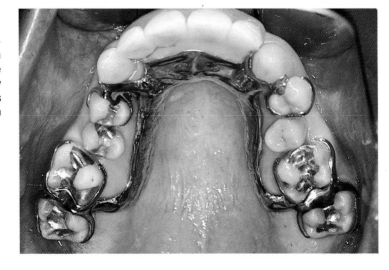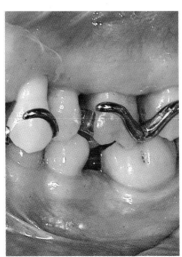

Problems Associated with Prosthetics in the Periodontal Patient

When is no replacement necessary?

Dental caries is diminishing slowly but steadily in all Western countries. Periodontal disease, on the other hand, does not enjoy such a trend as yet. Thus, especially in older persons, teeth are being lost due to periodontal disease and not to caries. This means that most efforts to replace missing teeth will, *a priori,* be through use of periodontally compromised teeth as abutments. The primary goal of *all* dental treatment must be the maintenance of the natural teeth by means of regular *preventive measures* and, when necessary, *early detection* and *treatment of periodontal disease.* Only in this way can the costly prosthetic measures, which more often than not injure the remaining teeth instead of helping maintain their health, be avoided.

If teeth are lost despite preventive and periodontal measures, the question arises: Should the lost teeth be replaced? It was once believed that only a dentition with at least 28 functional teeth could be considered "healthy." This notion has been discarded in recent years. It is generally acknowledged that a dentition whose most distal teeth are bicuspids is wholly acceptable, particularly so in elderly individuals and in persons who have lost molars due to furcation involvement (Helkimo et al. 1978; Käyser 1981; Lang 1982; De Boever 1978, 1984). This concensus may be modified by TMJ problems and the distribution of remaining teeth in an arch.

Possibilities and limits of fixed prosthodontics

When several teeth are lost, especially in the anterior, cuspid and bicuspid regions, function becomes severely compromised. Esthetic problems also occur. In such cases, prosthetic treatment borders on mandatory.

When planning fixed bridgework for a periodontally compromised dentition, some old dogmas have to be ignored. For example, the classical "Ante's Law" (*Ante* 1926, 1936, 1938) has been discarded in light of more recent investigations. *Ante's* concept was that a fixed bridge is indicated only if the periodontal support (root surface anchored in bone) of the proposed abutment teeth is at least as extensive as that of the teeth to be replaced. Use of multiple abutments was advocated to satisfy Ante's Law. Although this concept was never supported by any scientific evidence, it nevertheless was propagated for decades and influenced the thinking of many teachers and practitioners (some yet today). The potential for harm appears never to have been considered. For example, preparing a healthy tooth to receive a full crown may lead to loss of vitality; periodontal tissues may be injured by subgingival crown margins; plaque accumulation may be enhanced by such unnecessary "splinting."

The clinical investigations by the Gothenburg school (Nyman & Lindhe 1976; Nyman & Ericsson 1982) clearly demonstrated that extensive fixed bridgework seated on only a few periodontally compromised but healthy abutment teeth can remain fully functional for many years. The prerequisites for this type of treatment, however, must be fulfilled:

1. Periodontal disease must have been successfully treated
2. The patient must practice optimum oral hygiene
3. The fixed bridge must be periodontally "friendly"
4. The recall interval must be short (see Maintenance Therapy – Recall, p. 267).

The limitations of fixed bridgework are certainly reached when only 3–5 teeth remain as potential abutments. Of course, "heroic" bridgework may be attempted, but little is known about the prognosis for such constructions, or about the occlusal relationships required by them.

The Gothenburg school recommends "freedom in centric" to enhance periodontal health of compromised abutment teeth, as well as bilateral equilibration (i.e., balancing side contact, as in full denture prosthetics). On the other hand, De Boever (1984) warns against balancing side contact for functional reasons, stating that dysfunctional loading of the TMJ and parafunctions may result.

Removable replacement

It is without doubt preferable, in late stage periodontitis, to use the few remaining teeth as abutments for a removable partial denture (Geering & Kundert 1985) utilizing telescope crowns, stud retainers and interdental bars. This type of treatment makes plaque control much easier for the patient.

In patients who can only be treated palliatively (see Treatment Planning, p. 103), and in those for whom financial considerations play a major role in a final decision, the cast framework partial denture may be the option of choice.

The patient's own desires should never be exceeded ("overtreatment"). If a patient with advanced periodontal disease desires or is willing to accept a full denture, this option should not be kept from him.

Conclusion – Periodontology, quo vadis?

The evolution of knowledge in periodontology has moved forward rapidly in recent years. Critical consideration of this progress, however, reveals that significant problems associated with periodontitis and its treatment remain unsolved. Nevertheless, today we do have at our disposal *scientifically supported* and *clinically proven* treatment concepts with which the disease can be effectively prevented or treated.

But we are still a long, long way from our ultimate goals of true causal prevention and therapy: Immunization against the disease and *Restitutio ad integrum* after periodontal therapy. The paragraphs that follow relate how the profession of periodontics stands today, and consider which problems urgently require solutions in the immediate future.

State of knowledge – today and tomorrow

Etiology/disease types:
The microbial etiology of gingivitis was proven in 1965 (Löe et al.). A specific periodontopathic flora consisting primarily of *gram negative anaerobes* (e.g., Bacteroides species) appears to play an important role in the progression of periodontitis.

The *invasion* of periodontal tissues by microorganisms – typical for any infection – has been unequivocally demonstrated, but *no specific microorganism* fulfills the classic Koch's postulates as *sole* cause of the infectious disease. Socransky (1977) therefore modified and redefined the postulates specifically for periodontitis as a "chronic" local (opportunistic) infection.

Three types of periodontitis are acknowledged today (AP, RPP, LJP), based on their differing clinical courses in the permanent dentition and differences in the microbial colonization of the pockets. A prepubertal form of periodontitis is known, but it is exceedingly rare. Knowledge of its etiology and pathogenesis is wholly lacking; treatment of this disease process is seldom successful.

All types of periodontitis in the permanent dentition traverse extended periods of inactivity or quiescence, which are occasionally interrupted by periods of activity (exudate, pus) that are relatively short. This *cyclical course* of the disease appears to be due either to the pocket flora, which may undergo a change to a more virulent mixture of microorganisms, or to reduced host defense (immune status).

Pathogenesis:
The enormous importance of the immune status of an individual is undisputed. In terms of the pathogenesis of periodontitis, the concept of *host response* as one of the most important determining factors in susceptibility and disease progression is being acknowledged. Extreme clinical examples such as resistance to periodontitis despite long-standing massive gingivitis, or the dramatically rapid destruction of periodontal tissues in some individuals with systemic disorders characterized by reduced immune status (e.g., Chediak-Higashi syndrome) support this concept. Locally inadequate host resistance may represent the oft cited *Locus minoris resistentiae.*

Up until now, only the normal cellular and humoral immune reactions and interactions that occur everywhere in the body are partially understood. The recognition of immune deficiencies, e.g., a PMN defect, is in its infancy. It is premature even to discuss future possibilities such as enhancing host response by means of drugs, vaccination, or genetic manipulation.

Diagnosis – Prognosis:
Throughout past decades, clinical observations, diagnostic measurements (probing depths, indices) and radiographs provided the practitioner with an overview of the *momentary* condition of the patient's periodontium. These were *static* measurements, but the experienced clinician was often able to use such findings to predict the course of disease, its dynamics and a reasonable prognosis.

By evaluating the tendency to hemorrhage (e.g., PBI), the practitioner today attempts to determine the *activity* of a lesion at the time of the examination, because pocket activity is a critical factor in disease prognosis. Scientists continue to search for methods that will make it possible to measure current and future disease dynamics. Microscopic (morphologic) and microbiologic (culturing, metabolic studies) *examination of pocket flora* may represent a first step in this direction.

Therapy:
In earlier times, it was primarily the *symptoms* of periodontitis that were treated. The goal was radical elimination of the periodontal pocket; the means were gingivectomy, flap procedures, apical repositioning and osseous surgery. These *resective methods* were often successful, because by eliminating a pocket one also eliminated the pathogenic pocket microflora. The disadvantages were the massive sacrifice of periodontal tissues, lack of regeneration, clinically elongated teeth, cervical hypersensitivity, as well as problems of esthetics, phonetics and root caries.

Today, our treatment is *causal*. The primary goal is total elimination of the subgingival plaque (the "cause"). This is accomplished as always, mechanically using hand instruments, but may be supported in some cases by systemic administration of medicaments. The latter are and should be limited to treatment of severe or life-threatening situations, and not for the elimination of "insignificant" pocket flora.

The most important aspect of today's modern concept of periodontal therapy remains the mechanical cleansing of affected root surfaces, i.e., removal of endotoxin-containing layers of cementum. Without this, no regeneration of periodontal tissues can be expected. Treatment of the root surface can be accomplished "closed" (scaling, root planing) or "open," with direct vision (modified Widman procedure, flap surgery). Which treatment modality is selected depends less upon the diagnosis than upon the morphologic/anatomic circumstances such as localization and access to the pockets, technical difficulties and the dexterity of the practitioner.

Regeneration after periodontal therapy usually occurs in the form of a long junctional epithelium with epithelial attachment, although a connective tissue attachment with formation of new cementum and new collagen fibers would be preferable. Recent efforts to "condition" the root surface, e. g., by application of citric acid (pH 1), are targeted toward promoting such a connective tissue regeneration. Experiments are also being performed to prevent the downgrowth of epithelium, which seems to hinder the formation of new connective tissue attachment. For example, millipore filters have been used to maintain planed root surfaces free of epithelium for a long enough time to permit proliferation of PDL connective tissue cells.

The regeneration of bone in infrabony pockets can be enhanced in some cases by implanting or transplanting various materials. To date, however, it has been difficult to predict the outcome of such procedures, and successes have been of limited magnitude. Furthermore, osseous regeneration often occurs spontaneously after root planing and debridement.

Maintenance therapy, recall:
If periodontal healing occurs with formation of a long junctional epithelium, reinfection and recurrence of pocket formation must be permanently prevented by rigorous mechanical plaque control by the patient (home care) and by the professional dental team. In special cases, topical agents (e.g., chlorhexidine) may provide plaque control for a limited time, but a routinely applicable "chemical toothbrush" is unlikely to become available for general use in the near future.

Functional treatment:
Functional disturbances can lead to increased tooth mobility, which can be alleviated by selective occlusal grinding or "camouflaged" by splinting. The term functional therapy signifies treatment of the traumatized periodontal ligament, but *not treatment of periodontitis.*

Reconstruction, splinting:
Consideration of the patient's periodontal condition must become a routine part of prosthetic planning. Recent research has led to the rejection of old dogma (e.g., Ante's Law). Principles of prosthetic construction and occlusion have become simpler today (long centric, cuspid guidance). Periodontal pretreatment and follow-up (recall) are as important for the prosthetic patient as the particular prosthetic solution itself.

"Supply and Demand"

Epidemiology, need for treatment:
The very high prevalence of periodontitis in adults in Western industrialized countries, and the ever-increasing life expectancy will make it impossible to treat all patients who need treatment, using the methods available to us today. There are simply too few practitioners trained in periodontics to accomplish such a task.

Even a healthy patient requires 1 hour of a professional's time each year just for *preventive measures.*

●

A patient who has been treated for periodontitis should be seen 3–4 times per year...

> "... die ich rief, die Geister,
> werd ich nun nicht los"!

> "... these ghosts I summoned,
> will I never be free of them...!"
> Johann Goethe (*The Sorcerer's Apprentice*)

Without qualified auxiliary personnel (DH), it would be impossible even to provide sufficient *supervision.*

●

In 1978, the World Health Organization (Technical Report Series 621) projected that treatment for simple gingivitis requires approximately 1 hour per patient, early periodontitis, 3 hours; moderate periodontitis, 5 hours and advanced periodontitis, 7 hours. These are conservative estimates, and both Europe and North America have over 300 million inhabitants.

When one considers that an advanced case of periodontitis demands many times this number of treatment hours for restorative and reconstructive dentistry, it becomes absolutely clear that the only way to approach the public health problem is via *prevention in healthy individuals* and *early detection and treatment in persons with disease.* For this, we do not require any new treatment concepts; those we already possess are wholly adequate!

"The road away from reparative, towards preventive..."

It is quite true that preventive measures are expensive but these costs are tiny in comparison to the grotesque fees associated with periodontal and reconstructive treatment in an advanced case of disease. In the future, not only the treatment *provider* but also the treatment *recipient* and especially the treatment *payer* should ponder these facts.

Acknowledgements for Figures

The following individuals generously provided *illustrative material* for this book. The Figures are listed by number, with L and R to indicate their exact locations.

All *histological sections,* except those acknowledged below, were graciously provided by Dr. A. Kallenberger, Department of Histology, Dental Institute, University of Basle, Switzerland.

Diagrams and illustrations were prepared by Mr. Struchen & Partners in the Atelier for Scientific Illustrations, Zurich, Switzerland, from drafts prepared by co-author H. F. Wolf.

All Figures not listed below derived from the collections of the authors, their departments and private practices.

The authors used NIKON cameras and the MEDICAL NIKKOR lens for all *intraoral color photography.* Other NIKON lenses of 25–200 mm focal distance were used for photographing objects, and for reproductions.

Universities/Institutes

Dental Institute, University of Basle, Switzerland

Prof. B. Maeglin, Department of Stomatology and Oral Surgery:
111 R, 113 R, 115, 116 R, 117 L, 117 R

and his coworker:
Dr. C. Bassetti,
296, 297

Clinics for Dental Medicine, University of Berne, Switzerland

Prof. H. Graf, Department of Periodontology:
724 L, 724 R, 725 L, 725 R, 726 L, 726 R; 728 R, 752 L, 752 R

Prof. N. P. Lang, Department of Crown and Bridge Prosthetics:
13 R, 15, 16 L, 118, 219, 378 L, 767 R

Dental Institute, University of Geneva, Switzerland

Prof. G. Cimasoni, Department of Periodontology:
26 R, 214, 586 L, 587 L, 588 L

Prof. J.-M. Meyer, Department of Dental Materials:
272 L; 300 (background)

University of Pennsylvania, Philadelphia

Prof. M. A. Listgarten, Center of Oral Health Research:
24 R, 25 L, 25 R, 27 L

Dental Institute, University of Zurich, Switzerland

Prof. B. Guggenheim, Department of Oral Microbiology and General Immunology:
29 L, 29 R, 30 R, 31 L, 31 R, 32, 40, 41, 43, 44

Prof. H. R. Mühlemann, Department of Cariology, Periodontology and Preventive Oral Medicine:
4 R, 112 L, 112 R, 114 R

and his coworkers:

Prof. F. Lutz:
36 L, 724 R

Dr. A. Bachmann:
441, 442, 443

Dr. W. H. Mörmann:
270 L, 271 L, 645, 646, 647, 679 R, 680 R, 681 R

Dr. U. P. Saxer:
194, 196

Dr. Ch. Schweizer-Hirt:
270 R, 271 R, 273 L, 274 L

Prof. H. E. Schroeder, Department of Oral Structural Biology:
10 L, 10 R, 11 R, 14 L, 33 R, 50, 616

Prof. P. Stöckli, Department of Orthodontics:
757 L, 757 R, 758 L, 759 L, 759 R, 760 L, 760 R, 761 L, 761 R, 762 L, 762 R, 763, 764 L, 764 R, 765, 766, 768, 769

Private practitioners

Dr. M. Ebneter, Zurich
205

Dr. M. Leu, Zurich
388, 389, 798 L, 798 R

Dr. F. Wolgensinger, Kilchberg/ZH
3 L

References

This list contains only those citations relating directly to the procedures and problems discussed in this book.

References preceded by an asterisk (*) are not cited in the text, but provide additional information. This list is by no means offered as a complete literature review.

At the end of the References section are listed numerous *textbooks* and the most relevant *periodicals* that are recommended for further study of periodontology.

A

* **Addy, M., Dowell, P.:** Dentine hypersensitivity – A review. II. Clinical and in vitro evaluation of treatment agents. J. Clin. Periodont. 10: 351, 1983

Ainamo, J.: Relationships between malalignment of the teeth and periodontal disease. Scand. J. Dent. Res. 80: 104, 1972

Ainamo, J., Bay, J.: Problems and proposals for recording gingivitis and plaque. Int. Dent. J. 25: 229, 1975

Ainamo, A., Ainamo, J., Poikkeus, R.: Continuous widening of the band of attached gingiva from 23 to 65 years of age. J. Periodont. Res. 16: 595, 1981

* **Allenspach-Petrzilka, G. E., Guggenheim, B.:** Bacteroides melaninogenicus ss intermedius invades rat gingival tissue. J. Periodont. Res. 17: 456, 1982

Allenspach-Petrzilka, G. E., Guggenheim, B.: Bacterial invasion of the periodontium; an important factor in the pathogenesis of periodontitis. J. Clin. Periodont. 10: 609, 1983

Ante, I. H.: The fundamental principles of abutments. Thesis. Mich. St. Dent. Soc. Bull. 8: 14, 1926

Ante, I. H.: Abutments. J. Canad. Dent. Ass. 2: 249, 1936

Ante, I. H.: The fundamental principles, design and construction of bridge prosthesis. J. Canad. Dent. Ass. 10: 1, 1938

Armitage, G. C., Svanberg, G. K., Löe, H.: Microscopic evaluation of clinical measurements of connective tissue attachment levels. J. Clin. Periodont. 4: 172, 1977

Ash, M. M., Ramfjord, S. P.: An Introduction to Functional Occlusion. Saunders, Philadelphia 1982

Atkinson, D. R., Cobb, Ch. M., Killoy, W. J.: The effect of an air-powder abrasive system on in vitro root surfaces. J. Periodont. 55: 13, 1984

Axelsson, P., Lindhe, J.: The effect of a plaque control program on gingivitis and dental caries in school children. J. Dent. Res., spec. issue C 56: C 142, 1977

Axelsson, P., Lindhe, J.: Effect of controlled oral hygiene procedures on caries and periodontal disease in adults. Results after 6 years. J. Clin. Periodont. 8: 239, 1981a

Axelsson, P., Lindhe, J.: The significance of maintenance care in the treatment of periodontal disease. J. Clin. Periodont. 8: 281, 1981b

Axelsson, P.: Periodontal diseases. Can they be prevented? Dtsch. zahnärztl. Z. 37: 540, 1982

B

* **Badersten, A., Nilvéus, R., Egelberg, J.:** Effect of nonsurgical periodontal therapy. I. Moderately advanced periodontitis. J. Clin. Periodont. 8: 57, 1981

Bainton, D. F.: The cells of inflammation: a general view. In: Weissmann, G.: The Cell Biology of Inflammation. Elsevier/North-Holland. Biomedical Press, Amsterdam 1980

* **Baiorunos, J. R., Robbins, F. E.:** Root demineralization as a new-attachment procedure: A review of the literature. J. West. Soc. Periodont., Periodont. Abstr. 28/3: 84, 1980

Barrington, E. P.: An overview of periodontal surgical procedures, part II. J. Periodont. 52: 518, 1981

Bass, C. C.: An effective method of personal oral hygiene, part II. J. La. Med. Soc. 106: 100, 1954

Bassetti, C., Kallenberger, A.: The influence of chlorhexidine rinsing on the healing of oral mucosa and osseous lesions. A histomorphometric study on experimental animals. J. Clin. Periodont. 7: 443, 1980

Bauer, A., Gutowski, A.: Gnathologie. Einführung in Theorie und Praxis. Quintessenz, Berlin 1975

* **Bell, L. A., Valluzzo, Th. A., Garnick, J. J., Pennel, B. M.:** The presence of "creeping attachment" in human gingiva. J. Periodont. 49: 513, 1978

Bergmann, B., Hugoson, A., Olsson, C.: Caries, periodontal and prosthetic findings in patients with removable partial dentures. A ten year longitudinal study. J. Prosth. Dent. 48: 506, 1982

Bernimoulin, J.-P., Lange, D. E.: Freie Gingivatransplantate – klinische Aspekte und Zytologie ihrer Einheilung. Dtsch. zahnärztl. Z. 27: 357, 1972

Bernimoulin, J.-P.: Deckung gingivaler Rezessionen mit koronaler Verschiebungsplastik. Dtsch. zahnärztl. Z. 28: 1222, 1973

Bernimoulin, J.-P., Lüscher, B., Mühlemann, H. R.: Coronally repositioned periodontal flap. J. Clin. Periodont. 2: 1, 1975

Bernimoulin, J.-P., Curilović, Z.: Gingival recession and tooth mobility. J. Clin. Periodont. 4: 107, 1977

Björn, H.: Free transplantations of gingiva propria. Symposium in Periodontology in Malmö. Odont. Revy 14: 323, 1963

* **Bössmann, K.:** In-vitro Experimente zur Plaquebildung. Dtsch. zahnärztl. Z. 34: 437, 1979

*Bowers, G. M., Schallhorn, R. G., Mellonig, J. T.: Histologic evaluation of new attachment in human intrabony defects. A literature review. J. Periodont. 53: 509, 1982

Breitenmoser, J. Mörmann, W., Mühlemann, H. R.: Zahnfleischverletzung durch Zahnbürstenborsten. Acta parodont., in: Schweiz. Mschr. Zahnheilk. 88: 79/1, 1978

*Bridges, R. B., Kraal, J. H., Huang, L. J. T., Chancellor, M. B.: The effects of tobacco smoke on chemotaxis and glucose metabolism of polymorphnuclear leucocytes. Infect. Immun. 15: 115, 1977

Buckley, L. A.: The relationship between malocclusion and periodontal disease. J. Periodont. 43: 415, 1972

Buckley, L. A.: The relationships between malocclusion, gingival inflammation, plaque and calculus. J. Periodont. 52: 35, 1981

*Budtz-Jörgensen, E.: Bruxism and trauma from occlusion. An experimental model in Macaca monkeys. J. Clin. Periodont. 7: 149, 1980

*Budtz-Jörgensen, E.: A 3-month study in monkeys of occlusal dysfunction and stress. Scand. J. Dent. Res. 88: 171, 1980

C

*Caffesse, R. G., Burgett, F. G., Nasjleti, C. E., Castelli, W. A.: Healing of free gingival grafts with and without periosteum. Part. I. Histologic evaluation. J. Periodont. 50: 586, 1979

Carter, H. G., Barnes, G. P.: The gingival bleeding index. J. Periodont. 45: 801, 1974

Caton, J., Nyman, S.: Histometric evaluation of periodontal surgery. I. The modified Widman flap procedure. J. Clin. Periodont. 7: 212, 1980

Caton, J., Nyman, S., Zander, H.: Histometric evaluation of periodontal surgery. II. Connective tissue attachment levels after four regenerative procedures. J. Clin. Periodont. 7: 224, 1980

*Caton, J., Proye, M., Polson, A.: Maintenance of healed periodontal pockets after a single episode of root planing. J. Periodont. 53: 420, 1982

*Cerra, M. B., Killoy, W. J.: The effect of sodium bicarbonate and hydrogen peroxide on the microbial flora of periodontal pockets. A preliminary report. J. Periodont. 53: 599, 1982

Chaikin, R. W.: Elements of Surgical Treatment in the Delivery of Periodontal Therapy. Quintessenz, Berlin 1977

*Choung Pyoung, Ch., Nisengard, R. J., Slots, J., Genco, R. J.: Bacterial IgG and IgM antibody titers in acute necrotizing ulcerative gingivitis. J. Periodont. 54: 557, 1983

*Ciancio, S.: Chemotherapeutics in periodontics. Dent. Clin. N. Amer. 24: 813, 1980

*Cimasoni, G.: Mechanisms of soft tissue destruction in periodontal disease. J. Clin. Periodont. 7: 332, 1980

Cimasoni, G.: Crevicular Fluid Updated. Karger, Basel 1983

Cohen, B.: Morphological factors in the pathogenesis of periodontal disease. Brit. Dent. J. 107: 31, 1959

Cohen, B.: A study of the periodontal epithelium. Brit. Dent. J. 112: 55, 1962

*Cole, R. T., Crigger, M., Bogle, G., Egelberg, J., Selvig, K. A.: Connective tissue regeneration to periodontally diseased teeth. A histological study. J. Periodont. Res. 15: 1, 1980

Cole, R., Nilvéus, R., Ainamo, J., Bogle, G., Crigger, M., Egelberg, J.: Pilot clinical studies on the effect of topical citric acid application on healing after replaced periodontal flap surgery. J. Periodont. Res. 16: 117, 1981

*Coverly, L., Toto, P., Gargiulo, A.: Osseous coagulum: A histologic evaluation. J. Periodont. 46: 596, 1975

Curilović, Z.: Die Epidemiologie parodontaler Erkrankungen bei Schweizer Jugendlichen und prognostische Konsequenzen. Habilitationsschrift (Thesis), Zürich 1977

Curilović, Z., Mazor, Z., Berchtold, H.: Gingivitis in Zurich school children. A re-examination after 20 years. Helv. Odont. Acta in: Schweiz. Mschr. Zahnheilk. 87: 801/41, 1977

D

*Davenport, R. H., Simpson, D. M., Hassell, T. M.: Histometric comparison of active and inactive lesions of advanced periodontitis. J. Periodont. 53: 285, 1982

Davies, G. E., Francis, J., Martin A. R., Rose, F. L., Swain, G.: 1:6-di-4-chlorophenyl-diguanidohexane (Hibitane). Laboratory investigation of a new antibacterial agent of high potency. Brit. J. Pharmacol. 9: 192, 1954

Dayoub, M. B.: A new filter for osseous coagulum collection. J. Periodont. 52: 4, 1981

De Boever, J. A.: Prinzipien der prothetischen Versorgung nach systematischer Parodontalbehandlung. Quintessenz H. 11: 101. 1978

De Boever, J. A.: Basis und Grenzen der rationalen Paro-Prothetik. Acta parodont., in: Schweiz. Mschr. Zahnheilk. 94: 355/59, 1984

Dorfmann, H. S., Kennedy, J. E., Bird, W. C.: Longitudinal evaluation of free autogenous gingival grafts. A four-year report. J. Periodont. 53: 349, 1982

*Dowell, P., Addy, M.: Dentine hypersensitivity – A review. I. Aetiology, symptoms and theories of pain production. J. Clin. Periodont. 10: 341, 1983

E

Eaton, K. A., Kieser, J. B., Davies, R. M.: The removal of root surface deposits. J. Clin. Periodont. 12: 141, 1985

Edlan, A., Mejchar, B.: Plastic surgery of the vestibulum in periodontal therapy. Int. Dent. J. 13: 593, 1963

Eichenberger, M.: Zur Frage der Knochenregeneration nach operative Entfernung von verlagerten und retinierten Weisheitszähnen. Diss., Basel 1979

Ellegaard, B., Löe, H.: New attachment of periodontal tissues after treatment of intrabony lesions. J. Periodont. 42: 648, 1971

Emerson, T. G.: Hereditary gingival hyperplasia. Oral. Surg. 19: 1, 1965

Engelberger, Th., Hefti, A., Kallenberger, A., Rateitschak, K. H.: Correlations among papilla bleeding index, other clinical indices and histologically determined inflammation of gingival papilla. J. Clin. Periodont. 10: 579, 1983

*Erpenstein, H.: Die Realisierung der Nachsorge in der Praxis. Dtsch. zahnärztl. Z. 37: 625, 1982

Evian, C. I., Rosenberg, E. S., Listgarten, M. A.: Bacterial variability within diseased periodontal sites. J. Periodont. 53: 595, 1982

F

Feneis, H.: Gefüge und Funktion des normalen Zahnfleischgewebes. Dtsch. zahnärztl. Z. 7: 467, 1952

*Fesseler, A., Poksawad, N.: Über die Zuverlässigkeit dreier Mundhygiene-Indizes unter dem Einfluß verschiedener Plaque-Färbungen. Dtsch. zahnärztl. Z. 37: 572, 1982

*Fesseler, A.: Die Effektivität der medikamentösen Behandlung bei Parodontalbehandlungen. Dtsch. zahnärztl. Z. 38: 829, 1983

Flores de Jacoby, L., Sluka, H., Preusse, G.: Über die Verwendung von Bindegewebe des Gaumens und Trikalziumphosphat (TCP) zur Knochenbildung sowie der „Swaging-Methode" im Bereich des Parodontalknochens. Dtsch. zahnärztl. Z. 36: 322, 1979

*Flores de Jacoby, L., Lobeck, Chr.: Die Auswirkung kontrollierter, systematischer Mundhygiene auf entzündliche Parodontalerkrankungen Erwachsener. Dtsch. zahnärztl. Z. 36: 414, 1981

*Frank, R. M., Voegel, J. C.: Bacterial bone resorption in advanced cases of human periodontitis. J. Periodont. Res. 13: 251, 1978

Frank, R. M.: Bacterial penetration in the apical pocket wall of advanced human periodontitis. J. Periodont. Res. 15: 563, 1980

*Frank, R. M., Fiore-Donno, G., Cimasoni, G.: Cementogenesis and soft tissue attachment after citric acid treatment in a human. J. Periodont. 54: 389, 1983

Fröhlich, F.: Die okklusionsbedingten Schmerzen im Kiefergesichtsbereich. Schweiz. Mschr. Zahnheilk. 76: 764, 1966

*Froum, S. J., Kushner, L., Stahl, S. S.: Healing responses of human intraosseous lesions following the use of debridement, grafting and citric acid root treatment. I. Clinical and histologic observations six months postsurgery. J. Periodont. 54: 67, 1983

G

Galler, C., Selipsky, H., Phillips, C., Ammons, W. F.: The effect of splinting on tooth mobility. II. After osseous surgery. J. Clin. Periodont. 6: 317, 1979

Geering, A. H., Lang, N. P.: Die Michigan-Schiene, ein diagnostisches und therapeutisches Hilfsmittel bei Funktionsstörungen im Kausystem. I. Herstellung im Artikulator und Eingliederung am Patienten. Schweiz. Mschr. Zahnheilk. 88: 32, 1978

Geering, A. F., Kundert, M.: Atlas der Total- und Hybridprothetik, Thieme, Stuttgart 1985, im Druck

Geiger, A. M., Wassermann, B. H., Turgeon, L. R.: Relationship of occlusion and periodontal disease. Part VI. Relation of anterior overjet and overbite to periodontal destruction and gingival inflammation. J. Periodont. 44: 150, 1973

Geiger, A. M., Wassermann, B. H., Turgeon, L. R.: Relationship of occlusion and periodontal disease. Part VII. Relationship of crowding and spacing to periodontal destruction and gingival inflammation. J. Periodont. 45: 43, 1974

Genco, R. J., Taichmann, N. A., Sadowski, C. A.: Precipitating antibodies to Actinobacillis actinomycetemcomitans in localized juvenile periodontitis. Ann. Meet. AADR, Abstr. 246, Los Angeles 1980

*****Genco, R. J.:** Antibiotics in the treatment of human periodontal diseases. J. Periodont. 52: 545, 1981

Genco, R. J. Slots, J.: Host responses in periodontal diseases. J. Dent. Res. 63: 441, 1984

Germann, M.: Eine einfache Methode zur Quasi-Standardisierung der Parodontalfotografie. Parodontologie 25: 16, 1971

Gillett, R., Johnson, N. W.: Bacterial invasion of the periodontium in a case of juvenile periodontitis. J. Clin. Periodont. 9: 93, 1982

Goldman, H. M., Cohen, D. W.: Periodontal Therapy, 6th ed. Mosby, St. Louis 1980

*****Goodson, J. M., Tanner, A. C. R., Haffajee, A. D., Sornberger, G. C., Socransky, S. S.:** Patterns of progression and regression of advanced destructive periodontal disease. J. Clin. Periodont. 9: 472, 1982

*****Gordon, J. M., Walker, C. B., Murphy, J. C., Goodson, J. M., Socransky, S. S.:** Concentration of tetracycline in human gingival fluid after single doses. J. Clin. Periodont. 8: 117, 1981

Gorman, W. J.: Prevalence and etiology of gingival recession. J. Periodont. 38: 316, 1967

*****Götte, H.:** Zahnbeweglichkeit vor und nach Wurzelkanalbehandlungen an Zähnen mit apikalen Veränderungen. Dtsch. zahnärztl. Z. 34: 461, 1979

*****Graber, G.:** Psychosomatik und Okklusion. In: Schön, F., Singer, F.: Europäische Prothetik heute. Quintessenz, Berlin 1977 (S. 169)

Graf, H.: Bruxism. Dent. Clin. N. Amer. 13/3: 659, 1969

*****Graf, H.:** Physiologie der Zahnbeweglichkeit. Dtsch. zahnärztl. Z. 35: 678, 1980

Graf, H.: Analysis of human jaw movement patterns by graphic computer display. In: Kawamura, Y., Dubner, R.: Oral-facial Sensory and Motor Function. Quintessenz, Berlin 1981 (p. 323)

Grau, P., Lutz, F.: Intrakoronale, durch Polyesterfäden verstärkte, semipermanente Kompositschienen: klinische Erfahrungen nach 4 Jahren. Acta parodont., in: Schweiz. Mschr. Zahnheilk. 92: 83/19, 1982

*****Greene, J. C., Vermillon, J. R.:** Oral hygiene index: a method for classifying oral hygiene status. J. Amer. Dent. Ass. 61: 172, 1960

*****Griffiths, G. S., Addy, M.:** Effects of malalignment of teeth in the anterior segments on plaque accumulation. J. Clin. Periodont. 8: 481, 1981

Grupe, H. E., Warren, R. F.: Repair of gingival defects by a sliding flap operation. J. Periodont. 27: 92, 1956

*****Guggenheim, B.:** Gedanken zur Pathogenese der Parodontopathien. Acta parodont., in: Schweiz. Mschr. Zahnheilk. 91: 529.79, 1981

Guldener, P., Langeland, K.: Endodontologie. Thieme, Stuttgart 1982

H

Hammer, B., Hotz, P.: Nachkontrolle von 1- bis 5jährigen Amalgam-Komposit- und Goldgußfüllungen. Schweiz. Mschr. Zahnheilk. 89: 301, 1979

Hamp, S. E., Nyman, S., Lindhe, J.: Periodontal treatment of multirooted teeth. Results after 5 years. J. Clin. Periodont. 2: 126, 1975

*****Hancock, E. B.:** Determination of periodontal disease activity. J. Periodont. 52: 492, 1981

Haneke, E.: The Papillon-Lefèvre syndrome: Keratosis palmoplantaris with periodontopathy. Hum. Genet 51: 1, 1979

Hansen, G. C.: An epidemiologic investigation of the effect of biologic aging on the breakdown of periodontal tissue. J. Periodont. 44: 269, 1973

*****Harndt, R.:** Beziehungen zwischen Endodont und Parodont. Dtsch. zahnärztl. Z. 34: 453, 1979

Hassell, T. M.: Epilepsy and the Oral Manifestations of Phenytoin Therapy. Karger, Basel 1981

Hefti, A., Widmer, B.: Reduktion des Keimpegels in der Mundhöhle vor zahnärztlichen Behandlungen durch Mundwässer und Mundantiseptika. Acta parodont., in: Schweiz. Mschr. Zahnheilk. 90: 73/1, 1980

Hefti, A., Engelberger, T., Büttner, M.: Gingivitis in Basel school children. Helv. odont. Acta, in: Schweiz. Mschr. Zahnheilk. 91: 1087/25. 1981

Helkimo, E., Carlsson, G. E., Helkimo, M.: Chewing efficiency and state of dentition. Acta Odont. Scand. 36: 33, 1978

*****Herforth, A.:** Der laterale Verschiebelappen – modifizierte Operationstechnik. Dtsch. zahnärztl. Z. 35: 750, 1980

Herrmann, D.: Gingivostomatitis herpetica (Stomatitis aphthosa) bei Erwachsenen. Dtsch. zahnärztl. Z. 27: 870, 1972

Himmel, G. K., Marthaler, Th. M., Rateitschak, K. H., Mühlemann, H. R.: Experimental changes of diurnal periodicity in the physical properties of periodontal structures. Helv. Odont. Acta 1: 16, 1957

*****Hofstetter, H. W., Lang, N. P.:** Metronidazol – ein Antibiotikum für die subgingivale chemische Plaquekontrolle. Acta parodont., in: Schweiz. Mschr. Zahnheilk. 93: 282/44, 1983

Hug, H. U.: Periodontal status and its relationship to variations in tooth position. An analysis of the findings reported in the literature. Helv. Odont. Acta, in: Schweiz. Mschr. Zahnheilk. 92: 1073/11, 1982

*****Hull, P. S.:** Chemical inhibition of plaque. J. Clin. Periodont. 7: 431, 1980

I

Ingerwall, B., Jacobsson, U., Nyman, S.: A clinical study of the relationship between crowding of teeth, plaque and gingival condition. J. Clin. Periodont. 4: 212, 1977

J

Jankelson, B.: Technique for obtaining optimum functional relationship for the natural dentition. Dent. Clin. N. Amer. 4: 131, 1960

Joss, A., Graf, H.: A method for analysis of human mandibular occlusal movement. Helv. Odont. Acta, in: Schweiz. Mschr. Zahnheilk. 89: 1211/41, 1979

K

Käyser, A. F.: Shortened dental arches and oral function. J. Oral Rehabil. 8: 457, 1981

Keyes, P. H., Wright, W. E., Howard, S. A.: The use of phase-contrast microscopy and chemotherapy in the diagnosis and treatment of periodontal lesions – an initial report. I. Quintess. Int. 1, Report 1590: 1, 1978 a

Keyes, P. H., Wright, W. E., Howard, S. A.: The use of phase-contrast microscopy and chemotherapy in the diagnosis and treatment of periodontal lesions – an initial report. II. Quintess. Int. 2, Report 1590: 7, 1978 b

Khatiblou, F. A., Ghodssi, A.: Root surface smoothness or roughness in periodontal treatment. J. Periodont. 54: 365, 1983

King, J. D.: Gingival disease in Dundee. Dent. Rec. 65: 9, 1945

Knight, G. M., Wade, A. B.: The effects of hormonal contraceptives on the human periodontium. J. Periodont. Res. 9: 18, 1974

Knowles, J. W., Burgett, F. G., Nissle, R. R., Shick, R. A., Morrison, E. C., Ramfjord, S. P.: Results of periodontal treatment related to pocket depth and attachment level. Eight years. J. Periodont. 50: 225, 1979

Knowles, J., Burgett, F., Morrison, E., Nissle, R., Ramfjord, S. P.: Comparison of results following three modalities of periodontal therapy related to tooth type and initial pocket depth. J. Clin. Periodont. 7: 32, 1980

Koivuniemi, J., Savoff, K., Rateitschak, K. H.: Gingivitis- und Plaquebefall bei Schulkindern in städtischen und ländlichen Gemeinden. Acta parodont., in: Schweiz. Mschr. Zahnheilk. 90: 682/74, 1980

*****Kraal, J. H., Kenney, E. B.:** The response of polymorphnuclear leukocytes to chemotactic stimulation for smokers and non-smokers. J. Periodont. Res. 14: 383, 1979

*****Krekeler, G., Düker, J., Fabinger, A.:** Der Einfluß von lyophilisiertem Kollagen auf die Heilung der parodontalen Knochentasche. Dtsch. zahnärztl. Z. 35: 758, 1980

*****Krekeler, G., Pelz, K.:** Die juvenile Parodontitis – eine spezifische Infektion? Dtsch. zahnärztl. Z. 38: 928, 1983

*****Kremers, L., Daliemunthe, S. H., Lampert, F.:** Zahnsteinreduktion mit HEDP? Eine klinische Langzeitstudie. Dtsch. zahnärztl. Z. 35: 729, 1980

Krüger, E.: Operationslehre für Zahnärzte. Quintessenz, Berlin 1977

L

Lang, N. P., Löe, H.: The relationship between the width of keratinized gingiva and gingival health. J. Periodont. 43: 623, 1972

Lang, N. P., Cumming, B. R., Löe, H.: Toothbrushing frequency as it relates to plaque development and gingival health. J. Periodont. 44: 396, 1973

*****Lang, N. P.:** Chemische Plaquekontrolle. In Peters, S.: Prophylaxe. Quintessenz, Berlin 1978 (S. 245)

Lang, N. P., Ramseier-Grossmann, K.: Optimal dosage of chlorhexidine digluconate in chemical plaque control when applied by the oral irrigator. J. Clin. Periodont. 8: 189, 1981

Lang, N. P.: Was heißt funktionelle Rekonstruktion im parodontal reduzierten Gebiß? Acta parodont., in: Schweiz. Mschr. Zahnheilk. 92: 365/41, 1982

Lang, N. P., Kiel, R. A., Anderhalden, K.: Clinical and microbiological effects of subgingival restorations with overhanging or clinically perfect margins. J. Clin. Periodont. 10: 563, 1983

Lang, D. E., Schroeder, H. E.: Cytochemistry and ultrastructure of gingival sulcus cells. Helv. Odont. Acta 15: 65, 1971

Lange, D. E.: Parodontologie in der täglichen Praxis. Quintessenz, Berlin 1981

*****Lange, D. E., Plagmann, H.-Ch., Spickenheier, H.:** Experimentelle Studie über zwei Edlan-Mejchar-Operationsmodifikationen im Halbseitenvergleich. Dtsch. zahnärztl. Z. 36: 458, 1981

*****Lange, D. E.:** Mißerfolge bei der Parodontaltherapie durch diagnostische Fehler. Dtsch. zahnärztl. Z. 37: 604, 1982

*****Lekovic, V., Kenney, E. B., Carranza, F. A., Jr., Endres, B.:** The effect of metronidazole on human periodontal disease. A clinical and bacteriological study. J. Periodont. 54: 476, 1983

*****Leu, M.:** Nachsorge parodontalbehandelter Patienten. Dtsch. zahnärztl. Z. 32: 38, 1977

Lindhe, J. Björn, A. L.: Influence of hormonal contraceptives on the gingiva of woman. J. Periodont. Res. 2: 1, 1967

*****Lindhe, J., Socransky, S. S.:** Chemotaxis and vascular permeability produced by human periodontopathic bacteria. J. Periodont. Res. 14: 138, 1979

*****Lindhe, J.:** Treatment of periodontosis/juvenile periodontitis. Abstract, J. Clin. Periodont. 7: 334, 1980

Lindhe, J., Ericsson, J.: The effect of elimination of jiggling forces on periodontally exposed teeth in the dog. J. Periodont. 53: 562, 1982

Lindhe, J., Haffajee, A. D., Socransky, S. S.: Progression of periodontal disease in adult subjects in the absence of periodontal therapy. J. Clin. Periodont. 10: 433, 1983

Lindhe, J.: Textbook of Clinical Periodontology. Munksgaard, Copenhagen 1983

Lindhe, J., Westfelt, E., Nyman, S., Socransky, S. S., Haffajee, A. D.: Long-term effect of surgical/non-surgical treatment of periodontal disease. J. Clin. Periodont. 11: 448, 1984

Listgarten, M. A.: Electron microscopic observations on the bacterial flora of acute necrotizing ulcerative gingivitis. J. Periodont. 36: 328, 1965

Listgarten, M. A., Lewis, D. W.: The distribution of spirochetes in the lesion of acute necrotizing ulcerative gingivitis: an electron microscopic and statistical survey. J. Periodont. 38: 379, 1967

Listgarten, M. A.: Normal development, structure, physiology and repair of gingival epithelium. Oral Sci. Rev. 1: 3, 1972

Listgarten, M. A., Mayo, H. E., Tremblay, R.: Development of dental plaque on epoxy resin crowns in man. A light and electron microscopic study. J. Periodont. 46: 10, 1975

Listgarten, M. A.: Structure of the microbial flora associated with periodontal health and disease in man. A light and electron microscopic study. J. Periodont. 47: 1, 1976a

Listgarten, M. A.: Ultrastructural features of repair following periodontal surgery. In Stahl, S. S.: Periodontal Surgery. Thomas, Springfield/Ill. 1976b (p.189)

*****Listgarten, M. A., Mao, R., Robinson, P. J.:** Periodontal probing and the relationship of the probe tip to periodontal tissue. J. Periodont. 47: 511, 1976

*****Listgarten, M. A., Helldén, L.:** Relative distribution of bacteria at clinically healthy and periodontally diseased sites in humans. J. Clin. Periodont. 5: 115, 1978

Listgarten, M. A., Rosenberg, M. M.: Histological study of repair following new attachment procedures in human periodontal lesions. J. Periodont. 50: 333, 1979

Listgarten, M. A.: Periodontal probing: What does it mean? J. Clin. Periodont. 7: 165, 1980

*****Listgarten, M. A., Lai, C.-H., Evian, C. I.:** Comparative antibody titers to Actinobacillus actinomycetemcomitans in juvenile periodontitis, chronic periodontitis and periodontally health subjects. J. Clin. Periodont. 8: 155, 1981

Listgarten, M. A., Schifter, C. C., Laster, L.: 3-year longitudinal study of the periodontal status of an adult population with gingivitis. J. Clin. Periodont. 12: 225, 1985

Löe, H., Silness, J.: Periodontal, disease in pregnancy. Prevalence and severity. Acta Odont. Scand. 21: 533, 1963

Löe, H., Theilade, E., Jensen, S.: Experimental gingivitis in man. III. The influence of antibiotics on gingival plaque development. J. Periodont. 36: 177, 1965

*****Löe, H.:** Periodontal changes in pregnancy. J. Periodont. 36: 209, 1965

*****Löe, H., Theilade, E., Jensen, S. B., Schiött, C. R.:** Experimental gingivitis in man. J. Periodont. Res. 2: 282, 1967

Löe, H., Schiött, C. R.: The effect of suppression of the oral microflora upon the development of dental plaque and gingivitis. In McHugh, W. D.: Dental Plaque. Livingstone, Edinburgh 1970

Löe, H., Anerud, A., Boysen, H., Smith, M.: The natural history of periodontal disease in man. The degree of periodontal destruction before 40 years of age. J. Periodont. 49: 607, 1978

*****Loesche, W. J., Syed, S. A., Morrison, E. C., Laughon, B. E., Grossman, N. S.:** Treatment of periodontal infections due to anaerobic bacteria with short-term treatment with metronidazole. J. Clin. Periodont. 8: 29, 1981

*****Loesche, W. J., Syed, S. A., Laughon, B. E., Stoll, J.:** The bacteriology of acute necrotizing ulcerative gingivitis. J. Periodont. 53: 223, 1982

Lutz, F., Leuthard, P.: Verschleißfeste MOD-Kompositfüllungen durch Einpolymerisation von zentrischen Stops aus Keramik – 4-Jahres-Resultate. Schweiz. Mschr. Zahnheilk. 88: 739, 1978

Lutz, F., Leuthard, P., Imfeld, T.: Wear-resistant MOD composite restorations with ceramic centric stops - results after four years. Quintess. Int. 5, Report 1878: 1, 1980

M

Magnusson I., Runstad, L., Nyman, S., Lindhe, J.: A long junctional epithelium – A locus minoris resistentiae in plaque infection? J. Clin. Periodont. 10: 333, 1983

*****Marggraf, E.:** Die einzeitige Operationsmethode zur Deckung gingivaler Rezessionen und zur Gingivaextension. Dtsch. zahnärztl. Z. 35: 747, 1980

*****Marggraf, E.:** Vaskuläre Immunkomplexe bei der Parodontitis marginalis profunda. Dtsch. zahnärztl. Z. 37: 680, 1982

Marthaler, Th., M., Engelberger, B., Rateitschak, K. H.: Bone loss in Ramfjord's index: Substitution of selected teeth. Helv. Odont. Acta 15: 121, 1971

Marxer, M. A., Rateitschak, K. H., Hefti, A.: Freies Schleimhauttransplantat – Edlan-Mejchar-Operation. Ein Vergleich. Acta parodont., in: Schweiz. Mschr. Zahnheilk. 92: 75/11, 1982

Massler, M., Schour, J.: The P-M-A-Index of gingivitis. J. Dent. Res. 28: 634, 1949

*** Matter, J., Cimasoni, G.:** Creeping attachment after free gingival grafts. J. Periodont. 47: 574, 1974

Matter, J.: Free gingival graft and coronally repositioned flap. A 2-year follow-up report. J. Clin. Periodont. 6: 437, 1979

Matter, J.: Creeping attachment of free gingival grafts. A five-year follow-up study. J. Periodont. 51: 681, 1980

*** Matter, J.:** Free gingival grafts for the treatment of gingival recession: A review of some techniques. J. Clin. Periodont. 9: 103, 1982

*** Mayer, R.:** Rasterelektronenmikroskopische Untersuchungen von Zahnoberflächen nach manueller Zahnstein- und Konkrementenfernung. Dtsch. zahnärztl. Z. 37: 644, 1982

*** Mellonig, J. T., Bowers, G. M., Cotton, W. R.:** Comparison of bone graft materials. Part II. New bone formation with autografts and allografts. A histological evaluation. J. Periodont. 52: 297, 1981

*** Meyer, G., Krüger, W.:** Eine neue Methode zur rationellen Messung der horizontalen Zahnbeweglichkeit. Dtsch. zahnärztl. Z. 36: 440, 1981

*** Meyer, K., Lie, T.:** Root surface roughness in response to periodontal instrumentation studied by combined use of microroughness measurements and scanning electron microscopy. J. Clin. Periodont. 4: 77, 1977

*** Mierau, H. D., Hering, B.:** Der Turgor in unterschiedlichen Regionen der gesunden Gingiva und Alveolarmukosa. Dtsch. zahnärztl. Z. 36: 317, 1981

*** Mierau, H. D., Spindler, T., Strössenreuther, B.:** Die Wirkung eines Wasserstrahlgerätes auf den Volumenpuls der Gingiva (4. Mitteilung). Dtsch. zahnärztl. Z. 38: 930, 1983

*** Moozeh, M. B., Suit, S. R., Bissada, N. F.:** Tooth mobility measurements following two methods of eliminating nonworking side occlusal interferences. J. Clin. Periodont. 8: 424, 1981

Mörmann, W., Bernimoulin, J. P., Schmid, M. O.: Fluorescein angiography of free gingival autografts. J. Clin. Periodont. 2: 177, 1975

Mörmann, W., Schmid, M. O., Bernimoulin, J. P.: Fluoreszenzangiographische Untersuchung der Blutzirkulation im Mucosa-Spaltlappen bei der Vestibulumplastik nach Edlan und Mejchar. Dtsch. zahnärztl. Z. 31: 560, 1976

Mörmann, W., Lutz, F., Curilović, Z.: Die Bearbeitung von Gold, Keramik und Amalgam mit Composhape®-Diamantschleifern und Proxoshape®-Interdentalfeilen. Quintessenz 8, Referat 6524, Aug. 1983

*** Morrison, E. C., Ramfjord, S. P., Burgett, F. G., Nissle, R. R., Shick, R. A.:** The significance of gingivitis during the maintenance phase of periodontal treatment. J. Periodont. 53: 31, 1982

Mühlemann, H. R.: Das weibliche Parodont unter dem Einfluß geschlechtsspezifischer Hormone. Stoma 3, 1952

Mühlemann, H. R., Herzog, H., Vogel, A.: Occlusal trauma and toothmobility. Schweiz. Mschr. Zahnheilk. 66: 527, 1956

Mühlemann, H. R., Mazor, Z. S.: Gingivitis in Zurich school children. Helv. Odont. Acta 2: 3, 1958

Mühlemann, H. R., Herzog, H.: Tooth mobility and microscopic tissue changes produced by experimental occlusal trauma. Helv. Odont. Acta 5: 33, 1961

*** Mühlemann, H. R.:** Parodontale Gesichtspunkte in der zahnärztlichen Chirurgie. Schweiz. Mschr. Zahnheilk. 73: 106, 1963

Mühlemann, H. R.: Tooth mobility: A review of clinical aspects and research findings. J. Periodont. 38: 686, 1967

Mühlemann, H. R., Son, S.: Gingival sulcus bleeding – a leading symptom in initial gingivitis. Helv. Odont. Acta 15: 107, 1971

Mühlemann, H. R.: Patientenmotivation mit individuellem Intensivprogramm für orale Gesundheit. In Peters, S.: Prophylaxe. Quintessenz, Berlin 1978 (S. 137)

Mühlemann, H. R.: Klinische Innovationen in der präventiven Parodontologie. Acta parodont., in: Schweiz. Mschr. Zahnheilk. 93: 559/87, 1983

Müller-Glauser, W., Schroeder, H. E.: The pocket epithelium: a light- and electron-microscopic study. J. Periodont. 53: 133, 1982

*** Murray, P. A., Patters, M. P.:** Gingival crevice neutrophil function in periodontal lesions. J. Periodont. Res. 15: 463, 1980

*** Mutschelknauss, R.:** Methodisch bedingte Mißerfolge bei der Parodontaltherapie. Dtsch. zahnärztl. Z. 37: 610, 1982

*** Mutschelknauss, R.:** Verschiedene Methoden der Taschentherapie im klinischen Vergleich. Dtsch. zahnärztl. Z. 38: 816, 1983

Mutschelknauss, R., von der Ohe, H.-G.: Behandlung und Prognose der Parodontitis im Bereich von Bi- und Trifurkationen. Dtsch. zahnärztl. Z. 37: 805, 1982

Mutschelknauss, R., von der Ohe, H.-G.: Nachuntersuchungen behandelter Bi- und Trifurkationen bei Parodontitis profunda. Dtsch. zahnärztl. Z. 38: 891, 1983

N

Newman, M. G., Socransky, S. S.: Predominant cultivable microbiota in periodontosis. J. Periodont. Res. 12: 120, 1977

*** Newman, H. N.:** Update on plaque and periodontal disease. J. Clin. Periodont. 7: 251, 1980

*** Nisengard, R. J., Alpert, A. M., Krestow, V.:** Desquamative gingivitis: Immunologic findings. J. Periodont. 49: 27, 1978

*** Noble, R. C., Penny, B. B.:** Comparison of leucocyte count and function in smoking and non-smoking young men. Infect. Immun. 12: 550, 1975

Nyman, S., Lindhe, J.: Prosthetic rehabilitation of patients with advanced periodontal disease. J. Clin. Periodont. 3: 135, 1976

Nyman, S., Lindhe, J., Rosling, B.: Periodontal surgery in plaque-infected dentitions. J. Clin. Periodont. 4: 240, 1977

*** Nyman, S., Lindhe, J., Ericsson, I.:** The effect of progressive tooth mobility on destructive periodontitis in the dog. J. Clin. Periodont. 5: 213, 1978

Nyman, S., Lindhe, J.: A longitudinal study of combined periodontal and prosthetic treatment of patients with advanced periodontal disease. J. Periodont. 50: 163, 1979

*** Nyman, S., Lindhe, J., Karring, T., Rylander, H.:** New attachment following surgical treatment of human periodontal disease. J. Clin. Periodont. 9: 290, 1982

Nyman, S., Gottlow, J., Karring, T., Lindhe, J.: The regenerative potential of the periodontal ligament. An experimental study in the monkey. J. Clin. Periodont. 9: 257, 1982

Nyman, S., Ericsson, J.: The capacity of reduced periodontal tissue to support fixed bridgework. J. Clin. Periodont. 9: 409, 1982

O

O'Leary, T. J. Drake, R. B., Naylor, J. E.: The plaque control record. J. Periodont. 43: 38, 1972

P

Page, R. C., Schroeder, H. E.: Pathogenesis of inflammatory periodontal disease. A summary of current work. Lab. Invest. 33: 235, 1976

*** Page, R. C., Schroeder, H. E.:** Current status of the host response in chronic marginal periodontitis. J. Periodont. 52: 477, 1981

Page, R. C., Schroeder, H. E.: Periodontitis in Man and Other Animals. A Comparative Review. Karger, Basel 1982

*** Page, R. C., Bowen, Altman, L., Vandesteen, E., Ochs, H., Makkenzie, P., Osterberg, S., Engel, D., Williams, B. L.:** Prepubertal periodontitis. I. Definition of a clinical disease entity. J. Periodont. 54: 257, 1983

Page, R. C., Altman, L. C., Ebersole, J. F., Vandesteen, G. E., Dahlberg, W. H., Williams, B. L., Osterberg, S. K.: Rapidly progressive periodontitis. A distinct clinical condition. J. Periodont. 54: 197, 1983

Palenstein-Helderman, W. H. v.: Microbial etiology of periodontal disease. J. Clin. Periodont. 8: 261, 1981

Pankhurst, C. L., Waite, I. M., Hicks, K. A., Allen, Y., Harkness, R. D.: The influence of oral contraceptive therapy on the periodontium – duration of drug therapy. J. Periodont. 52: 617, 1981

*** Perrier, M., Polson, A.:** The effect of progressive and increasing tooth hypermobility on reduced but healthy periodontal supporting tissues. J. Periodont. 53: 152, 1982

Pindborg, J. J., Hjörting-Hansen, E.: Atlas of Diseases of the Jaws. Munksgaard, Copenhagen 1974

Pindborg, J. J.: Manifestations of systemic disorders. In Lindhe, J.: Textbook of Clinical Periodontology. Munksgaard, Copenhagen 1983

*Plagmann, H.-Chr.: Klinische Studien und Langzeitbeobachtungen nach der Deckung von freiliegenden Wurzeloberflächen durch koronale Verschiebeplastik. Dtsch. zahnärztl. Z. 35: 743, 1980

Playfair, J. H. L., Hurn, B. A. L., Schulster, D.: Production of antibodies and binding reagents. Brit. Med. Bull. 30: 42, 1974

Plüss, E. M., Engelberger, P. R., Rateitschak, K. H.: Effect of chlorhexidine on dental plaque formation under periodontal pack. J. Clin. Periodont. 2: 136, 1975

Polson, A. M., Meitner, S. W., Zander, H. A.: Trauma and progression of marginal periodontitis in squirrel monkeys. III. Adaption of interproximal alveolar bone to repetitive injury. J. Periodont. Res. 11: 279, 1976a

Polson, A. M., Meitner, S. W., Zander, H. A.: Trauma and progression of marginal periodontitis in squirrel monkeys. IV. Reversibility of bone loss due to trauma alone and trauma superimposed upon periodontitis. J. Periodont. Res. 11: 290, 1976b

Polson, A. M., Heijl, L. C.: Osseous repair in infrabony periodontal defects. J. Clin. Periodont. 5: 13, 1978

*Polson, A. M., Kantor, M. E., Zander, H. A.: Periodontal repair after reduction of inflammation. J. Periodont. Res. 14: 520, 1979

*Polson, A. M., Caton, J.: Factors influencing periodontal repair and regeneration. J. Periodont. 53: 617, 1982

*Polson, A. M., Adams, R. A., Zander, H. A.: Osseous repair in the presence of active tooth hypermobility. J. Clin. Periodont. 10: 370, 1983

Polson, A. M., Proye, M. P.: Fibrin linkage: A precursor for new attachment. J. Periodont. 54: 141, 1983

Posselt, U.: Studies in the mobility of the human mandible. Acta. Odont. Scand. 10, Suppl. 10: 19, 1952

*Proye, M., Caton, J., Polson, A.: Initial healing of periodontal pockets after a single episode of root planing monitored by controlled probing forces. J. Periodont. 53: 296, 1982

Q

*Quigley, G., Hein, J. W.: Comparative cleansing efficiency of manual and power brushing. J. Amer. Dent. Assoc. 65: 26, 1962

R

Ramfjord, S. P.: Indices for prevalence and incidence of periodontal disease. J. Periodont. 30: 51, 1959

Ramfjord, S. P., Nissle, R. R.: The modified Widman flap. J. Periodont. 45: 601, 1974

Ramfjord, S. P., Knowles, J. W., Nissle, R. R., Burgett, F. G., Shick, R. A.: Results following three modalities of periodontal therapy. J. Periodont. 46: 522, 1975

Ramfjord, S. P.: Present status of the modified Widman flap procedure. J. Periodont. 48: 558, 1977

Ramfjord, S. P., Ash, M. M. Jr.: Significance of occlusion in the etiology and treatment of early, moderate and advanced periodontitis. J. Periodont. 52: 511, 1981

Ramfjord, S. P., Morrison, E. C., Burgett, F. G., Nissle, R. R., Shick, R. A., Zann, G. J., Knowles, J. W.: Oral hygiene and maintenance of periodontal support. J. Periodont. 53: 26, 1982

Ramfjord, S. P., Ash, M. M.: Occlusion, 3rd ed. Saunders, Philadelphia 1983

*Ranney, R. R., Yanni, N. R., Burmeister, J. A., Tew, J. G.: Relationship between attachment loss and precipitating serum antibody to Actinobacillus actinomycetemcomitans in adolescents and young adults having severe periodontal destruction. J. Periodont. 53: 1, 1982

*Rateitschak, K. H.: Mißerfolge in der Paradontalbehandlung. Schweiz. Mschr. Zahnheilk. 87: 861, 1977

Rateitschak, K. H., Egli, U., Fringeli, G.: Recession: A 4-year longitudinal study after free gingival grafts. J. Clin. Periodont. 6: 158, 1979

Rateitschak, K. H.: Indikation, Wert und Unwert der Schienung. Dtsch. zahnärztl. Z. 35: 699, 1980

Rateitschak-Plüss, E. M., Hefti, A., Rateitschak, K. H.: Gingivahyperplasie bei Cyclosporin-A-Medikation. Acta parodont., in: Schweiz. Mschr. Zahnheilk. 93: 57/1, 1983a

Rateitschak-Plüss, E. M., Hefti, A., Lörtscher, R., Thiel, G.: Initial observation that cyclosporin-A induces gingival enlargement in man. J. Clin. Periodont. 10: 237, 1983b

Rateitschak-Plüss, E. M., Schroeder, H. E.: History of periodontitis in a child with Papillon-Lefèvre syndrome. A case report. J. Periodont. 55: 35, 1984

Renggli, H. H.: Auswirkungen subgingivaler approximaler Füllungsränder auf den Entzündungsgrad der benachbarten Gingiva. Habilitationsschrift (Thesis), Zürich 1974

*Renvert, S., Egelberg, J.: Healing after treatment of periodontal intraosseous defects. II. Effect of citric acid conditioning of the root surface. J. Clin. Periodont. 8: 459, 1981

Riethe, P.: Die Quintessenz der Mundhygiene. Quintessenz, Berlin 1974

Ririe, C. M., Crigger, M., Selvig, K. A.: Healing of periodontal connective tissues following surgical wounding and application of citric acid in dogs. J. Periodont. Res. 15: 314, 1980

Robinson, R. W.: Osseous coagulum for bone induction. J. Periodont. 40: 503, 1969

Roitt, J. M., Lehner, Th.: Immunology of Oral Diseases. Blackwell Scientific Publications, Oxford 1980

Rosling, B., Nyman, S., Lindhe, J.: The effect of systemic plaque control on bone regeneration in infrabony pockets. J. Clin. Periodont. 3: 38, 1976a

Rosling, B., Nyman, S., Lindhe, J., Jern, B.: The healing potential of the periodontal tissues following different techniques of periodontal surgery in plaque-free dentitions. A 2-year clinical study. J. Clin. Periodont. 3: 233, 1976b

*Roulet, J. F., Roulet-Mehrens, T. K.: The surface roughness of restorative materials and dental tissues after polishing with prophylaxis and polishing pastes. J. Periodont. 53: 257, 1982

*Rozanis, J., Johnson, R. H., Haq, M. S., Schofield, I. D.: Spiramycin as a selective dental plaque control agent. J. Periodont. Res. 14: 55, 1979

S

Saglie, R., Newman, M. G., Carranza, F. A., Jr., Pattison, G. L.: Bacterial invasion of gingiva in advanced periodontitis in humans. J. Periodont. 53: 217, 1982

Sauerwein, E.: Alterzahnheilkunde, 2. Aufl. Thieme, Stuttgart 1983

Saxén, L.: Juvenile periodontitis. J. Clin. Periodont. 7: 1, 1980

Saxer, U. P., Mühlemann, H. R.: Motivation und Aufklärung. Schweiz. Mschr. Zahnheilk. 85: 905, 1975

Schallhorn, R. G., Hiatt, W. H., Boyce, W.: Iliac transplants in periodontal therapy. J. Periodont. 41: 566, 1970

Schallhorn, R. G.: Postoperative problems associated with iliac transplants. J. Periodont. 43: 3, 1972

*Schallhorn, R. G.: Present status of osseous grafting procedures. J. Periodont. 28: 570, 1977

Schijatschky, M. M.: Lebensbedrohliche Zwischenfälle in der zahnärztlichen Praxis, 3. Aufl. Quintessenz, Berlin 1979

Schmid, M. O., Mörmann, W.: Die subperiostale Vestibulumextension. Acta parodont., in: Schweiz. Mschr. Zahnheilk. 86: 495/13, 1976

Schmid, M. O.: The subperiostal vestibule extension. Literature review, rationale and technique. J. West. Soc. Periodont., Periodont. Abstr. 24: 3, 1976

Schroeder, H. E., Listgarten, M. A.: Fine Structure of the Developing Epithelial Attachment of Human Teeth, 2nd ed. Karger, Basel 1977

Schroeder, H. E.: Orale Strukturbiologie. Entwicklungsgeschichte, Struktur und Funktion normaler Hart- und Weichgewebe der Mundhöhle, 2. Aufl. Thieme, Stuttgart 1982

Schroeder, H. E., Rateitschak-Plüss, E. M.: Focal root resorption lacunae causing retention of subgingival plaque in periodontal pockets. Acta parodont., in: Schweiz. Mschr. Zahnheilk.: 93: 1033/179, 1983

Schroeder, H. E.: Pathobiologie oraler Strukturen: Zähne, Pulpa, Parodont. Karger, Basel 1983

*Schroeder, H. E., Seger, R. A., Keller, H. U., Rateitschak-Plüss, E. M.: Behavior of neutrophilic granulocytes in a case of Papillon-Lefèvre syndrome. J. Clin. Periodont. 10: 618, 1983

*Schwartz, H., Flores de Jacoby, L.: Die Auswirkungen kontrollierter, systematischer Mundhygiene auf entzündliche Parodontalerkrankungen Erwachsener. 2. bakteriologische Studie. Dtsch. zahnärztl. Z. 36: 418, 1981

Schwarz, J. P.: Maschinelle Wurzelglättung. Acta parodont., in: Schweiz. Mschr. Zahnheilk. 93: 592/120, 1983

Schwarz, J. P., Hefti, A., Rateitschak, K. H.: Vergleich der Oberflächenrauhigkeiten des Wurzeldentins nach Bearbeitung mit Diamantschleifkörpern und Handinstrumenten. Acta parodont., in: Schweiz. Mschr. Zahnmed. 94: 343/47, 1984

Schweizer, B., Rateitschak, K. H.: Zur Topographie des Knochenschwundes und der Zahnfleischtaschen bei Parodontitis. Acta parodont., in: Schweiz. Mschr. Zahnheilk. 82: 1075/101, 1972

Schweizer, Ch.: Erosion und Abrasion des Schmelzes. Eine experimentelle Studie. Schweiz. Mschr. Zahnheilk. 88: 497, 1978

*****Schwenzer, N.:** Die medikamentöse Unterstützung bei zahnärztlich-chirurgischen Eingriffen. Prax. Zahnheilk. 31, Verlegerdienst München 1981

Scott-Metsger, D., Driskell, T. D., Paulrud, J. R.: Tricalciumphosphate ceramic – a resorbable bone implant: review and current status. J. Amer. dent. Ass. 105: 1035, 1982

Seymour, r. A.: Efficacy of paracetamol in reducing post-operative pain after periodontal surgery. J. Clin. Periodont. 10: 311, 1983

Sheiham, A.: Prevention and control of periodontal disease. In: International Conference on Research in the Biology of Periodontal Disease. June, 12–25, 1977 (p.308)

*****Shenker, B. J., Tsai, Ch.-Ch., Taichman, N. S.:** Suppression of lymphocyte responses by Actinobacillus actinomycetemcomitans. J. Periodont. Res. 17: 462, 1982

Silness, J., Löe, H.: Periodontal disease in pregnancy. II. Correlation between oral hygiene and periodontal condition. Acta Odont. Scand. 22: 121, 1964

Singletary, M. M., Crawford, J. J., Simpson, D. M.: Dark-field microscopic monitoring of subgingival bacteria during periodontal therapy. J. Periodont. 53: 671, 1982

*****Skach, M.,Zábrodský, S., Mrklas, L:** A study of the effect of age and season on the incidence of ulcerative gingivitis. J. Periodont. Res. 5: 187, 1970

Skougaard, M. R.: Turnover of the gingival epithelium in marmosets. Acta Odont. Scand. 23: 623, 1965

Skougaard, M. R.: Cell renewal, with special reference to the gingival epithelium. Advanc. Oral Biol. 4: 261, 1970

Slots, J.: The predominant cultivable organisms in juvenile periodontitis. Scand. J. Dent. Res. 84: 1, 1976

Slots, J.: Subgingival microflora and periodontal disease. J. Clin. Periodont. 6: 351, 1979

Slots, J., Rosling, B. G., Genco, R. J.: Suppression of penicillin-resistant oral Actinobacillus actinomycetemcomitans with tetracycline. Considerations in endocarditis prophylaxis. J. Periodont. 54: 193, 1983

*****Slots, J., Rosling, B. G.:** Suppression of the periodontopathic microflora in localized juvenile periodontitis by systemic tetracycline. J. Clin. Periodont. 10: 465, 1983

Socransky, S. S.: Microbiology of periodontal disease – present and future considerations. J. Periodont. 48: 497, 1977

Socransky, S. S., Haffajee, A. D., Goodson, J. M., Lindhe, J.: New concepts of destructive periodontal disease. J. Clin. Periodont. 11: 21, 1984

*****Spranger, H.:** Die Versorgung approximaler Kavitäten aus parodontologischer Sicht. Dtsch. zahnärztl. Z. 36: 251, 1981

Stahl, S. S.: The need for orthodontic treatment: A periodontist's point of view. Int. Dent. J. 25: 242, 1975

*****Stahl, S. S.:** Repair or regeneration following periodontal therapy? J. Clin. Periodont. 6: 389, 1979

Stahl, S. S., Froum, S. J., Kushner, L.: Periodontal healing following open debridement flap procedures. II. Histologic obervations. J. Periodont. 53: 15, 1982

Stahl, S. S., Froum, S. J., Kushner, L.: Healing responses of human intraosseous lesions following the use of debridement, grafting and citric acid root treatment. J. Periodont. 54: 325, 1983

Strub, J. R., Gaberthüel, T. W. Firestone, A. R.: Comparison of tricalcium phosphate and frozen allogenic bone implants in man. J. Periodont. 50: 624, 1979

Sullivan, H. A., Atkins, J. H.: Free autogenous gingival grafts. I. Principle of successful grafting. Periodontics 6: 121, 1968a

Sullivan, H. C., Atkins, J. H.: Free autogenous gingival grafts. III. Utilization of grafts in the treatment of gingival recession. Periodontics 6: 152, 1968b

Suomi, J. D., Smith, L. W., McClendon, B. J.: Marginal gingivitis during a sixteen-week period. J. Periodont. 42: 268, 1971

Svanberg, G., Lindhe, J.: Vascular reactions in the periodontal ligament incident to trauma from occlusion. J. Clin. Periodont. 1: 58, 1974

*****Syed, S. A., Morrison, E. C., Lang, N. P.:** Effects of repeated scaling and root planing and/or controlled oral hygiene on the periodontal attachment level and pocket depths in beagle dogs. II. Bacteriological findings. J. Periodont. Res. 17: 219, 1982

T

*****Tanner, A. C. R., Haffer, C., Bratthall, G. T., Visconti, R. A., Socransky, S. S.:** A study of the bacteria associated with advancing periodontitis in man. J. Clin. Periodont. 6: 278, 1979

Tarnow, D., Flechter, P.: Classification of the vertical component of furcation involvement. J. Periodont. 55: 283, 1984

*****Tenenbaum, H.:** A clinical study comparing the width of attached gingiva and the prevalence of gingival recessions. J. Clin. Periodont. 9: 86, 1982

Thornton, S., Garnick, J.: Comparison of ultrasonic to hand instruments in the removal of subgingival plaque. J. Periodont. 53: 35, 1982

Totti, N., McCusker, K. T., Campbell, E. J., Griffin, G. L., Senior, R. M.: Nicotine is chemotactic for neutrophils and enhances neutrophil responsiveness to chemotactic peptides. Science 233: 169, 1984

*****Trefz, H.:** Modifizierte Operationsmethode nach Edlan-Mejchar. Dtsch. zahnärztl. Z. 34: 338, 1979

*****Tsai, Ch.-Ch., McArthur, W. P., Baehni, P. C., Evian, C., Genco, R. J., Taichman, N. S.:** Serum neutralizing activity against Actinobacillus actinomycetemcomitans leukotoxin in juvenile periodontitis. J. Clin. Periodont. 8: 338, 1981

V

Van der Velden, U.: Probing force and the relationship of the probe tip to the periodontal tissues. J. Clin. Periodont. 6: 106, 1979

*****Van der Velden, U.:** Influence of periodontal health on probing depth and bleeding tendency. J. Clin. Periodont. 7: 129, 1980

Van der Velden, U., de Vries, J. H.: The influence of probing force on the reproducibility of pocket depth measurements. J. Clin. Periodont. 7: 414, 1980

*****Van der Velden, U.:** Location of probe tip in bleeding and non-bleeding pockets with minimal gingival inflammation. J. Clin. Periodont. 9: 421, 1982

Vollmer, W. H., Rateitschak, K. H.: Influence of occlusal adjustment by grinding on gingivitis and mobility of traumatized teeth. J. Clin. Periodont. 2: 113, 1975

W

Waerhaug, J.: Healing of the dento-epithelial junction following subgingival plaque control. II. As observed on extracted teeth. J. Periodont. 49: 119, 1978

*****Waerhaug, J.:** The angular bone defect and its relationship to trauma from occlusion and downgrowth of subgingival plaque. J. Clin. Periodont. 6: 61, 1979

*****Waerhaug, J.:** The furcation problem. Etiology, pathogenesis, diagnosis, therapy and prognosis. J. Clin. Periodont. 7: 73, 1980

*****Waerhaug, J.:** Effect of toothbrushing on subgingival plaque formation. J. Periodont. 52: 30, 1981

Watts, T. L. P., Combe, E. C.: Periodontal dressing materials. J. Clin. Periodont. 6: 3, 1979

Wennström, J. L., Lindhe, J.: Effect of hydrogen peroxyde on developing plaque and gingivitis in man. J. Clin. Periodont. 6: 115, 1979

*****Wennström, J. L., Heijl, L., Lindhe, J., Socransky, S.:** Migration of gingival leukocytes mediated by plaque bacteria. J. Periodont. Res. 15: 363, 1980

Wennström, J. L.: Keratinzed and attached gingiva. Regenerative potential and significance for periodontal health. Thesis, Göteborg 1982

Wennström, J. L., Lindhe, J.: Role of attached gingiva for maintenance of periodontal health. Healing following excisional and grafting procedures in dogs. J. clin. Periodont. 10: 206, 1983

*West, Th. L., King, W. J.: Toothbrushing with hydrogen peroxide-sodium bicarbonate compared to toothpowder and water in reducing periodontal pocket suppuration and darkfield bacterial counts. J. Periodont. 54: 339, 1983

Westfelt, E., Nyman, S. Socransky, S., Lindhe, J.: Significance of frequency of professional tooth cleaning for healing following periodontal surgery. J. Clin. Periodont. 10: 148, 1983

WHO: Epidemiology, etiology, and prevention of periodontal diseases. Wld Hlth Org. Techn. Rep. Ser. 621, 1978

Widman, L.: The operative treatment of pyorrhea alveolaris. A new surgical method. Svensk tandläk.-T. Dec. 1918

*Wirthlin, M. R.: The current status of new attachment therapy. J. Periodont. 52: 529, 1981

Wolf, H. F., Rateitschak, K. H.: Einfache temporäre Schienungsmöglichkeiten. Dtsch. Zahnärzteblatt 17: 525, 1965

Z

Zambon, J. J., Christersson, L. A., Slots, J.: Actinobacillus actinomycetemcomitans in human periodontal disease. Prevalence in patient groups and distribution of biotypes and serotypes within families. J. Periodont. 54: 707, 1983

Textbooks

Baer, P. N., Morris, M. L.: Textbook of Periodontics. Lippincott, Philadelphia 1977

Carranza, F. A., Jr.: Clinical Periodontology. Saunders, Philadelphia 1979

Goldman, H. M., Cohen, D. W.: Periodontal Therapy, 6th ed. Mosby, St. Louis 1980

Lindhe, J.: Textbook of Clinical Periodontology. Munksgaard, Copenhagen 1983

Manson, J. D.: Periodontics, 3rd ed. Kimpton, London 1975

Page, R. C., Schroeder, H. E.: Periodontitis in Man and Other Animals. A Comparative Review. Karger, Basel 1982

Pindborg, J. J., Hjörting-Hansen, E.: Atlas of Diseases of the Jaws. Munksgaard, Copenhagen 1974

Prichard, J. F.: The Diagnosis and Treatment of Periodontal Disease. Saunders, Philadelphia 1979

Ramfjord, S. P., Ash, M. M.: Periodontology and Periodontics. Saunders, Philadelphia 1979

Ramfjord, S. P., Ash, M. M.: Occlusion 3rd ed. Saunders, Philadelphia 1983

Schroeder, H. E., Listgarten, M. A.: Fine Structure of the Developing Epithelial Attachment of Human Teeth, 2nd ed. Karger, Basel 1977

Schluger, S., Yuodelis, R. A., Page R. C.: Periodontal Disease. Lea & Febiger, Philadelphia 1977

Stahl, S. S.: Periodontal Surgery. Thomas, Springfield 1976

Ward, H. L., Simring, M.: Manual of Clinical Periodontics, 2nd ed. Mosby, St. Louis 1978

Atlas for Patient Information

Ebneter, M., Wolf, H. F., Wolgensinger, A.: Dental Atlas. Quintessence Publishing Co., Inc., Chicago, London, Tokyo, Rio de Janeiro and Berlin 1984

Periodicals

Journal of Periodontology (American Academy of Periodontology)
Periodontal Case Reports (Northeastern Society of Periodontists)
Periodontal Abstracts (Western Society of Periodontology)

Journal of Clinical Periodontology (Munksgaard, Copenhagen)
Journal of Periodontal Research (Munksgaard, Copenhagen)
Acta Parodontologica in: Schweizerische Monatsschrift für Zahnmedizin

Index

A

Abrasion facets 282
Actinobacillus actinomycetem-
  comitans (Aa) 17, 56
Acute necrotizing ulcerative
  gingivitis (ANUG) 41
Acute reaction 22
Adult periodontitis (AP) 55, 66
Alveolar bone 6
– Cribriform plate 6
Alveolar process 6
Anesthesia 158
– Block anesthesia 158
– Direct infiltration 158
– Superficial anesthesia 158
– Terminal anesthesia 158
– Vasoconstrictors 158
Anomalites of keratinization 52
Autoimmune diseases 52
Antibiotics, use prior to
  periodontal therapy 263
ANUG, acute necrotizing
  ulcerative gingivitis 41
AP, adult periodontitis 55, 66
Aphthous ulcer, isolated 54
Apical flap repositioning 196
Attachment loss 23, 64, 88, 93
Autoimmune diseases 52
Axelsson study 267
– Maintenance therapy 267

B

Bacteria 9, 16
– Actinobacillus actinomycetem-
  comitans (Aa) 17
– Actinomyces 11, 12, 16
– Anaerobes 16
– Antigens 9
– Bacteroides gingivalis 17
– Bacterial products 9
– Capnocytophaga 16, 17
– Chemotaxins 9
– Cocci 17
– Enzymes 9
– Fusiformes 17, 42
– Gram-negative 11, 16, 17
  (Table)
– Gram-positive 11, 16, 17
  (Table)
– Infection 9

– Invasion 9, 13
– Mitogens 9
– Motile 12
– Quality 16
– Quantity 16
– Rods 17
– Spirochetes 17, 43
– Streptococci 11, 16
– Toxins 9
– Types of disease 16
Bacterial invasion 13
Balancing side 281
Basal lamina, internal 4
– Lamina densa 5
– Lamina lucida 5
Bass technique 114
Bite guard 283
Bite guard, occlusal 283
– Michigan splint 283
Bone destruction 23
– Mechanisms of 23
Bone loss 57
– Horizontal 57
– Vertical 57
Bone regeneration 220
Bone resorption 23
Bony pockets 58, 89
– Combined 58
– Infrabony 58
– Interdental crater 59
– One-wall bony pocket 58
– Three-wall bony pocket 58
– Two-wall bony pocket 58
Bruxism 271

C

Calculus 10, 14, 137
– Subgingival 14
– Supragingival 14
Calculus removal 121, 135
– Gross debridement 132
– Scaler 122
– Subgingival 121, 135
– Supragingival 121
Charting 96
Chemical plaque control 119
Chlorhexidine (CHX) 119
– Digluconate 119
– Dihydrochloride 120
– Indications 120
– Side effects 120

– Plaque inhibition 119
Chlorhexidine powder 162, 264
– Periodontal dressing 162
Citric acid 150
Clenching 95
Col 3
Combined operative procedure
  197
– Extraction, revision 204
– – Operative procedure 204
– Facial flap, GV and oral flap
  198
– – Operative procedure 199
– Flap, gingivectomy 201, 203
Composite resin splint 293
– Acid etch technique 293
– Semipermanent 291, 293, 295
– Temporary 292
– With cavity preparations 293
– Without preparations 292
Connective tissue supporting
  structures 6
Coronal repositioning 255, 258
– First operation 255
– Operative procedure 255
– Second operation 256
Correction of alveolar ridge 206
Corticosteroid 106, 264
Course of therapy 102
– Basic 102
– Checklist 102
– Time course 103
Covering denuded areas
  (recession) 253
– Contraindications 253
– Coronal repositioning after
  FGG 253
– "Creeping attachment" 253
– Direct coverage with FGG 253
– Indications 253
– Operative procedure 253
– Repositioned flaps 253
– Sliding flap 253
Creation of hygienic relationship
  121, 126
– Hoes 138
– Hygienic relationship 121
Creeping attachment after free
  gingival graft 254
Crowding 14
Curettage (root planing) 121,
  135
– Advantages 136
– Anesthesia 141

– Attachment gain 151
– Checking the surface 143
– Closed 135
– Curettes 122, 138, 143
– Dentist's position 140
– Disadvantages 136
– Endotoxin-containing cement
  137
– Ergonomics 140
– Finger rest 140
– Goal of treatment 137
– Granulation tissue 144
– Healing 145
– Indication 136
– Instruments 138
– Open 135, 148
– Position of the operator 140
– Pocket epithelium 137
– Pocket measurement 135
– Pocket reduction 151
– Pocket rinsing 144
– Operative procedure 141
– Root planing 136, 143
– Systematic approach 139
– Soft tissue adaptation 144
– Soft tissue curettage 135, 144
– Working angle for curette
  blade 143
Curettes 122, 138, 143
– Sharpening 138
– Use 139
Cuticula dentis 4
Cyclosporine-A hyperplasia 49
– Therapy 49
Cytotoxicity 20

D

Data gathering 87
Debris 10
– Food debris 10
– Food impaction 10
– Plaque 10
Defense against infection 21
Dental assistant 267
Dental floss 116
Dental hygienist 267
Dentifrice 113
– Components 113
– Enamel abrasion 113
Diagnosis 87
Diagnostic charting 96

– Bleeding Index 96
– Charts 96
– Functional findings 97
– Hygiene Index 96
– Periodontal findings 97
– Periodontal status 96
– Photographic survey 96
– Probing depths 97
– Radiographic survey 96
– Single tooth diagnosis 97
– Specific findings 97
– Tooth mobility 97
– Treatment planning 97
Disclosing agents 111
– Demonstration of plaque 111
Dystrophic disease 57

E

Edlan-Mejchar Operation
    (vestibuloplasty) 245
– Contraindication 245
– Disadvantages 245
– Indication 245
– Operative procedure 246
– Principles of operation 245
– Preprosthetic surgery 245
– Problems 248
– Wound healing, fluorescence
    angiography 251
– – Clinical 250
Electromyography 283
Electrosurgery 160
– Tips 160
Elevator 176
Emergencies 105
Emergency treatment 104
– Acute stage 105
– Gingivitis ulcerosa 104, 106
– Medicinal treatment 105
– Pocket abscess 105
Endodontics – Periodontics 259
Epidemiology 25
– Gingivitis 25
– Periodontitis 26
– Tooth loss 26
Epithelial attachment 4
Epithelial attachment structures 4
Epithelium, oral 4
Epulis 48, 51
– Fibromatosa 51
– Giant cell 51
– Granulomatosa 51
– Gravidarum 48
– Therapy 49
Etiology 9
– Bacteria 9, 16
– – Bacterial products 9
– – Calculus 14
– – Debris 10
– – Gram-positive (Table) 17
– – Gram-negative (Table) 17
– – Microorganisms 9
– – Plaque 10
– Cofactors 24
– – Actinic irritant 24
– – Age 24
– – Allergic reaction 24
– – Burns 24
– – Chemical irritant 24
– – Clenching 24

– – Exogenous irritant 24
– – Functional disturbance 24
– – Hormonal situation 24
– – Mechanical injury 24
– – Mouth breathing 24
– – Nutrition 24
– – Saliva 24
– – Side effects of medica-
    ments 24
– – Stress 24
– – Systemic diseases 24
– Host defense 9
EVA polishing files 127
EVA system 127
Extension operation 228
Extraction, periodontal revision
    of adjacent teeth 204
– Osseous regeneration 207
– Ridge correction 206

F

Failure 270
Fiber apparatus 6
– Course of fiber bundles 7
– Gingival 6
– Periodontal 6
Fibrosis, idiopathic 49
– Therapy 49
Findings 87
– Compulsory 87
– Facultative 87
– Functional 97
– Hygiene index 96
– Periodontal 97
– Photographic survey 96
– Radiographic survey 96
Fixed prostheses 300
– Ante's law 303
– Bridges 300
– Crowns 300
– Limitations 303
– Pontics 300
– Possibilities 303
– Precision attachments 300
Flap – Gingivectomy 201, 203
Flap surgery 175
– Advantages 175
– Apical flap repositioning 196
– Completely reflected flaps 199
– Contraindications 170
– Disadvantages 175
– Indications 175
– Instruments 176
– – Bone bur 176
– – Bone file 176
– – Curettes 176
– – Explorers 176
– – Forceps 176
– – Gingival scissors 176
– – Needle holder 176
– – Needles 178
– – Rasps 176
– – Scapels 176
– – Suture material 178
– – Use 177
– Modified Widman flap 175
– Mucoperiosteal flap 175, 196
– Ostectomy 196
– Osteoplasty 196
– Partially reflected flap (see

modified Widman, Ramfjord
technique) 179
– Ramfjord technique 179
– Suture technique 178
– Split thickness flap 170
– Thinning the flap 205
Flora, subgingival 11, 92
Free gingival graft (FGG) 229
– Contraindications 229
– Donor site 232
– Fixation of the graft 237
– Healing 240
– – Clinical 238
– – Fluorescence angiography
    240
– – FGG histology 232
– Indication 229
– Instruments 230
– – Gingivectomy knife 230
– – Hand mucotome 230
– – Motor driven mucotome
    230
– – Scalpels 230
– Mesh graft 242
– Operation planning 234
– Operative procedure 233
– Palatal wound 236
– Principles of operation 229
– Recipient site 229
– Revascularization 240
– Single teeth 241
– Stent for wound protection
    236
– Stillman's clefts 242
– Taking the graft 236
– Thickness and shape 232
– Thinning 232
– Trimming 232
Frenectomy 228, 244
Frenotomy 228, 244
Fully reflected flaps 190
– Advantages 190
– Apical flap repositioning 194
– Contraindication 190
– Vertical incisions 192, 194
Function 95, 271
Functional analysis 272
Functional disturbances 271
– Afunction 271
– Bruxism 271
– Consequences 272
– – Attrition, abrasion 272
– – Muscle pain 272
– – Muscle spasms 272
– – Neuralgiform disorder 272
– – Occlusal periodontal trauma
    272
– – Temporomandibular joint
    disturbances 272
– – Tooth mobility increase 272
– Dysfunction 271
– General causes 271
– Oral, local causes 271
– Parafunction 271
– Therapy 271
Furcation diagnosis 91
Furcation involvement 60, 90
– Severity 60, 90
– – Class F0 60, 90
– – Class F1 60, 90, 146, 221
– – Class F2 60, 90, 147, 221
– – Class F3 60, 90, 221
Furcation treatment 146, 221, 224

– Ability to clean 147
– Curettage 146
– Furcation-plasty 147
– Hemisection 221
– Indication 221
– Resection 221
– Root resection 224, 226
– Surgical 221
– Techniques 221

G

Gingiva 2, 16, 37
– Attached 2
– Col 3
– Free marginal 2
– Gingival width 3
– Healthy 37
– Interdental 2
– Melanocytes 2
– Mucogingival junction 2
– Mucogingival line (MGL) 2
– Pigmentation 2
Gingiva extension 229
– Free gingival graft (FGG) 229
Gingival Bleeding Index (GBI) 29
Gingival Index (GI) 29
Gingival Index Simplified (GI–S)
    29
Gingival overgrowth 49
Gingival pocket, see pockets
Gingival width 3
Gingivectomy (GV) 159
– Advantages 159
– Anesthesia 164
– Contouring 167
– Contraindications 159
– Debridement 167
– Disadvantages 159
– Dressing removal 168
– Esthetics 173
– Endodontics 173
– Gingival enlargement 164
– Incision 165
– Indications 159
– Instruments 160
– Marking pocket depths 164
– Minor procedures 172
– Operative procedure 163
– Phenytoin-induced gingival
    overgrowth 49, 171
– Principles of operation 159
– Prosthetic reasons 172
– Pseudopockets 164
– Revealing preparation margins
    172
– Scaling 166
– Tooth cleaning 167
– Wound care 168
– Wound dressing 168
Gingivitis 9, 16, 18, 35
– Climacterica 46
– – Therapy 46
– Clinical symptoms 37
– – Bleeding 37
– – Edema 37
– – Gingival pockets 37
– – Pseudopockets 37
– – Swelling 37
– – Ulceration 37
– Definition 35

– Early 18
– Established 19
– Histopathology 36
– Histolopathology of development 18
– Hormonal modulation 46
– Hyperplasia 49
– Initial 18
– Initiation of 10
– Menstrualis and intermenstrualis 46
– – Therapy 46
– Mild 38
– Moderate 39
– Mouth breathing 40
– Severe 40
– Ulcerosa (ANUG, acute necrotizing ulcerative gingivitis) 41
– – Bacteria 42
– – Bacteroides 42
– – Clinical symptoms 43
– – Course 41
– – Etiology 41
– – – General factors 41
– – – Local factors 41
– – Fusiformes 42
– – Histopathology 42
– – Spirochetes 42
– – Therapy 41
Gingivoplasty 159, 169
– Hyperplastic gingivitis 163
– Instruments 160
Gingivosis 52
– Gingivitis desquamativa 52
– Therapy 52
Gingivostomatitis herpetica 52, 54
– Therapy 52
Gracey curettes 138
Granulocytes (PMN) 20, 22
– Acute reaction 22
– Chemotaxis 22
– Defects 22
– Function 22
– Left shift 22
– Opsonins 22
– Phagocytosis 22
– Phagolysosome 22
Gross debridement 121

H

Healing, see periodontal healing
Hemidesmosomes 4
Hemisection 222
– Flaps 222
– Operative procedure 222
– Plaque control 223
– Reconstruction 223
– Temporaries 223
Herpes 54
Hexetidine 264
Hoe scaler 138
Host defense 9
– Defects 9
– Positive 9
Hydantoin hyperplasia 49, 171
– Therapy 49
– Tray for topical application 171
Hygiene indices 96
– Hygiene Index (HI) 28

– Interdental hygiene index (HYG) 28, 96
Hyperplasia 49

I

Iatrogenic irritant 15
– Removal of 126
– – Amalgam overhangs 126
– – Bridge pontics 129
– – Contouring restorations 127
– – Correction of open margins 149
– – Diamond stones 129
– – EVA system 127
– – Metal pigmentation 130
– – Open crown margins 128
– – Plaque retention 128
– – Proxoshape files 127
– – Removal of overhangs 126
– – Subgingival crown margins 128
Immune reaction 20
Immune status 9
Immune system 20
Immunity 21
– Aquired 21
– Cellular 21
– Humoral 21
– Inherited 21
– Natural 21
Immunoglobulin 21
Implants 201, 215
– Allogenic 215
– Alloplastic 215
– Apatite 215
– Autologous 215
– Bioglas 215
– Bone 215
– Bone chips 215
– Calcitite 215
– Calcium phosphate 215
– Calcium sulfate 215
– Cartilage 215
– Collagen 215
– Durapatite 215
– Frialite 215
– Heterologous 215
– Homologous 215
– Hydroxyapatite (HA) 215
– Isologous 215
– Lyophilized bone 215
– Osseous regeneration 215
– Periograf 215
– Syngeneic 215
– Synthograft 215
– Spongiosa (trabecular bone) 215
– Tricalcium phosphate (TCP) 215
– Xenogenic 215
Indices 225, 27
– Gingival Index (GI) 29
– – Gingival Bleeding Index (GBI) 29
– – Gingival Index Simplified (GI-S) 29
– – Papilla Bleeding Index (PBI) 29
– – Sulcus Bleeding Index (SBI) 29

– Gingival indices 27, 29
– Periodontal indices 27, 32
– – Periodontal Disease Index (PDI) 32
– Plaque indices 27
– – Hygiene Index (HI) 28
– – Interdental Hygiene Index (HYG) 28, 96
– – Plaque Index (PI) 28
– "Ramfjord teeth" 32
Infection 13
– Abscess 13
– Bacterial invasion 13
– Exacerbation 13
– Micronecrosis 13
– Necrosis 13
– Pus 13
– Viral 52
Information 108
Initial therapy 107, 151
– Definition 107
– General 107
– Limitations 151
– Possibilities 151
– Success of treatment 152
Interdental brushes 116
– Spiral brush 116
Interdental hygiene 116
– Dental floss 116
– Spiral brush 116
– Superfloss 116
– Toothpicks 116
Irrigators 118
Irritation, iatrogenic, see iatrogenic irritation
Jaw musculature 283
– Relaxation 283
– Spasm 283

J

Junctional epithelium 4
– Attachment epithelium 4
– Basal lamina 4
– Epithelial attachment 4
– Hemidesmosomes 4
– Stratum basale 5
– Stratum suprabasale 4
Juvenile Periodontitis (LJP, localized juvenile periodontitis) 55, 72
– Advanced stage 74
– Initial stage 72

L

Labial frenum 244
Lateral movement 280
Leukocyte 20
Leukotoxin 13
Lichen planus 52
– Therapy 52
Lip biting 95
LJP (localized juvenile periodontitis) 55, 72
Lugol solution 93
Lymphocytes 20
– B lymphocytes 21
– T lymphocytes 20

M

Macrophages, monocytes 20
– Lymphocyte mitogenic factor (LMF) 20
– Macrophage activation factor (MAF) 20
– – Chemotactic factor (MCF) 20
– – Migration inhibition factor (MIF) 20
Maintenance therapy 267
– Goals 267
– Prevention of caries 267
– Prevention of new infection 267
– Prevention of reinfection 267
Mandibular border movements 273
– Frontal 273
– Horizontal 273
– Posselt figure 273
– Sagittal 273
Mandibular movements 274
– At tooth contact 274
– Computer plots 274
– Contact areas 275
– In abraded dentition 274
– Normal bite 274
– Overbite 274
McCall's festoons 83
Medical history 87
– General 87
– Special 87
Medicament carriers 171
Medicaments 263
– Chlorhexidine 263
– Contraindications 264
– General medicine 263, 266
– Gingivitis therapy 263
– Hexetidine 263
– Indications 264
– Local periodontitis therapy 264
– – Achromycin ophthalmic ointment 264
– – Amosan 264
– – Aureomycin ointment 264
– – Chlorhexidine (CHX) 264
– – – Digluconate 264
– – – Dihydrochloride 264
– – Chlorhexamed 264
– – Corsodyl 264
– – Corticosteroid with antibiotic 264
– – Dontisolon P 264
– – Hexetidine 264
– – Hextril 264
– – Hydrogen peroxide 264
– – Kavosan 264
– – Keyes technique 264
– – Locacorten 264
– – Plak-Out 264
– – Sodium bicarbonate 264
– – Terracortril 264
– – Tetracycline 264
– Pain alleviation 266
– Pain therapy 263
– Periodontitis therapy 263
– Pre- and post-treatment 263
– Prophylactic coverage 263, 266
– Reduction of swelling 263, 266

– Side effects 264
– Systemic periodontitis therapy 265
– – Combination preparations 265
– – Flagyl 265
– – Hostacycline 265
– – Ledermycine 265
– – Metronidazole 265
– – Ornidazole 265
– – Rodogyl 265
– – Rovamycine 265
– – Spiramycine 265
– – Tetracycline 265
– – Tiberal 265
– – Vibramycine 265
– Treatment of acute conditions 263
– Wound treatment 263, 266
Mesh graft 242
Mesiotrusion 281
Metal pigmentation 130
Metronidazole 68
Michigan long-term study 151
Microorganisms 17
– Classification (table) 17
Microscopic diagnosis 92
Michigan splint 283
Michigan studies 151, 157
Modified Widman procedure 279
– Advantages 179
– Contraindication 179
– Disadvantages 179
– First incision 180, 184
– Flap adaptation 180, 182
– Healing 179
– Indication 179
– Interdental defect closure 179
– Long-term result 179, 181
– Operation planning 184
– Operative procedure 183
– Partially reflected flap 182
– Principles 180, 182
– Root planing with direct vision 180
– Schematic 182
– Second incision 180, 185
– Sutures 182
– Systematic procedure 183
– Third incision 181, 185
– Tooth cleaning 188
Monocytes, see macrophages 20
Motivation 108
– Case presentation 109
– Plaque 109
– Descriptive brochures 109
– Motivation aids 109
– Motivation mirror 108
– Papilla bleeding index (PBI) 108
Mouth breathing 14
Mucogingival surgery 228
– Coronal repositioning 228
– Covering recession (denuded areas) 228
– Edlan-Mejchar 245
– Free gingival graft (FGG) 228
– Halting recession 228
– Lateral repositioning 228
– Sliding flap 228
Muscle spasms 283

N

Needle holder 176
Needles 178
– Atraumatic 178
– Cross sectional profile 178
– Degree of curvature 178
– Sizes 178
Negative results of treatment 262
– Desensitization 262
– Esthetics 262
– Gingival mask 262
– Hypersensitive areas 262
– "Long teeth" 262
– Phonetics 262
– Sensitivity 262
New attachment 260

O

Occlusal bite guard, see bite guard, occlusal 283
Occlusal periodontal trauma 272
Odontoplasty 121
Open curettage, see curettage, open 135, 148
Operations, combined, see combined surgical techniques
Opsonins 22
Oral epithelium, see epithelium, oral
Oral hygiene 110
– By the dentist 121
– Dentifrices 113
– Dental floss 116
– Disclosing agents 111
– Flossing aides 118
– Interdental brushes 116
– Interdental hygiene 116
– Irrigators 118
– Marginal brushes 118
– Oral irrigation by the patient 111, 125
– Oral irrigators 118
– Polishing materials 113
– Special hygiene aides 118
– Stimulators 118
– Superfloss 118
– Systematic 115
– Toothbrushes 112
– Toothpicks 116
Oral photography 96
Ornidazole 68
Orthodontics 285
– Bone loss and regeneration 289
– Crowding 285
– Fixed appliances 287
– General 285
– Periodontitis and abnormal tooth position 285
– Plate with labial bow 287
– Protusion of canine 290
– Removable appliances 286
– Retention 286
– – Attached anterior retainer 287
– – Bridge treatment 288
– – Composite splint 286

– – Night guards 286
– – Space closure 286
– – Tooth tipping 285
– – Torsion 285
– – Treatment for protrusion 287
– – Treatment using bridges 288
– – Uprighting the second molar 288
Ostectomy 191, 196
Osteoclast 23
Osteoplasty 191, 196
– Instruments 191
– – Bone burs 191
– – Bone files 191
– – Bone forceps 191
– – Burs 191
– – Rongeur 191

P

Papilla Bleeding Index (PBI) 30
– Technical procedure 31
– Motivation 30
Papillon-Lefèvre Syndrome 78
– Course of disease 80
– Deciduous teeth 78
– Prognosis 79
Parafunctions 95, 271
– Habits 95
– Professional 95
– Occlusal 95, 271
Partially reflected flaps 179
Pathogenesis 9
Pellicle 4, 11
Pemphigoid 52
– Therapy 52
Pemphigus vulgaris 52
– Therapy 52
Penicillin 266
Periodontal abscess 64
Periodontal Disease Index (PDI) 32
Periodontal diseases 33
– Epithelial regeneration 260
– Gingivitis 33
– – Ulcerosa 33
– In combination with general systemic diseases 34
– Local etiology 33
– Periodontitis 33
– – Ulcerosa 33
– Recession 33
– Healing 260
– – Connective tissue accumulation 261
– – New bone formation 261
– – New attachment 260
– – Regeneration 260
– – Reattachment 260
– – Shrinkage 261
Periodontal dressings 162
– Carrier for medicaments 171
– Coe-Pak 162
– Eugenol-free 162
– Patient comfort 162
– Peripac 162
Periodontal indices 27, 32
Periodontal probes 88
Periodontal status 97
Periodontal surgery 155
– Drug pre-treatment 157

– Goals 155
– Indications 155
– Operation methods 157
– Preparation 157
– Re-evaluation following initial therapy 156
Periodontium 1, 6
– And endodontics 259
– – Class I 259
– – Class II 259
– – Class III 259
– – Combined problems 259
– – Endodontic problems 259
– – Periodontal problems 259
– Marginal 4
Periodontitis 9, 17, 23, 55
– Adult periodontitis (AP) 16, 55, 66
– Clinical symptoms 63
– – Attachment loss 63
– – Bleeding 63
– – Bone loss 63
– – Exudate 63
– – Fistula 63, 65
– – Furcation abscess 63, 65
– – Pocket abscess 63
– – Pocket activity 63
– – Pus 63
– – Shrinkage 63
– – Swelling 63
– – Tooth mobility 63, 65
– – Tooth drifting 63, 65
– Course of disease 55
– Cyclic course of disease 23
– Definition 56
– Histopathology 18, 62
– Localized juvenile periodontitis (LJP) 17, 55, 72
– Prepubertal 78
– Rapidly progressive periodontitis (RPP) 17, 55, 68
– Ulcerosa 76
Phagocytosis 20
Phase contrast microscope 92
Phenytoin gingival overgrowth 49
– Therapy 49
Photographic survey 96
"Pill" gingivitis 46
– Therapy 46
Plaque 10
– Accumulation 10
– Adherent 10, 12
– Bacterial 10
– Composition 11, 16
– – Healthy gingiva 16
– – Gingivitis 16
– – LJP 17
– – RPP 17
– Corn cob 11
– Expanse 11
– Extracellular polysaccharides 10
– Formation 11
– Iatrogenic factors enhancing plaque retention 15
– – Crown margins 15
– – Restorations 15
– Natural factors 14
– – Calculus 14
– – Crowding 14
– – Curves 14
– – Enamel projections and pearls 14

– – Furcations 14
– – Mouth breathing 14
– Non adherent 10, 12
– Pellicle 11
– Subgingival 12
– Supragingival 10
Plaque indices 27
Plaque removal (see also curettage) 121, 135
– Subgingival 135
– Supragingival 121
Plaque retentive area 131
Plaque retentive areas, removal of 121, 131, 134
Plaque smear 92
Plasma cells 20
Plate with labial bow (see orthodontics) 286
Pocket depth 88
Pocket implant, see implants
Pocket measuring probe 88
Pockets 57, 64
– Activity 92
– Diagnosis 89
– – Microscopic 92
– Gingival 11
– Infrabony 57, 62
– Pseudopocket 57
– Suprabony 57, 62
– True 57
Polymorphonuclear leukocytes (PMN), see granulocytes
Polysaccharide, extracellular 10
– Dextrans 10
– Fructans 10
– Glucans 10
– Levans 10
– Matrix 10
– Mutans 10
Pregnancy gingivitis 46
– Therapy 46
Premature contacts 277
Prevention 99
Probing depths 64, 88
Prognosis 87
– General prognostic factors 98
– Local prognostic factors 98
– Single tooth prognosis 98
Prophy-Jet 124
Prophylactic paste 127
– RDA (relative dentin abrasion) 124
Prophylaxis 99, 267
– Initial therapy 107
– Prevention of caries 99
– Prevention of gingivitis 99
– Prevention of periodontitis 99
– Oral 99
Prophylaxis spray 124
Prostaglandin 23
Prosthesis, removable 301
– Cast framework partial denture 302
– Telescope primary anchorage 301
– Telescoping bridge 301
– Telescoping partial denture 301
Prosthetics 297
– Esthetics 297
– Ante's law 303
– Cast framework partial denture 297, 302

– Clasp guidance 297
– Crown contour 297
– Crown margin 297
– Definitive treatment 297
– Fixed replacement 300
– Interdental space contouring 297
– No replacement? 303
– Occlusion 297
– Pontic shape 297
– Precision attachments 297
– Premolar occlusion 303
– Problems 303
– Prosthesis base 297
– Removable replacement 297, 301
– Splinting 297
– Telescope construction 297
Proxoshape files 127
Pseudopockets 35, 57
Puberty gingivitis 46
– Therapy 46

R

Radiographic status 96
Radiology 94
– Long cone 94
– Right angle technique 94
Ramfjord Technique (see also modified Widman procedure) 179, 182, 186
Rapidly progressive periodontitis (RPP) 55, 68
Re-evaluation 87
Reattachment 260
Recall 267
– Dental assistant 268
– Dental hygienist 268
– Effect 268
– Findings 268
– Frequency 269
– Maintenance therapy 269
– Organization 268
– Plaque and calculus removal 268
– "Prophy hour" 269
– Recall appointments 269
– Re-instruction 268
– Re-motivation 268
Recession 81, 93
– Clinical picture 81
– Clinical pictures resembling recession, shrinkage 86
– Definition 81
– Dehiscence 82
– Diagnosis 93
– Etiology 81
– – Improper toothbrushing 81
– – Mild inflammation 81
– – Frenum attachment 81
– Fenestration 82
– Generalized 85
– Localized 84
– McCall's festoons 82
– Osseous dehiscence 82
– Radiology 81
– Roll test 93
– Secondary inflammation 81
– Stillman's cleft 83
– Symptoms 83

– Therapy 81
Reconstruction, see prosthetics
Relative Dentin Abrasion 124
Resistance 9
Resting muscle tone 283
Restorations 15
Rodogyl 265
Root cementum 6
Root conditioning 150
– Citric acid 150
Root fusion 90
Root irregularities 90
Root planing (see also curettage) 121, 135, 140, 145, 149
– Cleaning the root surface 135
– Dentin, smoothing of 150
– Diamonds 150
– Endotoxin-containing cement layer 135
Root resection 224, 226
– Buccal root 224
– Furcation involvement 224
– Hygiene 227
– Odontoplasty 226
– With reconstruction 224
– Without reconstruction 226
Rovamycine 265

S

Scaler 122
Scapels 176
Schiller iodine solution 293
– IPI solution 93
– Iodine potassium iodide 93
Selective grinding 121, 276
– Balance side 281
– Balancing side interferences 281
– "BULL" rule 276, 280
– Freedom in centric 277, 279
– Goals 276
– Instruments 277
– Lateral mandibular movement 280
– Long centric 280
– Morphologic 121
– Position of intercuspation 276
– Premature contacts 277
– – Anterior area 279
– – Cusp-fossa 279
– – Mesiodistal 277
– – Orofacial 278
– Protrusive interferences 282
– "PUBL" rule 276
– Reduction of abrasion facets 282
– Retruded contact position 276
– Slide in centric 277
– "Tapping test" 276
– Working side 280
Sharpey's fibers 6
Single tooth diagnosis 97
Soft tissue curettage 131, 135
Spirochetes 17, 43
Splinting 291
– Amalgam "stops" 296
– Biological stabilization 291
– Fixed 291
– Indications 291
– Intracoronal 294

– Reinforcement with ligatures 294
– Removable 291
– Wire reinforcement 295
– Wire splint 292
Stabilization, see splinting
Stillman's cleft 83, 154
Stillman technique 115
Structural biology 1
Subgingival flora, see flora, subgingival
Sulcus 4, 57
– Sulcular epithelium 5
Sulcus Bleeding Index (SBI) 29
Supragingival plaque removal 121
Suture materials 178
Suture technique 178

T

Temporaries 207, 298
– Fixed 298
– Immediate temporary 298
– Long-term temporary 298
– Removable 299
Tetracycline 264, 265
Therapy 101
– Course of treatment 102, 103
– Emergency treatment 104
– General 101
– Goals of therapy 101
– Initial therapy 101, 107
– Maintenance therapy (recall) 267
– Orthodontics 285
– Prosthetics 297
– Reconstruction 297
– Splinting 291
– Surgical treatment 101, 155
– Treatment planning 102
Third molar extraction 209
– Atraumatic 209
– Early 209
– Late 209
Tissue adhesive 162
– Bucrylate 162
– Histoacryl 162
Tongue thrust 95
Tooth cleaning 121, 124
– Fine debridement 124
– Gross debridement 112
– Polishing strips 125
– Prophy-Jet 125
– Prophylactic paste 124
– – RDA (relative dentin abrasion) 124
– Tooth polishing 123, 125
– Ultrasonic scaler 124
Tooth loss 26
– Causes 2
Tooth mobility 8, 95
– Degrees of 95
– Increased 95
– Periodontal 8
– Physiologic 8
– Progressive 95
– Stable 95
– Unstable 95
Tooth polishing (see also tooth cleaning) 123, 125

Tooth supporting apparatus 6
Toothbrushes 112
– Electric 112
– Hand 112
Toothbrushing techniques 114
– Bass technique 114
– Stillman technique 115
– Vertical-rotatory method 114
Toothpick 116
Transplant (see also implants) 215
– Autologous 215
– Collection of bone chips 217
– Instruments 216
– Removal of bone 216
Transplantation of bone 218
– Autologous 218
– – Operative procedure 218
– Bone removal 218
Trauma, occlusal, see occlusal periodontal trauma
Treatment planning 102
Tumors 49
– Therapy 49
Types of disease 216
Types of periodontal diseases 33

U – Z

Ultrasonic instruments 124
Vertical-rotatory brushing 114
Vincent's gingivitis, see Gingivitis ulcerosa, ANUG
Wedge excisions 210, 213
– According to Chaikin 210
– "Classic" 210
– Distal wedge 214
– Incisions 212
– Lingual nerve 210
– Lone standing tooth 214
– Mesial wedge 214
– Modified incision 210
– Most distal tooth 211
– – Operative procedure 211
– Principles of operation 210
– Recurrence 210
– Root planing 212
Widman operation, see modified Widman procedure
Working side 280